Berelson on Population

Berelson on Population

Editors

John A. Ross
Columbia University
Center for Population and Family Health
New York, New York 10032, USA

W. Parker Mauldin
The Population Division
The Rockefeller Foundation
New York, New York 10036, USA

With 38 Illustrations

Springer-Verlag
New York Berlin Heidelberg
London Paris Tokyo

Library of Congress Cataloging-in-Publication Data
Berelson, Bernard, 1912–1979
Berelson on Population.
Bibliography: p.
1. Population policy. 2. Birth control.
I. Ross, John A, 1934– II. Mauldin, W. Parker
(Wayman Parker) III. Title.
HB8883.5.B47 1988 304.6 81-3150

Softcover reprint of the hardcover 1st edition 1988

Typeset by Publishers Service, Bozeman, Montana.

9 8 7 6 5 4 3 2 1

ISBN-13:978-1-4612-8382-9 e-ISBN-13:978-1-4612-3868-3
DOI: 10.1007/978-1-4612-3868-3

Acknowledgments

We are grateful to The Ford Foundation, The Population Council, and The Rockefeller Foundation for providing financial assistance for this book. Their support of Berelson's population work dates from the early 1960s, notably from 1965, when all three joined him in launching the historic Geneva conference on population programs, the first of its kind ever held. Over the years, the collaboration continued and helped measurably to shape the development of the population movement. Our special appreciation to Oscar Harkavy at The Ford Foundation, George Zeidenstein at The Population Council, and Sheldon Segal at The Rockefeller Foundation for their personal encouragement.

For assistance in assembling the full corpus of Berelson's population writings and for their work on the Bibliography, we thank Janet Molzan, Marjorie Rich, and Tessa Wardlaw. Susan Pasquariella and her staff at the library of Columbia's Center for Population and Family Health were most helpful to our literature searches.

Our special thanks to the staff at Springer-Verlag for their fine editorial work and extraordinary efforts to speed the manuscript through publication.

To Ruth Berelson, our deep appreciation for suggestions regarding Chapter 1 and, well beyond that, for all she did in support of the original writings.

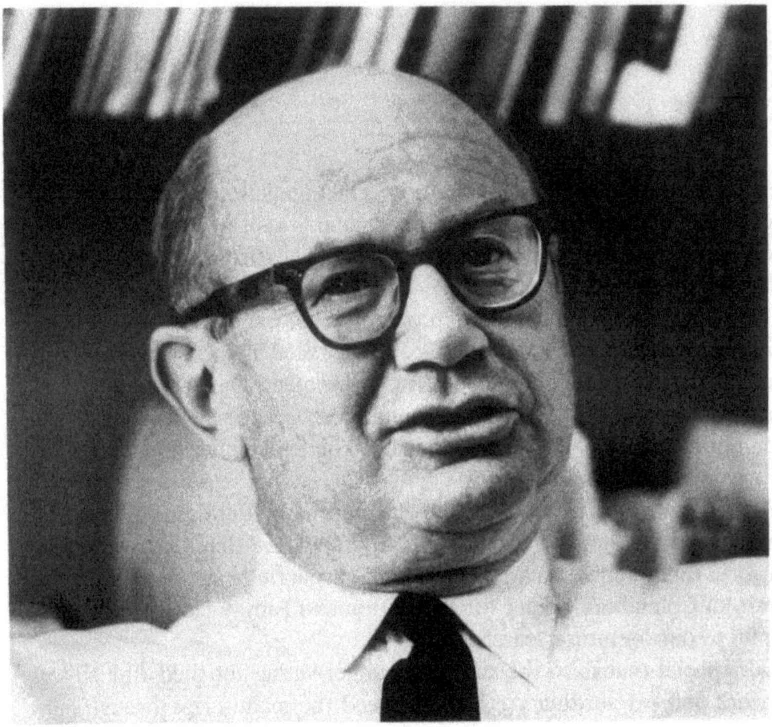

Bernard Berelson, 1912-1979

Foreword

Bernard (Barney) Berelson had a major influence in the application of social science concepts and methods to population policy during the period from 1962 to 1980. This was the period when concern with population problems spread from a relatively small group of scholars and population activists to a much larger, diverse, international group of political and intellectual leaders and to the general public as well. There was an exponential growth in the number of scholars and service personnel in various population and family specialities in this period.

Barney came into the field with his appointment as Director of the Communication Research Program of The Population Council in 1962. He had no previous training or experience in demography. Frank Notestein, President of The Population Council at the time, had the wisdom to appreciate the value and relevance of Barney's impressive background in communication research and other social science areas, as well as his creative mind and leadership qualities. His influence on the Council's rapidly expanding program was so immediate and impressive that within a year, he was named Vice President. When Frank Notestein retired in 1968, Barney became President, a post he held for 6 very productive years.

John Ross and Parker Mauldin, in Chapter 1 of this volume, provide an excellent systematic review of the place of Barney's many important publications in the field. Therefore, in this foreword, I only present my impressions of Barney from our interaction on joint projects and in other ways.

Like many other demographers, when I first heard of Barney's appointment, I was skeptical about what an "outsider" could contribute. I quickly revised this view as I worked with him, beginning in 1962. I found that he brought to the field imaginative and creative applications from his extensive experience in behavioral science research. As far demography was concerned, he was a "quick study," learning from his demographic colleagues and his extensive reading. In this, as in so many other areas, he had the capacity to ask the right questions focusing on central problems and concepts. He did not become, or ever claim to be, a skilled demographer. Nevertheless, I believe that he did more to increase general knowledge of important policy-relevant demographic concepts than many of us who were his technical mentors.

I had the good fortune to read many of his publications in draft form. Although almost invariably his ideas were excellent and his writings of exceptional clarity, he was open to advice and suggestions. He was also good enough to read much of my writing in draft. I, like others who worked with him, gained greatly in this exchange. Frequently, his comments led me in new directions. In addition, he was a marvelous editor.

Soon after Barney joined the Council, we cooperated with Chinese officials in designing the Taichung experiment, a major trial of various aspects of a family planning program (see Chapter 13). Barney had told me early in our relationship that he was looking for an opportunity to help mount a large-scale quasi-experiment to evaluate as carefully as possible the potential of an intensive "state of the art" family planning program. I had begun to visit Taiwan under Population Council auspices to see in what ways we could assist with demographic studies as a baseline for the family planning initiative they were planning. On my second visit there, I called Barney and suggested that conditions for an experimental study in Taiwan were excellent. He flew over. In cooperation with the Chinese, the design for the Taichung experiment was developed rather quickly.

While in retrospect I cannot remember the origin of all the key elements, many of the ideas tested were Barney's: (1) the power of diffusion, given an early critical-mass center of acceptance; (2) the acceptability of the intrauterine device in a mass field study; (3) whether visiting both husbands and wives resulted in more new acceptors than visiting the wives only; (4) whether the poor and illiterate would accept family planning in significant numbers in a traditional Chinese society; (5) whether a large-scale program in one city involving tens of thousands of home visits, hundreds of group meetings, and mass mailings could be carried out without serious political problems, or difficulties in serving the needs of the population. Readers can judge for themselves the value of the study from the article in Chapter 13 and from the book[1] that followed it. It was Barney's idea also to make the project big enough so that if it succeeded, it would allay the fears of government leaders in Taiwan and elsewhere that large-scale family planning programs would be politically risky.

Those who fund such pilot projects often have the view that basic social science research is expensive and unnecessary for program purposes. Barney supported my view that we should spend the money and time to document the demographic, social, and programmatic aspects of the study to meet high social science standards. But, at the same time, it was his view that we should give priority to early analysis of those aspects of the study which would provide the action program with the guidance it needed without too much delay for the next steps. This strategy, as we followed it, made it possible for the program to increase its momentum and scope without delay, based to a significant extent on what we and the Chinese thought were the lessons of the study. Our ability to serve the program with timely and reliable data helped to convince the Chinese that basic research was a part of the program, rather than excess baggage. Research on the program intervention became a legitimate and necessary part of the study of population in Taiwan. This strategy of serving the program needs as part of

[1] Ronald Freedman, John Takeshita and others, *Family Planning in Taiwan, An Experiment in Social Change*. Princeton: Princeton University Press, 1969.

the basic research program made it possible to publish the article in Chapter 13 within 2 years after the study began.

Barney's concerns about the ethical aspects of population policy, apparent in many of his publications, were evident also in the Taichung program. Thus, before the major Taichung study, there was a smaller pilot project to learn about what Taiwanese couples wanted and about cultural values to which the larger study should be sensitive. There was also a substantial medical backup for the program from the beginning. With the assistance of Dr. Sheldon Segal, then of The Population Council, all acceptors in the Taichung program were followed up for 7 years to check on possible side-effects and also to monitor their fertility and fertility control histories after their first contact with the program. They were followed up whether or not they continued to use program methods.

The Taichung study was a large and complex operation—one of the largest carefully monitored social science experiments ever carried out. Its execution was an achievement of Dr. S.C. Hsu, Dr. J.Y. Peng, Dr. T.C. Hsu, and many other Chinese public health and medical workers. A few Americans were consultants. Barney Berelson's vision and encouragement fired the enthusiasm and commitment that characterized the program.

In the years that followed the Taichung study, I observed many others whose work with Barney inspired respect for his ability to stimulate thinking about central issues and to state these issues with a simple clarity that captured the attention of a wide and diverse audience and led to major programmatic initiatives. The selected articles in this volume each had a significant effect in the field. They influenced a generation of scholars, officials, and activists. They are relevant for this generation as well.

Ronald Freedman
Roderick D. McKenzie Distinguished
Professor Emeritus of Sociology
University of Michigan

Contents

Acknowledgments v

Foreword vii

Part I – Overview

1 Berelson's Population Writings in Review
John A. Ross and W. Parker Mauldin 1

Part II – Population Policy

2 The Great Debate on Population Policy:
An Instructive Entertainment 11

3 Paths to Fertility Reduction: The 'Policy Cube' 33

4 Beyond Family Planning 42

5 Romania's 1966 Anti-Abortion Decree:
The Demographic Experience of the First Decade 59

Part III – Resource Allocation

6 On the Efficient Allocation of Resources
for Fertility Reduction
Written with Robert H. Haveman 71

Part IV – Action Strategies

7 National Family Planning Programs: A Guide 85

8 Maternity Care and Family Planning as a World Program
Written with Howard C. Taylor, Jr. 101

9 18–35 in Place of 15–45? 109

Part V – Contraceptive Technology

10 The Impact of New Technology 115

Part VI – Assessment of National Family Planning Programs

11 The Record of Family Planning Programs
Written with Ronald Freeman 123

Part VII – Ethical Considerations

12 Government Efforts to Influence Fertility:
The Ethical Issues
Written with Jonathan Lieberson 157

Part VIII – Specialized Investigations

13 A Study in Fertility Control
Written with Ronald Freedman 179

14 Prospects and Programs for Fertility Reduction:
What? Where? 190

15 Conditions of Fertility Decline in Developing Countries,
1965–75
Written with W. Parker Mauldin 217

Bibliography 261

Index 267

Part I—Overview

1
Berelson's Population Writings in Review

John A. Ross and W. Parker Mauldin

In his professional life, Bernard Berelson ranged widely and left his mark on many fields: library science, communications, behavioral sciences, and population. He had a great appreciation of the quest for knowledge and a great loyalty to the institutions that nurture intellectual development. Especially, it was the application of knowledge to the solution of societal problems that stimulated and guided his efforts.

He was an outstanding intellectual leader in the field of population. He was concerned with solutions, with what makes a substantial difference, and was impatient with efforts to refine data and analysis unnecessarily. His strength was in logic, relationships, and magnitudes, not in mathematics as such. But he had a keen "number sense," and a remarkable ability to remember the salient points of a broad range of experiments, programs, and analyses, and to apply these in new situations.

Berelson was a pragmatist, always asking what works, what doesn't work, what makes "a nontrivial difference." Although he viewed rapid population growth as a problem, he was always clear that it was not *the* problem, and that reduction of rapid growth rates was not an end in itself. Population problems need to be solved to promote the goals of increased equity and improved welfare. Ethical issues were always important to him.

More than any other person he helped to guide governments in the development of population policies and programs aimed at lowering rates of population growth. He established the journal *Studies in Family Planning*, the first in the field; he was the principal organizer of the first international conference on population programs, in 1965, and the senior editor of the volume *Family Planning and Population Programs*, a report on that conference; he developed with a colleague a large international program for offering family planning information and services in maternity hospitals in much of the developing world; he was the chief architect in collaboration with John D. Rockefeller 3rd of the World Leaders Declaration on Population, presented on Human Rights Day at the United Nations in 1966; and he sought ways "beyond family planning" to achieve the goal of reducing rates of population growth.

Berelson was constantly sought to participate in inquiries, commissions, review groups, and seminars. One domestic project occupying a great deal of his attention in the late 1960s and early 1970s was the U.S. Commission on Population Growth and the American Future, on which he served as an especially creative member. His ability to look for the applicable meanings and his capacity for synthesis were unique. He was the practical scholar.*

In this chapter, we discuss Berelson's writings on population—which, as the preceding remarks suggest, were only one of the several channels through which he so profoundly affected the field. All of the articles in this volume are discussed in this chapter, but not in the sequence in which they appear. Here we present them as they developed in Berelson's thought and career, roughly chronologically.

---

*The above passages are adapted from W. Parker Mauldin, "Bernard Berelson: A Personal Appreciation," *Studies in Family Planning* 10(10) October 1979.

Because Berelson began at The Population Council as a communications specialist, he examined programs closely at the field level. Thus, his early orientation was highly concrete, and he produced writings on communications strategies (see Bibliography), as well as a guide for large-scale programs and, with Ronald Freedman, the report on the famous Taichung experiment. He also spearheaded development of the postpartum strategy for family planning.

Meanwhile, he was appointed Vice-President of The Population Council and, in 1968, President. These leadership roles encouraged him toward a larger view of the field, and he then wrote also on general issues surrounding the family planning approach to fertility reduction, as in "The Great Debate on Population Policy" and "Beyond Family Planning" (Chapters 2 and 4). He also repeatedly reviewed the progress of national efforts, especially in "The Record of Family Planning Programs," written with Ronald Freedman (Chapter 11). He examined questions of population policy in numerous writings, editing a volume on developed nations and producing such pieces as the "Policy Cube" (Chapter 3) and "Population Policy: Personal Notes" (see Bibliography). He also did a remarkable analysis of Romania's experience in abolishing abortion. This study addressed in part the question of how the available contraceptive technology can affect fertility levels, a recurrent interest in his writings.

Berelson produced a number of these works in the final stage of his population career, after he had left the Council's presidency. In this period, he also dealt with such general questions as the proper allocation of resources and the ethical issues attending population action. He produced a major analysis, with W. Parker Mauldin, of the conditions of fertility decline; somewhat later, he did another on the prospects of attaining low fertility in the developing world by the year 2000. We recommend close attention to the Bibliography; it contains numerous items related to each of these subjects, which could not be included in this volume.

The Guide

In the early 1960s, relatively few countries had family planning programs, and there was but little experience to guide program administrators. In addition, there was a natural tendency for each country to regard its situation as unique and, consequently, not to look for lessons from other programs. Early experience from country efforts and pilot trials suggested how large-scale programs could be designed, and Berelson set these forth in a "Guide" (Chapter 7). He stressed the diffusion opportunity—that if programs would work outward from cities and in a checkerboard pattern across a population, information would probably spread through the grapevine to the untouched areas, and so save costs. Part of the basic plan was to approach couples who were already interested and assist them in carrying out the family limitation objectives they already had, as distinct from working to change motivational levels. "The primary aim, and the direct effort, should be to satisfy the existing interest in family planning." Berelson laid out communication strategies and calculated reasonable expectations as to response, considering that at the outset of a new program substantial percentages will be ineligible, such as the currently pregnant, those wanting more children, and those already sterile. Field-worker types were considered, and a variety of tactics set forth, along with likely budgetary needs. Berelson gave the essentials of a simple record-keeping system, and concluded with 25 summary ground rules that expressed most of the available practical wisdom. The "Guide" was well received and served as a valuable blueprint for program design.

The Taichung Experiment

Soon after he joined The Population Council, Berelson, with Ronald Freedman, cooperated with officials in Taiwan to design a major trial of a family planning program. There had always been serious doubts as to whether populations anywhere were ready, and the sense was that if a strong family planning effort would not work in Taiwan, it would not work anywhere. More optimistically, it was felt that the field badly needed a success. The new IUD had just been developed, and in clinical experience it had shown high acceptability and lengthy continuation; moreover, it cost only about 6¢ and was not dissimilar to the traditional Ota Ring already used by private doctors in Taiwan. Given this technology and the relatively advanced state of Taiwan's economic development, it seemed time for a decisive trial.

The experiment, done in Taichung City, tested four communication approaches crossed by three levels of intensity in home visiting. Each of these variations was evaluated by the proportion of couples adopting family planning, especially the IUD, and these results were posed against costs. It turned out that home visits in half of neighborhoods produced the most acceptances (greatest effectiveness), but the highest cost per acceptance (least efficiency); home visits in one-fifth of neighborhoods did the opposite. Thus, field-workers could visit that one-fifth of neighborhoods and use the saved time to cover a larger territory, with a sizable net gain. The results were published in a noted *Scientific American* article, "A Study in Fertility Control" (Chapter 13), in professional journals, and in the Chinese language in Taiwan.

Overall, the experiment was a breakthrough. It was indeed a success; it documented the popularity of the new IUD; and it showed the diffusion effect outward from such prime inputs as mass media messages and personal contacts by trained field-workers. Numerous acceptors came from unvisited neighborhoods and areas entirely outside the city, and most chose the IUD rather than traditional contraceptive methods. The experiment also gave important guidance on field strategies; for example, it showed that, in Taiwan at least, visits to both wife and husband did little better than visits to the wife alone. Another conclusion basic to much later thinking was that "the nature of the contraceptive method . . . has more of an effect on the success of a program than may have been generally recognized. A 'one-time' method requires far less field effort over a long-term than a method dependent on resupply and sustained motivation."

Postpartum

Searching persistently for better action methods, Berelson called early attention to the potential of postpartum programs (Chapter 8). He noted the efficiency of offering contraceptive education and methods to women seen in maternity facilities, many of whom want the present birth or abortion to be their last. These represent the core of the relevant population—couples who have attained their desired family size (or wish now to space), who are clearly part of the active childbearing subgroup, and who can act to initiate contraception before becoming pregnant again. Previous studies clearly showed that highly fecund, unprotected couples would conceive again quickly, so that prompt action was of the essence.

In the developing world, it was mainly cities that contained postpartum facilities; moreover, professionally attended births occurred only in cities and accounted for only a minority of all deliveries. Nevertheless, contraceptive services could be provided to at least that minority of women, and also to others hearing of the new services by word of mouth and coming in on their own. Further, such programs could engage the medical profession and establish another precedent to energize the family planning movement.

Berelson organized an internationally collaborative trial in some of the world's largest maternity hospitals (25 hospitals from 19 cities in 14 countries, handling about 300,000 deliveries and abortions per year). This project, called the International Postpartum Program, grew to include entire networks of hospitals in India, Colombia, Thailand, and other countries. Postpartum family planning spread to become a standard part of medical practice in much of the developing world.*

The Taylor-Berelson Proposal

An ambitious extension of the postpartum idea then seemed possible (also presented in Chapter 8). Berelson pursued it in collaboration with Howard C. Taylor, an eminent obstetrician who had directed the International Institute for the Study of Human Reproduction at Columbia University and had assisted with the International Postpartum Program. If large donor funding could be attracted to add to country monies, simple infrastructures might be built to give basic maternity care, with family planning, to rural populations.

*For documentation, see G.I. Zatuchni, "International Postpartum Family Planning Program: Report on the First Year," *Studies in Family Planning* Vol 1, No. 22, August 1967. Also R.G. Castadot et al., "The International Postpartum Family Planning Program: Eight Years of Experience," *Reports on Population/Family Planning*, No. 18, November 1975, and G.I. Zatuchni, ed., *Postpartum Family Planning: A Report on the International Program*, New York, McGraw-Hill, 1969.

A feasibility study was completed in 29 countries, and the plan was carried out in five demonstration projects in Asia and Africa. Large-scale applications were never undertaken, however, partly because donors felt that they should focus their funds upon fertility itself rather than upon high cost maternity care infrastructures. National governments, for their part, were already doing what they felt they could to extend buildings and personnel to rural areas, although economic planning boards seldom invested as much in this as the health ministries desired. Governments, in fact, did not take up the concept as such, though in principle many favored the extension of maternity services including family planning. Most real progress for extended family planning services came later, through simple village systems of contraceptive provision that came to be known as community-based distribution programs.

18–35 in Place of 15–45

Berelson's innovative bent appeared in his espousal of childbearing only within the age range 18–35.* He detailed the elevated risks to both mother and child from births at high parities and at very young and old ages, and he was one of the first to make the case for a childbearing range of about 17 years, rather than the biological maximum of about 30 (Chapter 9). Health risks were not the only consideration. The best indication of unwanted pregnancies (i.e., induced abortions) paralleled the ages and parities of high medical risks, reflecting similar profiles of medical, psychological, and social pressures.

Demographic advantages would follow a narrower childbearing range, since birthrates would decline, with the amount of the decrease depending upon the number of births postponed and the numbers permanently averted. There were also benefits to female status, as well as humanitarian gains. Berelson noted that "the girl who has an illegitimate child at the age of 16 suddenly has 90 percent of her life's script written for her . . . Her choices are few, and most of them are bad."

*Or 20–35 in the developed world.

Moreover he observed:

> For many poor women throughout the world, surely 20 years of producing tissue, milk, and children should be enough – 20 years of the "maternal depletion syndrome" that leaves them old before their time. At both the lower and the upper range, the lives of the mothers are particularly ruled by the fact of birth for a long period of years, with alternatives closed off or at best deferred – especially because such mothers tend to be disadvantaged on other scores as well.

He concluded:

> The idea of concentrating human reproduction in the "best years" for childbearing may have much to recommend it. If no children were . . . born to women below 18 or 20 or above 35, the benefits to mankind, and especially to womankind, would appear to be considerable.

Beyond Family Planning

Berelson was very much preoccupied with a central question of strategy in fertility reduction. Looking always for "the do-able," he saw the family planning route as the way to get something going, build consensus, and create a precedent for government involvement. In fact, it represented the only choice generally acceptable to governments and their constituencies. Other measures could come later, if and when they proved feasible, and by then new behavior would be in place that would itself create a new reality and bring some normative change. Norms and behavior interact; either may precede. The norms did not have to be worked on by totally separate approaches. Instead, encouragement and support of the existing interest in birth control would itself reinforce and enlarge that interest. Servicing the present market would enlarge the market.

Others disagreed.† The family planning approach seemed flawed by resting on whatever was acceptable to individuals. Merely helping people attain their desires might leave fertility disastrously high. Further measures were required. For direct attacks

†See, for example, an interesting exchange of letters in the February 23, 1968, issue of *Science*: the first by the Population Committee of the National Academy of Science, and the second a reply by Kingsley Davis.

upon high fertility, however, feasible alternatives to family planning were hard to devise; and historically it was development that had produced lower fertility, though never *replacement* fertility until some years afterward. In this respect, development and family planning alike could promise only intermediate gains. Even later, when much of Western fertility did fall below replacement, it could not be shown that development had caused it to do so. Development had existed long before and, in fact, the fall was unforeseen and unexplained.

Besides, development was hard to come by. Berelson once wrote that there was no puzzle about how to reduce fertility in India – simply elevate the standard of living, raise the marriage age, spread popular education, forbid child labor, and so on.* The problems, of course, were feasibility and costs, and pending solutions to those, it made sense to do the possible, which was to educate and encourage the population toward smaller families and make the means easily available. However, none of this reasoning quieted the controversy.

Berelson himself then wrote the best account ever done on the alternatives to family planning (Chapter 4). Compiling the various suggestions of the critics (and others), he subjected each option to six tests:

> "is the scientific/medical/technological base available or likely? will governments approve? can the proposal be administered? can the society afford the proposal? is it morally acceptable? and finally, will it work?"

He rated each proposal on each of the six criteria, and showed that family planning programs did not compare badly with alternatives. Moreover, if they did not exist they would have to be invented; in fact, they were embedded within many of the other proposals. He noted that it was not for lack of being known that the alternatives had failed to win broad acceptance; most of them had been discussed for years. He called for a more energetic use of what was already workable: "If the field did well what it knows how to do, that in itself would in all likelihood make a measurable difference – and one competitive in magnitude with other specific proposals." At the same time, he urged a persistent search for improvements.

*"Formulation of Population Policy," p. 454. (See Bibliography.)

The Record of Family Planning Programs

The "family planning vs. development" debate was very much sharpened by the United Nations Conference on Population held in 1974 in Bucharest. Because governments were represented officially, the views expressed there tended to subordinate population concerns to larger themes reflecting international political objectives. The focus was largely on development issues generally, in the context of the economic interests of the Third World. This had polarizing effects; it escalated the debate and tended to undermine programs devoted specifically to fertility reduction, which were meant in the first instance to hasten the development effort.

In response, Berelson and Ronald Freedman published "The Record of Family Planning Programs" (Chapter 11), which comprehensively reviewed programs of various types and intensity. They were the first to show the remarkable pattern across developing countries: that for each social setting, the stronger the family planning program, the lower the birthrate and the faster its decline. They looked at country examples and developed a comprehensive set of conclusions detailing the manner in which family planning programs had so far functioned and the ways in which they had contributed to fertility reduction.

The Great Debate

Berelson's efforts to sift out the best truths from the critics of the family planning approach produced a remarkable piece, "The Great Debate on Population Policy" (Chapter 2). There is nothing like it in the literature. It pits three protagonists against each other, each espousing one of the prominent positions and probing for weaknesses in the other two. There is FamPlan, who is convinced of the need to reduce fertility rates in the developing world and sees public family planning programs as the means of choice. There is DevDev, who sees development as the overriding need and the real solution to excessive fertility. Then there is AcCrit, a research-minded, academic type with an admixture of doomsaying. These three thrust and parry, each driven at points to making a lawyer's case for his own position. The arguments fly back and forth on a number of fronts that cover the chief points at issue in the field at large. The debate is lively and, through the generous use of quotations from the literature, reflective of a large cross-section of the best thinking on all sides.

The Policy Cube

In another analysis (Chapter 3), Berelson detailed 31 policy paths, or options, open to governments wishing to reduce their fertility levels. He organized these in seven categories (family planning programs of various types, improved contraceptive technology, socioeconomic determinants, public information, incentives/disincentives, community-level action, and sanctions), and rated each option on three scales (from 1 to 10) regarding their public acceptability, administrative feasibility, and effectiveness in reducing fertility.

Needless to say, no single option qualified as 10–10–10; had any done so, it would have emerged long ago as the dominant policy measure. Highly acceptable approaches tend to lack either feasibility or effectiveness, those possessing effectiveness often lack acceptability, and so on. Berelson arranged the results in a graphic cube to show the position of each choice on each of the three dimensions, and commented upon the resulting implications for the allocation of such resources as funds, staff, and facilities. In practice, policy decisions are indeed made within some such framework, even an unconscious one, to weigh some of the 31 options against criteria like those given, and then to balance the results against costs.

The Romanian Case

In 1966, the Romanian government decided that its population growth rate was too slow. It chose to manipulate the means of fertility control as an instrument to raise fertility, and thereby provided a natural experiment of great interest. At a time when the population placed heavy reliance on abortion as the principal method of birth control, the government suddenly declared abortion essentially illegal. In the 9–11 months following the decree, the birthrate shot up from 14.3, to as high as 39, and it was 27.4 for the year 1967. It then declined as the population turned to other means of fertility control. Many commentators regarded the peak as a temporary dislocation from a stable state that fundamentally reflected the desired family size of Romanians.

Berelson, however, showed that this interpretation was mistaken (Chapter 5). Over the 10 years following the decree, the birthrate never returned to its original level. It also remained above the average level recorded during those years in five nearby countries, whereas it had run below their rates before. During the decade in question, there were about 39% more births than the baseline rates would have produced, and the population grew by over 1 million more than it would have without the abortion decree.

At this writing, with over 20 years elapsed, the indications are that although Romania will fall short of its population goal of about 25 million by 1990, it has succeeded in shifting its level of fertility from the lowest to among the highest in Eastern Europe. It has used both incentives for childbearing and stringent control over access to birth control technology, with some variation in its abortion regulations.

Contraceptive Technology

A debate over the contribution of improved contraceptive technology arose quite early, almost simultaneously with the breakthroughs of the IUD and the pill. Berelson came down solidly on the side of the positive potential of better methods. He held that at any given motivational level and within any social setting, the easier the contraceptive technology was to use, the more it would be used. Various drags on contraceptive use could be relieved: costs could be reduced, coitus-dependent methods could be replaced, pelvic procedures could be avoided, and side effects could be ameliorated. If acceptability could be high, if effectiveness could be certain, and if continuation could be prolonged and automatic, surely that would help.

Those who differed claimed that people would avoid births if they "really wanted to," that "mere contraceptive supply" changed nothing, and that fertility in "the long run" was controlled by life conditions and socioeconomic factors. Berelson addressed the technology question most fully in the article reprinted in Chapter 10.*

In it, he pointed out that:

> Modernization is occurring throughout the developing world, but slowly: Do we wait for that to "solve" the problem of population growth through fertility reduction? If so we need improvements in neither program nor technology. Programs are improving too, but slowly and unevenly: Should we wait for them to carry the existing technology in a more effective manner, limited only by the socioeconomic thresholds? And the technology is improving, but that too is slow: Nothing really new in 10–15 years. The easy answer, and the correct one as far as it goes, is to work on all three simultaneously, as we now do.

That answer led to the question of how best to allocate resources among the three efforts. Time enters into the equation—improved technology deserves a large investment if it promises a better method soon, but not if it takes 50 years. The investment question, however, must be answered repeatedly, year by year. Fourteen years have passed since Berelson's analysis, and the only "breakthrough" method to be developed in that time (the implant) is just beginning to have field implementation. In retrospect, that would have argued for less investment in it. Yet today, most programs still stand badly in need of better technology, and investments are still needed in possibilities that promise to reach application within a reasonable time frame.

Berelson considered three areas in which technology could be improved, namely, effectiveness, acceptability, and continuation. Effectiveness of the pill, IUD, and sterilization (with abortion in some areas as backup for failures) was already sufficiently high that little improvement could be expected. Acceptability was vital; the more couples accepting a contraceptive method, the better. The value of acceptances, however, depended upon continuation, which analysis showed to be very important.

There was the question of trade-offs—a new method might offer good acceptability but mediocre continuation, or it might offer the reverse. While acceptance rates are important, their value rests heavily upon average continuation. Berelson found that:

> Demographically, improving the continuation of a method by 10 points within the current range is worth more than the entire acceptance level today in the largest most needy countries. From their standpoint, which is easier: to get twice as many acceptors or to improve continuation by 5–10 points? If a new method could do either one, that would double the demographic impact where it is most needed.

A new method might contribute in another way: it might transform the program's delivery system by extending its reach into the rural sector. The IUD did this in the early Taiwan and Korea programs by stimulating the addition of a new cadre of fieldworkers, who put interested women in touch with physicians who inserted IUDs. Later, when the pill was produced at low cost, Thailand permitted its delivery through a system of rural paramedics that radically enlarged the national program.

Berelson was a strong supporter of The Population Council's International Committee for Contraception Research, a group devoted to the rapid testing of promising contraceptive leads. Over the years, its work and that of others made it clear that no magic method would appear with all the advantages. Still, research could discover additional methods, each of which could better serve the needs of a particular subgroup. In addition, programs could make fuller use of methods already created, and the evidence seemed to show that where local views permitted their use, the addition of either sterilization or abortion significantly increased program effectiveness. Historically, better technology appeared to be helping to reduce fertility, as the pill, IUD, and simpler female sterilization became the world's leading birth control methods, and country after country found that contraceptive prevalence increased with each additional modern method introduced.

*He also set forth his basic position in "Demographic Requirements of Fertility Control Technology: 15 Propositions." (See Bibliography.)

Resource Allocation

Questions of resource allocation arose from two sources. One was the problem of what emphasis to give to the usual family planning programs, as opposed to others that included such alternatives as maternal and child health components, incentives, "development," and so on. The other was the problem of how to allocate funds among action programs, contraceptive development, social science research, and other such choices. Much of the difficulty stemmed from the very willingness of foundations, governments, and international donors to commit large funds in support of country efforts—in essence, a continuation of the humanitarian support of mortality control programs after World War II. Even in 1952, only 7 years after the war, the new imbalance of mortality and fertility had become clear. In that year, the International Planned Parenthood Federation was founded, India established the first national program, and a meeting of population specialists in Williamsburg, Virginia, where the presence of extraordinary growth rates was confirmed, led to the creation of The Population Council. Ten years later, when Berelson joined the Council, there were still relatively few donors; but by the late 1960s, they had become numerous, and Berelson took an increasing interest in the optimal allocation of the funding resources of the population field.

Aggregate funding grew into the 1970s, but the recession of 1973 and the global oil crisis caused drastic reductions in the funding strength of certain foundations and developing nations. Funding plateaued also for the two largest grant-making donors, the U.S. Agency for International Development and the United Nations Fund for Population Activities, moving them to set priorities among the various population activities they supported.

In 1979 Berelson, with Robert Haveman, published a study on resource allocation (Chapter 6). They took the novel tack of querying a panel of experienced professionals in the population field, directing them to give effectiveness ratings to 12 choices of how governments might approach fertility reduction—including such options as family planning programs of various types, incentives, information campaigns, and sanctions. The 12 options, however, were rated not simply in general, but for each of nine different situations, which crossed three social setting levels by three program strength levels. The result was a set of judgments as to the most effective ways to reduce fertility in these nine different situations.

Using the methods of applied welfare economics, Berelson and Haveman were able to translate the ratings into a rational allocation of donor funding. Money would be spent more effectively where the social setting was better and where implementation was stronger, regardless of which intervention was involved. And although the experts disagreed considerably, certain interventions were uniformly favored over others, with the greatest agreement on the family planning program variations. The panel members fell into five clusters as indicated by similarity of ratings, but nearly all responses implied the allocation of over half of available resources to the most favored social settings and the strongest implementation categories. In effect, this meant that most resources would go to smaller countries, with relatively few people; however, this imbalance could be reduced if resources were free to go to the least disadvantaged sectors within countries. The analysis, while exploratory, pointed to the need to assess effectiveness per unit of investment.

Ethics

Berelson had a sharp appreciation for what he called the time penalty—that anything not done now would be more difficult to do later. The discouraging reality of this penalty was confirmed in technical analyses that documented the terrible momentum of population growth, showing that even with an immediate decline to replacement fertility, the total population in most developing countries would grow by another two-thirds before stabilizing. The growth would, in fact, considerably exceed that, since an immediate change was impossible. Berelson was acutely aware of the need for action that was prompt, large-scale, and vigorous.

Yet this did not deter him from returning insistently to the ethical questions that attend population action. Upon receiving the Margaret Sanger

Award from The Planned Parenthood Federation of America,* he stressed that:

In the best of all possible worlds it would be enough to do three things: maximize the flow of full information about the consequences of fertility behavior both individual and collective, maximize the capacity of people to regulate their fertility by medically approved means in accordance with individual conscience, and minimize undue legal or cultural pressures on fertility behavior either way. Those conditions are met today for a small fraction of the world's population—and that fraction, incidentally, has very low fertility. If those conditions were met, then let the demographic chips fall where they may: the trade-off between childbearing and other ends in life would then have found their free and rational level. What we seek is human welfare, personal freedom, and the quality of life, and demographic trends and changes take on meaning only insofar as they contribute to such ends.

He added, in a major ethical inquiry (Chapter 12):

The trouble is, this is not the best of all possible worlds, so we must settle for less-than-optimal solutions in order not to get worse. This essay has been our effort to pick a way through the maze of ethical issues enmeshing "the population problem" and chart a decent and humane path.

His treatment of the ethical issues and his refusal to choose simple resolutions are best understood by reference to that chapter. He and coauthor Jonathan Lieberson identify three government policies that have raised ethical questions, give an appraisal and ethical assessment of each, and explain the general rationale that they themselves favor. They take an eclectic approach, refusing to embrace any single, rigid system. They also stick to those ethical concerns that fall into the domain of actions, taken on demographic grounds, by governments, to change fertility.

Certain concerns pertain to limitations placed on access to medically approved birth control methods (e.g., sterilization in many countries, abortion in yet more, and even the pill, as in Japan for some years). Other concerns revolve around both positive and negative incentives. Finally, some pertain to government-induced peer pressure and community pressures upon the individual.

In all cases, there are gray areas, exceptions, and refinements. The array of conflicting "goods" and multiple ethical desiderata put clear resolutions out of reach, but Berelson and Lieberson argue for proper *process* and proper *substance*: the former concerned with the citizens' participation in decisions affecting them, and the latter concerned with such values as personal freedom and collective welfare.

Conditions of Fertility Decline

Yet another investigation, undertaken with W. Parker Mauldin, looked at a comprehensive set of factors controlling fertility declines (Chapter 15). These included the effects of socioeconomic correlates, demographic factors, and family planning program strength. Going beyond previous analyses, Mauldin and Berelson applied six models of analysis to data from 94 developing countries, and found that the six approaches agreed rather closely. Given any social setting, stronger programs produced larger fertility declines; and given any program strength, the better social settings produced larger declines. Most fortunate of all were those countries with both high social settings and strong programs—they had the sharpest declines and the lowest levels of fertility.

From the action standpoint, it was a great advantage that the social settings were helping; in fact they explained about two-thirds of variance in fertility declines. It was also an advantage that the programs were in place as a hastening and reinforcing influence; they explained about 15–20% of the variance, beyond what the social settings could explain. The relative importance of the two could easily differ from one country to another—in some cases, the program was more the initiating force, working rather independently in the absence of much social change, while in others, rapid modernization was the key factor. But overall, the evidence was that both mattered, and each could help the other.

*See "1966–1977: A Look at the Record" for the acceptance address. See also "Population and Its Problems: A Plain Man's Guide." (See Bibliography.)

Prospects

Near the end of his life, Berelson stood back to take a measure of country prospects. Would countries after all experience significant fertility reduction? There were the Koreas and Taiwans, which were well on the way, showing every sign of coming to the desired balance of low fertility and low mortality. But there were also the Nigerias and Pakistans, for which less hope existed. What change was likely, and what programs might hasten it?

Berelson's attack on the prospects question (Chapter 14) was characteristically concrete. He asked how close developing countries would come to a crude birthrate of 20 by the year 2000, corresponding roughly to a one percent growth rate and a 2.5 child family. To answer this question for each of 29 countries (covering 85% of the developing world), he drew upon three bodies of information: demographic, socioeconomic, and program. Part of his assessment rested on "correspondence points" between fertility levels and the socioeconomic indicators, with attention to tentative "thresholds" of development, beyond which fertility change usually begins or accelerates. Although these assessments depended upon correlations from the past, and involved uncertainty about the nature of thresholds, Berelson showed what could be wrested from this material and how extensively the results would have to be contradicted if differing predictions were to be accepted.

Four groups of countries emerged in terms of their likelihood of meeting the target: the certain, the probable, the possible, and the unlikely, with 70% of people in the developing world (including the Chinese) falling into the middle two groups. The bottom group, however, included Bangladesh, Pakistan, and Nigeria. Overall, even an optimistic extrapolation of past fertility declines in the 29 countries showed a shortfall in reaching the year 2000 target.

This led naturally to the question of policy, whose purpose, as Berelson once wrote, is to change the future. He again reviewed measures advocated by the several protagonists, ranging across family planning programs of different types, various development strategies, new approaches at the community level, and official incentives and sanctions. He assessed the promise of each measure for each of the four groups and called for better ideas than had yet been contributed by the partisans of measures beyond family planning.

It is our pleasure to introduce you to *Berelson on Population*. Intellectually curious readers of this volume will also profit from reading *Voting*, his outstanding study of public opinion formation in a presidential campaign (written with Paul Lazarsfeld and William McPhee), published in 1954. *Graduate Education in the United States*, published in 1960, was an important scientific analysis in yet another field. In 1964, he published (with Gary Steiner) *Human Behavior: An Inventory of Scientific Findings*, which stands as a classic in the literature of the behavioral sciences.

Part II – Population Policy

2
The Great Debate on Population Policy: An Instructive Entertainment

Preface

This paper is a debate among three positions intended as prototypic. On any matter as complicated as population policy, there are probably as many positions as there are participants. Hence no one is likely to feel fully represented in this (or any other) typology: "That's not the way I see it." Several other prototypic participants could have been included, but I have made a conscious effort to incorporate various subpositions intended to reflect the breadth if not the richness of the debate. If some qualification is lost, that is after all the essence of prototypes—and, it must be added, public policy as well, where the decision-maker takes what he can from the contending parties.

In order to maximize faithful representation, the debate utilizes actual statements from the literature that has built up in recent years. That literature is quite large, so the selections are illustrative only, and in a double sense: there is much more where they came from and there are many more participants. In any case, no individual's view should be confused with that of the debater here who borrows his argument: individuals speak for themselves. Nor is there any reason to identify organizations with these prototypes: the major population organizations are all characterized by internal debate on these same issues, indeed accommodate the three debaters within.

Reprinted with permission from The Population Council, New York, NY, 1975.

I believe the main themes are here, given expression by their own advocates, and I trust that the content truly and fairly illustrates the present state of the discourse. The discussion does tend to concentrate on the dominant current strategies, and hence the debate is a little lopsided since the major actor tends to defend his efforts against the criticisms of the others. But that too is the way it is, perhaps inevitably in such situations.

I have taken the liberty of eliminating what would have been a jarring profusion of quotation marks, so frequent are the attributions. In virtually all cases, the passage preceding a numbered reference is verbatim from the indicated source; the beginning of the quotation is marked by the symbol ►. In the few cases where no symbol appears, the referenced passage is a paraphrase. Nowhere, to the best of my knowledge, is any selection misquoted or misrepresented. Naturally, I have provided the transition, summary, organization, and textual flow required by this form of exposition—in short, the orchestration.

It remains for me to acknowledge explicitly what in any case should be obvious—namely, that this is only one man's view of the matter, in selection and emphasis, in juxtaposition and conclusion. At least, this is how it all sounds to one participant. If what follows is not the debate as it really is, at least it is a perception of the debate that probably prevails in a major sector of the field. And in a major geographic sector too: this formulation of the debate is heavily, unduly, Western in origin—but then so is the debate itself.

In any case, here is an effort to hold the mirror up to nature, with a compressing mechanism: to distill the issues by having the major protagonists have at each other in frank exchange, and thus come closer to saying, in compacted form, what they really think. I trust it has the ring of verisimilitude to informed others, plus utility. For something may be gained by this device, if as intended it captures the essential elements for candid cross-appraisal. That something, in the end, is to clarify and advance the debate.

Finally, I trust that I may be forgiven for borrowing the form of this essay from myself, in "The great debate on cultural democracy," *Values in America*, Donald N. Barrett, editor (Notre Dame, Indiana: University of Notre Dame Press, 1961), pages 147–168; and that it is understood that to the extent I speak in these pages, I do so for myself, and not for the sponsoring organization.

Introduction

The past decade has been marked by debate on "population policy," within countries and among countries. Like most other debates dealing with public policy on complex social issues, it has been conducted on shifting grounds, under changing rules, by differing participants. Nevertheless, the double core of the debate has always been visible: *whether*, for human welfare now and later, the current rapid rates of population growth need to be slowed down; and if so, *how* that is to be done through deliberate action, mainly by governments.

In 1974, for the first time in man's history, a worldwide conference of governments was held on population policy under United Nations auspices. Far from being settled, the debate was if anything heightened thereby and now continues on a post-Bucharest basis.

This is a contribution to that debate. It is intended to distill the argumentation to essentials, to confront the contending positions directly with one another, to join the issues in a manner not customary in traditional modes. From such a review may come a re-view of where matters really stand.

The growth issue is not the only issue of population policy, but it is the central issue under debate in recent years and the central focus of national and international remedial action. A recent paper exploring the possibility of consensus [81] listed no fewer than 16 policy positions, and even that does not exhaust the distinctions insisted upon by various protagonists.

The debaters are spokesmen for three prominent viewpoints, clearly identifiable amid the rhetorical mosaic:

FAMPLAN persuaded of the validity of "the population problem," defined as the need to reduce growth rates and hence fertility rates throughout the world but primarily in the developing countries where they are now particularly high; further persuaded that a useful action to that end is public provision of information and services directed at the voluntary control of fertility among interested couples; typically of a public health or sociological orientation. (It might be fair to add that FamPlan can be seen as representing the Population Establishment in the elementary sense that most of the available resources for population activities are now allocated under this direction, at least in the applied field; thus he could have been called PopEst, but since family programs are near the heart of the policy controversy it seemed better to utilize the more proximate title.)

DEVDEV primarily interested in "development not population"; varies in his concern over the effect of demographic variables upon development but firmly convinced that the best way to attack population growth, perhaps the only way, is via economic development, social change, social/political revolution, "the new international economic order" . . . ; typically of an economic or political orientation.

ACCRIT primarily comes to the debate with deep specialized knowledge, theoretical identification, methodological sophistication, and perhaps the ingrained intellectual tendency toward commentary ranging across disciplinary interests but centering on professional demography; plus at some points the voice of another academic commentator, the voice of demographic doom, eco-catastrophe, population

[81] Teitelbaum.

bomb, the lifeboat ethic, triage—typically biological and ecological in origin.*

These three seem to represent major foci of views for a productive interchange, and there are three broad topics before the house: population in the context of development, the merit of family planning programs, and the strategies of intervention.

Population in the Context of Development

DEVDEV—I begin at the foundation: for the poor of the world, development is the thing, not population; population control is no panacea for development; more than that, development and only development will cure the ills of population. ► Lowering the birth rate will not in itself free developing countries from the need to search vigorously for means to achieve agrarian reform, to modernize industry and agricultural production, and to raise the level of education and culture [44]. As the nations of the world in congress assembled said, ► population policies are constituent elements of socio-economic development policies, never substitutes for them [89]. ► Population policy objectives cannot properly be set in isolation of other social and economic objectives [79]. ► As a matter of fact, Bucharest put population where it belonged—on the back seat of the development bus, and you fellows should feel lucky that you got on the bus at all [84]. ► It has truly been said that the best contraceptive is development [76]. ► Take Care of the People and the Population Will Take Care of Itself [1].

FAMPLAN—You are making several points at once, and they need separation. First is the point that lowering population growth is no panacea for development. I'm glad you began with that for I couldn't agree with you more. If population growth rates were halved tomorrow in the developing countries, that in itself would not solve the problems of poverty, education and illiteracy, sanitation and disease, food and nutrition, and all the rest. At the same time, it *would* provide a better opportunity for their solution. I have always believed that ► no population policy can be a substitute for economic development. Poverty can only be cured by enhanced production [60]. I thought we had agreed about ending the ► almost meaningless debate in recent years among the advocates of economic development, social change, and family planning.... The debate is unnecessary because, if one thing is more obvious than another, it is that all three are required and that no one is a substitute for the other [60]. ► While neither I nor most of my professional colleagues in the population establishment can be considered revolutionaries, it is always a surprise to us to learn that we are proposing population control *instead of* some other ingredients of modernization. We talk more about population than about the balance of trade, income equalization or revamping primary school education, not because we consider these to be of less importance, but because we prefer to talk about those things we know something about. At the very least, this should be judged as merciful [78]. Somehow the attention given population matters in recent years has boomeranged on this point, but those of us working in the field—except perhaps for a few zealots—haven't claimed that we have the magic key to the future, only one important element. It would be good to put that caricature to rest.

ACCRIT—Not so fast, and speak for yourself. ► The explosive growth of the human popula-

*The title does not imply, of course, that there are no critical academics in the other camps, for surely there are. And I appreciate that this title, unlike the others, does not represent a position in the population debate per se. However, in this as in other debates on public policy, the academic critic receives restitutional expression—the commentator on society's actions from outside the pit, the evaluator, the defender of intellectual and moral standards, and so on.

[44] Guzevaty, p. 22. [89] World Population Conference, para. 14d. [79] Tabbarah, p. 32. [84] United Nations. [76] Singh, p. 2.

[1] Action Pack. [60] Notestein, p. 2. [60] Notestein, p. 7. [78] Stycos, p. 162.

tion is the most significant terrestrial event of the past million millennia.... No geological event in a billion years . . . has posed a threat to terrestrial life comparable to that of human overpopulation [36]. ► It is now too late to "solve" the world's population problem. Much that has been destroyed or wasted can never be restored [32]. ► No technical solution can rescue us from the misery of overpopulation. Freedom to breed will bring ruin to all [45].

FAMPLAN—There speaks the California School of Population Crisis. But that is more an argument between you fellows, between those who think population is Nothing and those who think it is Everything. I am content to think it is a significant Something—as the US Commission said, a serious intensifier and multiplier of a whole range of social problems.

DEVDEV—I'm grateful for FamPlan's discovered moderation, but what I want to stress is that ► decision-making in population must be integrated in the decision-making process of development [79]. ► The message of Bucharest is not that development policy is a substitute for population policy but that the latter is a component of the former [79], and must be carried on, as the Plan of Action says, within the context of development.

FAMPLAN—I've heard that so often, without specification, that I'm beginning to think it's a slogan. We had thought that population or family planning "going it alone" represents simply a division of labor, an elementary recognition of specialized interests and talents. Yet somehow we are always criticized for not being located ► solidly within the context of general economic and social development . . . [71]. Is the point organizational, programmatic, political, propagandistic, or simply semantic? What exactly does it mean?

DEVDEV—To begin with, it means that population activities should be organized within national and international developmental efforts. Beyond that . . .

[1] Action Pack. [60] Notestein, p. 2. [60] Notestein, p. 7. [78] Stycos, p. 162. [36] Ehrlich and Ehrlich, p. 1. [32] Davis, p. 26. [45] Hardin, p. 1248. See also [43] Greene. [79] Tabbarah, p. 35. [79] Tabbarah, p. 16. [71] Rockefeller, p. 4.

FAMPLAN—Excuse me, but they already are and always have been. ► Family planning programs are, without exception, part of broader economic development plans [56]. Moreover, the United Nations Fund for Population Activities is the only specialized agency that operates *within* the United Nations Development Programme—not outside as with health or education or industry or employment or environment or food and agriculture. As it happens, population is the only one to be organizationally integrated.

DEVDEV—As I was about to say, beyond that, you should do three things. First, as a tactical improvement over the present situation, you should integrate your family planning efforts into ongoing programs of broader character, as, for example, health, maternal and child care, rural development, community development, agricultural modernization, small industry, and so on.

FAMPLAN—That must really be a question of efficiency. It's not at all clear that putting family planning into other efforts won't raise more problems than it solves, or work worse than the traditional models, especially when you take into account the administrative difficulties of implementing anything as well as the limitations in funding. We may be in for it, post-Bucharest, but if so, that's for political reasons not professional ones.

DEVDEV—As I said, that was only tactical. Second, and the major strategic issue, is to appreciate that development itself will bring about a fertility decline. And Bucharest agreed that basic ► development goals generally have an effect on the socio-economic context of reproductive decisions that tends to moderate fertility levels [89], to quote the Plan. Anyway, isn't that what history shows us?—not only in the great fertility gulf between developed and developing countries, as rationalized in the theory of the demographic transition, but before our very eyes in what's happening around the world today when, for example, you compare Taiwan with India. ► There is no need to take steps to affect fertility directly; all our resources should be directed

[56] Mauldin, p. 2. [89] World Population Conference, para. 32.

to accelerating development, not preventing births [58].

AcCrit–► To take this position is to ignore the fact that the explosively rapid population growth which will occur during the waiting period may well prevent the development of its cure [63].

FamPlan–Anyway, ► to call the promotion of economic and social change a population policy seems like letting the tail wag the dog [61]. ► Perhaps [we] have paid little attention to economic development as a specific population policy on the simple grounds that if development is not undertaken for itself, it will not be undertaken because it should help to reduce birth rates [60]. It is absurd to advocate development as a cure for a high birth rate: who cares about the birth rate if development is achieved? Then the rationale for fertility intervention diminishes–cart before the horse, defining away the problem. It's a Rube Goldberg solution par excellence.

AcCrit–Here I must agree. ► That population policy considerations somehow could speed up the overall level of such developmental efforts of governments seems to me an extremely far-fetched idea [33]. ► We are likely to be left with the platitudinous proposition that economic and social development will be helpful in solving the population problem–the more development, the better–but the structure of development measures, the real policy issue, remains determined without reference to demographic considerations [33]. ► Must we simply credit development in toto and not seek to analyze and encourage those aspects of the developmental process which are important [63]?

DevDev–But of course that is what I have in mind. The trouble is, FamPlan, that you fellows work on supply without sufficiently considering demand. For that, you must single out those factors in development that are most likely to have an impact on fertility and stress them–what some people call the threshold factors. ► What this actually says is that population policy should attempt to emphasize those aspects of development that have the maximum desirable effect on the achievement of its objectives [79], those ► development programmes and educational and health strategies which ... have a decisive impact upon demographic trends, including fertility [89].

AcCrit–Before you get very far over the threshold, I have to warn that the more we learn about the historical causes of fertility decline, the less we seem to know. The European transition now appears to be much more complicated, with the so-called threshold factors very blurred if indeed they exist at all. After close examination of such factors as industrialization, urbanization, infant mortality, and literacy, we find ► that there appears to be little in the statistical record for Europe which confirms the existence of an association between the beginning of the fertility decline and any specific level, or threshold, of economic and social development [85]. ► Examples can be found illustrating the presumed influence of [several] factors, but counter-examples or exceptions are nearly as prevalent [26]–the Austrio-Hungarians, the French peasants, the Hutterites, the Soviet republics in Asia. In short, ► research into particular threshold values of social and economic variables which might yield satisfactory predictions of when fertility falls could be expected to occur does not appear to have produced such predictions; rather the reverse–it has suggested such a diverse pattern of demographic transition as to cast significant doubt as to whether it will ever be possible to use historical experience to make such predictions [52]. Not to mention the dangers in equating the twentieth century Third World with the nineteenth century West.

DevDev–Academic caution, if not one-upmanship! There are surely a number of aspects of development that can reasonably be expected to have the effect of reducing fertility. We talk about them all the time: popular education [79, 46, 58, 70, 21, 22, 57, 89], equality for women [70, 21, 57, 58, 12, 89], income equalization [21, 12, 22, 70, 53, 89], improvements in employment espe-

---

[58] National Academy of Sciences et al., p. 95. [63] Oppenheimer, p. 75. [61] Ohlin, p. 159. [60] Notestein, p. 8. [33] Demeny, p. 4. [33] Demeny, p. 5. [63] Oppenheimer, p. 75.

[79] Tabbarah, pp. 34–35. [89] World Population Conference, para. 31. [85] van de Walle and Knodel, p. 18. [26] Coale, p. 18. [52] King, p. 7. [79] Tabbarah, p. 34; [46] Hauser, p. 412; [58] National Academy of

cially for women [79, 70, 22, 21, 57, 89], extension of social security and old-age benefits [53, 79, 70, 58, 57, 89], reduction of infant mortality [79, 57, 22, 89], encouragement of social mobility [79, 70, 57], rural modernization and increased agricultural productivity [70, 53, 46], extension of children's rights and the elimination of child labor [58, 70, 57, 89], increased incomes and living standards [22, 57, 70], improved health services [21, 70, 57], industrialization with special reference to employment of women [46, 11], reform of land-tenure systems [58, 57], better housing [57, 21], urbanization [57, 70], new roads [46], reform of inheritance laws [58], and elimination of polygamy [58]—and I may have overlooked a few. In short, those overall social policies that do most to promote social justice [21, 89].*

FAMPLAN—Well, if AcCrit doesn't know what they are, you certainly do! But what am I supposed to do about that impressive list—which, when you add it up, takes us back to development in toto, or very close to it. If you, DevDev, haven't been able to do "enough" on such factors with all your resources, where does that leave us in the population field? ► To think that manipulation of such variables adds significant new weaponry to population policies is almost certainly an exaggeration, and frequently amounts to, or fosters, wishful thinking [33]. Can nothing be done until these thresholds are reached?—which are pathetically out of reach where needed most. What are the programmatic specifics, not just the theoretical positions? Do you advocate simply incorporating the present allocation of population resources into that broad search?—putting the 2 percent now supporting population efforts in with the 98 percent devoted to general development, and forgetting about population?

DEVDEV—No, it would probably get lost there and population shouldn't be forgotten. The point is that selected efforts should get greater emphasis, and from far greater resources. Anyway, I don't mean to suggest that everything on this list is of equal importance. Start at the root, with income equalization and poverty reduction. ► In the absence of rural modernization, sustained overall fertility decline in rural areas *cannot* be anticipated [53]. ► Equality in the distribution of the development process and its benefits [53] is the thing. ► In most poor countries, large-scale fertility declines cannot be expected until the living conditions of the majority of the population improve enough so that they no longer consider large families necessary for *economic* reasons . . . [70]. Stress reduction of poverty rather than reduction of fertility. The former will lead to the latter, as it always has. Thus large social changes appear to be required before FamPlan's effort can be more than trivially effective. And to the extent that population growth holds back those very changes, then we have a chicken-egg problem of great magnitude on which only the edges can be attacked.

---

*These references should not be considered as exhausting the possible listing.

Sciences, p. 96; [70] Rich, pp. 10, 45; [21] Casey, p. 24; [22] Cassen, p. 238; [57] National Academy of Sciences, p. 85; [89] World Population Conference, para. 32d. [70] Rich, p. 44; [21] Casey, p. 24; [57] National Academy of Sciences, p. 86; [58] National Academy of Sciences, p. 96; [12] Black and Hankinson, p. 23; [89] World Population Conference, para. 32b. [21] Casey, p. 24; [12] Black and Hankinson, p. 23; [22] Cassen, p. 238; [70] Rich, p. 17; [53] Kocher, p. 89; [89] World Population Conference, para. 32c. [79] Tabbarah, p. 34; [70] Rich, pp. 16, 32; [22] Cassen, p. 238; [21] Casey, p. 24; [57] National Academy of Sciences, p. 86; [89] World Population Conference, para. 32b. [53] Kocher, p. x; [79] Tabbarah, p. 34; [70] Rich, p. 42; [58] National Academy of Sciences, p. 96; [57] National Academy of Sciences, p. 86; [89] World Population Conference, para. 32e. [79] Tabbarah, p. 34; [57] National Academy of Sciences, p. 86; [22] Cassen, p. 238; [89] World Population Conference, para. 32a. [79] Tabbarah, p. 34; [70] Rich, p. 15; [57] National Academy of Sciences, p. 85. [70] Rich, p. 29; [53] Kocher, p. 89; [46] Hauser, p. 412. [58] National Academy of Sciences, p. 96; [70] Rich, p. 45; [57] National Academy of Sciences, p. 85; [89] World Population Conference, para. 32e. [22] Cassen, p. 238; [57] National Academy of Sciences, p. 85; [70] Rich, p. 15. [21] Casey, p. 24; [70] Rich, p. 13; [57] National Academy of Sciences, p. 86. [46] Hauser, p. 412; [11] Bindary, pp. 193–194. [58] National Academy of Sciences, p. 96; [57] National Academy of Sciences, p. 85. [57] National Academy of Sciences, p. 87; [21] Casey, p. 24. [57] National Academy of Sciences, p. 85; [70] Rich, p. 14. [46] Hauser, p. 412. [58] National Academy of Sciences, p. 96. [58] National Academy of Sciences, p. 96. [21] Casey, p. 24; [89] World Population Conference, para. 32c. [33] Demeny, p. 4. [53] Kocher, p. x. [53] Kocher, p. 57. [70] Rich, p. 2.

ACCRIT—The trouble is that ► the spread of modernization is painfully slow [31], although at the same time I must acknowledge that, ► in actual fact, many developing countries have undergone enormous, if piecemeal, changes in recent years [13]. But still, a direct demographic attack is needed because ► modernization alone . . . has nowhere in the world to date had an abiding and drastically downward effect on family-size desires [13]. ► In any case, there is no ineluctable process at work here, as though a kind of mechanistic determinism will prevail—some peoples are more amenable to change than others, good operators get results where poor ones don't [48].

FAMPLAN—I agree that things are changing slowly, but they are changing. And that provides my rationale. ► To assert categorically that India or Indonesia or any other country "is not ready" for family planning or a fertility decline seems to assume that these countries are no different than they were twenty-five or fifty or one hundred years ago. . . . But . . . they have changed in many ways [40]. ► It is still plausible to argue that the transformations that have already occurred *may* be sufficient to support a reasonably successful family planning program, at least in the advanced sectors of most populations [40]. And the only way to find out is to try. As Justice Holmes said, "The way in which the inevitable comes to pass is through effort." In any case, we do seem to agree ► on two propositions: alleviate the plight of the poor (read: promote social and economic development) and at the same time make available modern means of fertility control . . . (read: provide family planning) [9].

DEVDEV—What we're trying to tell you is that development ► planning should focus on the diffusion of the material conditions of socio-economic change which accompany the demographic transition [22]. Despite this array, ► this is not the same as to say that development is a substitute for population policy [79].

ACCRIT—► These policies are socially beneficial as an integral part of modernization and can be so evaluated quite apart from any effects they may have on fertility. On the other hand, although they are statistically correlated with relatively low or declining fertility, the causal relations are not entirely clear. The quantitative magnitude of the impact on fertility and the time required for this impact are uncertain [57]. In any case, ► precisely because of [their] appeal . . . , it can be taken for granted that countries do their best to pursue policies aimed at achieving them regardless of fertility effects. . . . [Moreover,] the existing state of knowledge concerning the determinants of fertility behavior in general seems to dictate strong reservations as to the adequacy of a spontaneous adjustment of fertility in response to the process of economic and social development [35].

DEVDEV—► This seems to me precisely the opposite of the truth. Most of the things that might help fertility require doing things about poverty, and this is just what governments do *not* do. Family planning can only have a modest impact on poor, illiterate rural populations subject to high mortality, so improve socio-economic circumstances and, since it doesn't cost much, do whatever you can with family planning at the same time. But surely the point is to avoid pretense that there is any substitute for making poor people richer. When you get right down to it, more governments are pursuing family planning than income re-distribution [23].

FAMPLAN—So where does that leave us? The fact is, DevDev, that you and your colleagues don't think population pressures are sufficiently serious to warrant any shift in your own development plans. ► It is, in fact, doubtful whether arguments based on fertility effects of development policies are ever strong enough appreciably to modify the mix of development measures that planners would otherwise propose [35]. And despite what you think, AcCrit isn't sure which buttons should be pushed—except that family planning isn't one of them.

ACCRIT—All I can say is that ► the conceptualization of the determinants of fertility requires acceptance of the involvement of a multitude of factors that vary greatly in the intensity and

---

[31] Davis, p. 18. [13] Blake, p. 42. [13] Blake, p. 59. [48] Heaps. [40] Freedman and Takeshita, p. 359. [40] Freedman and Takeshita, p. 360. [9] Berelson, p. 27. [22] Cassen, p. 238. [79] Tabbarah, p. 34.

[57] National Academy of Sciences, p. 85. [35] Demeny, p. 8. [23] Cassen. [35] Demeny, p. 9.

direction of force they exert on fertility [49]. In other words, ► virtually all models of fertility decline involve assertions of multiple causation, that is, the view that several different factors make at least a non-trivial contribution to the process [18]. In short, ► existing theories of fertility decline leave the policy maker vast room for choice. Narrow policy prescriptions do not flow from [the] theory. If we wish to be doctrinaire, there must be some other basis for it [18].

The Merit of Family Planning Programs

The debaters turn to the major effort now being made to directly affect demographic considerations, namely, family planning programs.

AcCrit—► Will current programs succeed [30]? The answer is No. ► The world has yet to witness a family planning program which initiated a decline in fertility in a "traditional society" characterized by mass illiteracy and poverty. The examples of "successful" family planning programs to date . . . are in areas in which fertility declines had already set in before the advent of national family planning policies and programs . . . [47].

FamPlan—To initiate any broad social trend is quite a trick, but we do think we have expedited decline, and consider that a worthwhile accomplishment at the cost. In most settings it has proved impossible to actually carry out the intended program, except on a pilot basis. We probably overestimated the capacity of the administrative system to provide the indicated services, but that would be true of most field efforts, as DevDev surely knows from his own experience. Most programs are still quite weak [56], so we may not really know—is it lack of interest or lack of program?

DevDev—You still won't acknowledge failure, ► that the lowering of population growth rates is [really] dependent on such things as higher living standards, more equal income distribution, higher levels of employment, education, health care—and not by pills and loops alone. . . . ► The results [of your family planning programs] were a dismal and expensive failure [66].

FamPlan—In all fairness to both of us, what you meant to say was ► that population control, measured by the hopes and expectations of the neomalthusians in the mid-sixties . . . is unquestionably a considerable—and costly—failure [67]. I must say, "considerable" is not quite as painful as "dismal," but it still hurts. Maybe in hindsight we were too euphoric a decade ago—perhaps regrettable now but perhaps understandable for the first years of a social movement—and maybe we claimed or expected or simply talked too much.

DevDev—There is an important point buried there—namely, that you pushed family planning before the ground was prepared. You would have done better to send economists to planning boards in the 1960s than public health doctors to run programs.

FamPlan—You may well be right. And we had that other mistaken perception in the 1960s—an exaggerated idea of the administrative capacities of developing countries. As things turned out, that was a serious error, and one that affected various programs, not just population. All the same, it's always enlightening in such discussions to ask the alternative questions. What if we had not tried hard to spread family planning in the 1960s—when we had new policies, supporting surveys of interest, an improved contraceptive technology, and increasing funds? Could we really have known then that "it wouldn't work"? What would you have said then: that we had missed the boat?

AcCrit—You've continually been insensitive to any policy alternative to family planning. And you've pushed that unduly, to the point of antagonistic boomerang, as Bucharest documented so well. Worst irony of all—it doesn't work; so you're guilty not only of promising something under false pretenses but diverting attention from

[49] Interdisciplinary Communications Program, p. iii. [18] Burch, p. 12. [18] Burch, p. 19. [30] Davis, p. 730. [47] Hauser, p. 21. [56] Mauldin, for a recent review.

[66] Pradervand, p. 13. [67] Pradervand.

other efforts. ► The family planning movement is failing to insure itself against the failure of its present rationale and methods [46].

FAMPLAN—When you say that current programs cannot succeed, what is your definition of success? What is the goal, or at least the standard of judgment?

ACCRIT—► Zero population growth [32], of course. ► To achieve fertility and population control adequate to the need, the objective must be that of inducing couples to restrict their childbearing to the replacement level. That is, it is necessary to produce the desired number of children in order to achieve a zero-rate of growth [47]. Current measures do ► not provide population control for any collective purpose, least of all for population stability. . . . About all they could accomplish would be to help countries approaching a modern condition reach *an industrial level* of fertility, a level they would soon reach anyway [32].

FAMPLAN—If that is the goal—replacement fertility, or roughly the two-child family by, say, the year 2000—then I agree that "family planning" will probably fail. But that's your goal assigned to me, not mine. ► If the goal is to take one to one and a half points off the growth rate in the developing world in the next 20 years, or, say 15 to 18 points off the birth rate, then . . . we have a differential chance at that. . . . If the goal is to bring about the ultimate fertility decline faster than it would otherwise occur . . . [8].

ACCRIT—► The important question, however, is not whether the present campaign is somewhat hastening the downward trend in the birth rate but whether, even if it is, it will provide population control for the nation. Actually, the campaign is not designed to provide such control and shows no sign of doing so [30]. And where does that leave you?—you end up offering family planning as a panacea for population growth.

FAMPLAN—That's like the other panacea that DevDev attributed to me, and I don't accept this one either. I know as well as you that a policy of family planning isn't necessarily equivalent to a population policy. You speak of "population control." Well, that depends upon the definition of "control." Can we have a marginal effect, nontrivial?—that's my question. Just as I agree that lowering fertility will make a marginal but important contribution to development, so I think that family planning, if done well, could make a marginal but important contribution to lowering fertility. Is the controversy balanced on an adverb: *only* versus *fully*? A recent study found that in the famous Ceylon case, about 25 percent of the mortality decline could be ascribed to the program of malaria control and the remainder to "development"—nutrition, health services, economic factors [42]. Only 25 percent or fully 25 percent? You don't attack health programs that have made only a marginal contribution, or educational efforts or agricultural modernization. What you usually argue, DevDev, is that since they are only marginal they need more support not less, improvement and expansion of program not contraction. Why does population or family planning turn out to be the special case? ► Would an anti-TB campaign be regarded as a failure if "only" one-third of the decline in TB could be attributed to the campaign efforts? I would judge it a smashing success [78].

ACCRIT—Just as I thought: ► one can of course defend the programs by saying that the present goals and measures are merely interim ones [30]. ► If it is only a first step, it should be so labeled, and its connection with the next step (and the nature of that next step) should be carefully examined [30].

FAMPLAN—But, don't you see, I think of family planning as already a next step, after general development and the "threshold" factors, in line with the division of labor we discussed earlier. But I must add that if family planning could bring down the growth rate in the interested developing countries to 1 percent in 20 years or so—which is even more demanding than, for example, the goals recommended by the National Academy of Sciences committee [57]—I would settle, consider it a great historical achievement, call it "success," and leave the next steps to that next generation—since neither I nor the two of

[46] Hauser, p. 412. [32] Davis, p. 15. [47] Hauser, p. 26. [32] Davis, pp. 15–16. [8] Berelson, p. 7. [30] Davis, p. 735.

[42] Gray. [78] Stycos, p. 162. [30] Davis, p. 731. [30] Davis, p. 736. [57] National Academy of Sciences, p. 95.

you know what the world's situation would then be, nor could or should we set policy now for then. ► In order to act rationally, you don't need to know the ultimate goal, only the direction in which it is likely to be found [86]. ► Don't forget that in order to get from a growth rate of 2½% to 0, you have to go through 1 [38].

AcCrit—Then you admit that you don't have a full solution to the problem of population growth, that you offer a remedy not a cure [30].

FamPlan—I prefer "acknowledge" to "admit," but of course. Do you have one?—not on paper but for the real world?

DevDev—At least, then, we can agree on this: that ► family planning programs alone do not appear to be the answer to the population problem in developing societies [63], ► that family planning alone is not adequate . . . when compared to the magnitude of the problems [71].

FamPlan—That's called the mortal blow of Bucharest, I know. But ► it is a canard that any serious leader in the population or family planning fields has held the view that family planning "alone" will solve the population problem . . . They have been remarkably candid in acknowledging the limitations of their proposals [50].

AcCrit—Not all of them. Listen to this:

> ► Provision of improved means and information for control of fertility to people in developing countries ordinarily exerts a powerful effect upon fertility. . . . There appears to be a substantial basis for optimism that the major part of this work will be accomplished by the end of the current decade. . . . With continued vigorous action by the world community it should be possible to reduce the world crude birth rate to less than 20 and the world population growth rate to less than 1% per annum by the year 1980 [69].

Culminating in this flourish:

> ► As the spring sun erodes and finally breaks the icy grip of winter upon the Northland, so the increasing availability of knowledge and means for control of fertility is removing the mantle of ignorance which has combined with primaeval sexual passion to hold human reproduction at traditionally high levels . . . [69].

And the claim is still made post-Bucharest: ► Availability of Family Planning Services [is] the Key to Rapid Fertility Reduction [68]. But I know those little "fertility silhouettes," and I've already warned that ► these countries were selected because in general their data are reasonably reliable, which means that on the whole they are more advanced. . . . [with] the fastest declines in fertility. . . . This suggests that the declines are being caused by changing social and economic conditions rather than by family-planning policy [32]. So you can't expect me to take that kind of thing very seriously.

FamPlan—Actually, we may never know how well the purely family planning efforts did, for technical reasons, just as we do not know why the fertility decline in the West occurred when and as it did. You can always say that it would be happening anyway, and neither of us can prove his case beyond legitimate scientific doubt. ► Historians consider change to have been rapid when there was a perceptible difference in the behaviour of successive generations; some of our colleagues are impatient when change from year to year cannot plainly be discerned in the statistics. . . . Some draw the conclusion that little success means that there is little point in continuing to make efforts. The proper conclusion is almost certainly that the effort should increase; especially as success in the field is probably wedge-shaped—in fact ultimate rapid change may depend on a lot of effort now with little or no apparent result at this time [19].

AcCrit—But even there you are not faithful to your own creed. In turning away from abortion you have turned away from your own best method. ► Induced abortion . . . has been proved capable of reducing birth rates rapidly . . . yet this method is rejected in nearly all national and international population-control programs [30].

FamPlan—Well, I'm delighted to learn that you believe that family planning can work, if only it

[86] Wallis. [38] Freedman. [30] Davis, p. 737, for the remedy/cure apposition. [63] Oppenheimer, p. 54. [71] Rockefeller, p. 3. [50] Jaffe, p. 8. [69] Ravenholt, Chao, and Brackett, pp. 10, 26, 28.

[69] Ravenholt, Chao, and Brackett, p. 1. [68] Ravenholt and Chao, p. 217. [32] Davis, p. 25. [19] Caldwell, p. 6. [30] Davis, p. 732.

would include another method of fertility control. Actually, perhaps the two sharpest fertility changes in recent years were technological in character: the famous decline of fertility in Japan rested on the legalization of abortion [29] and the increase of fertility in Romania on the delegalization of abortion [80]. In any case, *I* haven't turned away, governments and cultures have—and you can't assign responsibility to me for all their policies. I'm under enough attack from you and DevDev now for "imposing" my views on them!

DEVDEV—What you must guard against is misleading the world by offering a purely technological solution to a basically structural problem. ► The population problem cannot be solved in a technical way . . . [45].

FAMPLAN—As the fellow says, all the intellectuals like to put down technology these days, but no one wants to give up his refrigerator—or birth control device, for that matter. Surely abortion as well as contraception is a technological matter, and surely the present methods of fertility control are hardly ideal for illiterate rural populations. And suppose we come up with an immunization against pregnancy—not inconceivable, if you'll pardon the expression—and ask yourself, what realizable social policy would affect fertility as much within a decade? ► The availability of such an inoculation would have more impact on population policy than anything else I have heard discussed. Political leaders are more likely to back programs that can succeed than programs that they believe will fail [74].

ACCRIT—But there you go again—obsessed with the technology of fertility control. By your own admission, all you could possibly do, if indeed that, is to eliminate unwanted fertility. That strategy is surely based on an article of faith—that there really is such a thing, that you have measured it correctly, and that it will disappear if services are offered. ► The assumption . . . is that the population problem is a function of unwanted births and therefore, if women have the means to limit births, the population problem will be solved [32]. The evidence is all to the contrary.

FAMPLAN—It is true that much of the rationale rests on "unwantedness." Those surveys have been and still are social scientific currency in good standing; why are they distinctively misleading here? Moreover, in all fairness, the question is still open as to how much the disparity between response and behavior is because ► we are measuring the demand incorrectly or not meeting it properly or some mixture. We can't just write off the fact that, in one study after another, sample strata representing millions of people say they are having more children than they want. It isn't enough to assert without proof that these responses are invalid [39], not to mention the actual demonstration of unwantedness made by the prevalence of illegal and life-risking abortions in much of the world.

DEVDEV—And I must say, AcCrit, that ► as long as the problem of unwanted births remains as large as it is . . ., it seems to constitute the biggest and most incontrovertible population problem [61].

FAMPLAN—As for cutting into *wanted* fertility, I confess that I don't realistically know how to do that, short of changing life conditions. But I must add that here as elsewhere satisfying the existing market may not be a bad way to extend the market. Anyway, both of you tend to end up your criticisms by saying, "But don't get me wrong, I'm all for family planning."

ACCRIT—But I am. ► There is no reason to abandon family-planning programs; contraception is a valuable technological instrument [30]. ► Family planning movements should not be condemned. . . . It makes sense to proceed with programs that appear to be the most direct [46].

DEVDEV—Me too. ► Family planning is a means to an end and its availability is desirable on many humanitarian, ethical, and utilitarian grounds. These programs provide a necessary service . . . [21]. ► This standpoint does not imply that we are opposed to family planning. On the contrary, we are of the opinion that free access to efficient

[29] Davis, for evidence. [80] Teitelbaum, for evidence. [45] Hardin, p. 1243. [74] Segal.

[32] Davis, p. 21. [39] Freedman. [61] Ohlin, p. 158. [30] Davis, p. 739. [46] Hauser, p. 413. [21] Casey, p. 24.

contraceptives and other means of birth control should be a human right and available to all . . . [59]. ► Family planning . . . can be an effective means of the liberation of the female half of mankind in all societies . . . [2]. Family planning should be recognized ► as an essential means to achieve national goals of the countries wishing to reduce population growth [83]. ► Family planning can be an effective means to fight against sterility, enhance the quality of health and the socioeconomic conditions of mothers and children, and liberate women. . . . Obviously, family planning can be a useful instrument of modernization [4]. ► This is not at all to deny the importance of continuing to step up both the provision of family planning services in most if not all countries, and research to improve birth control techniques. Nothing . . . should be construed as advocating reduced support for family planning assistance [70]. Finally, ► this is not to cast doubt on the virtue of family-planning programmes, which can and do produce worthwhile results. It is only to caution against expecting too much from them [22].

FAMPLAN–Your last point, DevDev, is a key one: what is to be expected. Population efforts may indeed have failed by your standards, but what does not, in any field involving the behavior of masses of people? You, AcCrit, have been advising all over the place on how to control inflation and eliminate racial discrimination and relieve urban congestion and educate the young and reduce poverty and sustain prosperity and eliminate crime and control drug addiction and bring peace, and how successful have you been? Not to mention, DevDev, the shortfalls in your own Development Decade. And incidentally, if development is supposed to bring down fertility, then it must have failed from this standpoint as well as in its own right; indeed, you can turn the point around–► the relative failure of economic development programs has hampered the attainment of family planning goals [37]. Yet you do not turn away from the renewed effort. On such large matters there are limits to what can be done by direct intervention.

DEVDEV–The picture is not quite so dark as AcCrit sometimes makes out. ► Careful attempts to disentangle the impact of these programs from that of changes in socio-economic conditions in several countries suggest that family planning programs have made a sizable contribution to the observed decline in fertility [88]. ► Much of the disappointment with the achievement of population programs can be traced not to their failure, but to the fact that too much has been expected from them. . . . Programs which have succeeded in protecting 15 per cent of eligible women . . . are adjudged to have failed. In any other aspect of the struggle to achieve economic and social development, such a percentage would be hailed as an outstanding success [12]. But you do tend to claim too much; you take up too much of the population stage; and your promise has outrun your performance.

FAMPLAN–From the experience to date, about all I would claim is that in the more favored of the developing countries modern family planning, *if done*, can contribute to a decline in the birth rate of about ten points in a decade; and in the less favored, *if done*, to about half that.

DEVDEV–The irony is that ► it is likely that the answers will only come retrospectively when they will be too late to influence either policy or programs [12].

Strategies of Intervention

The debaters now turn to the strategies beyond family planning and beyond development. What should be done now to hasten a fertility decline?

FAMPLAN–The record will show that we have been searching for additional ways to reduce fertility, beyond family planning [7], but without much success. We've scrutinized the inventory but have not come up with many actionable ideas. ► The measures which are generally discussed by advocates of "beyond family planning"

---

[59] Nikolinakos et al., p. 2. [2] Amin, p. 190. [83] United Nations, p. 18. [4] Bahri et al., p. 7. [70] Rich, p. 2. [22] Cassen, p. 221. [37] Finnigan, p. 9.

[88] World Bank, p. 137. [12] Black and Hankinson, p. 29. [12] Black and Hankinson, p. 22. [7] Berelson.

policies are almost uniformly vague, or are politically or ethically unacceptable, or technically or administratively infeasible [50].

AcCrit—The first thing to do is the obvious one. ► Support and encouragement of research on population policy other than family planning is negligible [30]. ► Such programs must be supplemented with equal or greater investments in research and experimentation to determine the required socioeconomic measures [30]. ► The specific measures required for developing [attractive] substitutes [for family interests] are not easy to determine in the absence of research on the question [30]. ► The most immediate barriers to effective programs today are the ignorance of the social sciences . . . and . . . of the biomedical sciences . . . [46]. In short, ► an incremental, piecemeal, or band-aid approach to global problems is no substitute for judicious investigation and systematic analysis [25].

FamPlan—"More research" is of course the last, and first, refuge of the academic, on anything. But you cannot assure us of settled and practicable answers; you do not spell out how the research will feed into the determination of policy; you are reluctant to work on issues defined by the policymaker; and your results, quite properly, are always limited in application and often qualified away, judged from a practical standpoint. I'd be more sympathetic if the studies were tied more closely to the decisions presented to those who have to act. If I may say so, AcCrit, ► just as a university professor may learn a subject rapidly and efficiently (although at the cost of occasional embarrassment) through being suddenly thrust into teaching a course in it, the need for giving policy advice *now* will reveal the most obvious weaknesses and gaps in knowledge . . . [34]. But I do support AcCrit's call for more research—like family planning, it can't hurt and it might, probably will, help.

AcCrit—The demographer ► is constantly told, "Tell us what can be done about population," with the implication that if he cannot come up with a satisfactory answer, he is a failure. . . . The demand is for "a solution that will work" [32]. ► In calling for approval in advance, the family-planning movement confuses the issues. The question of whether a policy, *if adopted*, would succeed is different from the question of whether, *if proposed*, it would be accepted [32]. Anyway I repeat: what the field really needs is more research. Hardly any resources are going into that compared with what FamPlan is getting for programs that are clearly inadequate to the task.

FamPlan—I confess that I do tend to consider what is workable, since it's easy to think of policies that would be effective but are impractical. In many situations it is less a question of knowing than of doing; it's the implementation that is lacking, not the knowledge. For example, if India could educate all the children through eight years of school, employ 35–40 percent of the women for money outside the home, lower infant mortality to below 25, raise the per capita income to $800, increase nonagricultural employment by four-fold, and so on—if India could do all that, its birth rate would fall to the low 20s or so [10]. We know what to do, more or less; we just can't do it.

DevDev—Another channel is incentives, and not just "bribing" people to practice family planning. ► It is important for every government to carefully examine the total structure of incentives regarding family size which its laws and institutions present to the individual. The object must be to design a broad framework of positive inducements to limit family size, and negative incentives to discourage large families [17]. For example, ► among the devices to be considered . . . are: (1) incentives for deferment of marriage; (2) incentive payments for childless periods . . . ; (3) incentive payments for sterilization; (4) old age pension plans . . . [47]. And one might also mention raising the legal age of marriage, easy divorce, establishment of a youth corps [58], military and national service, village financing of services [57], putting ► people

[50] Jaffe, p. 5. [30] Davis, p. 737. [30] Davis, p. 739. [30] Davis, p. 739. [46] Hauser, p. 410. [25] Choucri, p. 96. [34] Demeny, pp. 10–11.

[32] Davis, p. 27. [32] Davis, p. 22. [10] Berelson, p. 144. [17] Brown, p. 170. [47] Hauser, p. 27. [58] National Academy of Sciences et al., p. 96. [57] National Academy of Sciences, p. 87.

back into closed ecological systems . . . where there is little opportunity to escape the ecological consequences of one's own actions [37], and other community-level programs [54].

AcCrit—All of that is fine as far as it goes. What's basically needed is the removal of pronatalist pressures, legal and cultural, that have been so imbedded in the human consciousness across the centuries that we do not even notice they are there. That's where the real compulsion now is—*pro*natalist not anti-. And beyond that is an historical novelty that is now "unacceptable," to some people "unthinkable"—namely, that the state may have to impose involuntary controls on fertility [7] in the public welfare, as it now does on so many other things. ► Coercion is a dirty word to most liberals now, but it need not forever be so. . . . The only kind of coercion I recommend is mutual coercion, mutually agreed upon by the majority of the people affected [45]. The state now says that you can have only one spouse at a time; why can't it tell you that you can have only two children? ► Why not simply limit each couple to two births, with sufficient penalties to discourage three [32]? Alternatively, ► I have suggested, a little tongue in cheek, my "green stamp plan" of marketable licenses for having babies [15], with transferable coupons which add up to replacement fertility. China, by report, uses community pressure backed by the political apparatus to allocate the children within quotas, and Bangladesh speaks of ► formulat[ing] a set of bold and, if necessary, drastic policies for vigorous action [5] and of ► consider[ing] the imposition of progressively increasing punitive measures against additional children after the second child . . . [5]. There are no two ways about it: population control does not come easy. Even ► in countries where contraception is used, a realistic proposal for a government policy of lowering the birth rate reads like a catalogue of horrors . . . [30]. ► In the famous words of Chairman Mao, adapted rather liberally to this context, a demographic revolution is no picnic [14].

DevDev—In that case, we may not want it. I prefer the disease to the cure, particularly since you haven't proved beyond a reasonable doubt that the blessings of slower growth will be so very large. ► The social consequences of population growth do not seem either so clear-cut or so terrifying to me as to warrant emergency measures [61]. ► Quite apart from the fact that it does not have a shred of political acceptability in the present world, is there a strong enough case to press for a coercive regime of fertility [61]? Why should people let themselves in for your catalogue of horrors and deprive themselves of one of the few values that life holds out for them, all for an uncertain benefit? Would you?

FamPlan—I agree. Most of that isn't acceptable, to either the people or the governments.

AcCrit—Then down with the governments. You mean the likelihood of proposed programs ► to gain acceptance by *existing* governments . . . [3]. "Acceptability" is a trap. ► Virtually all proposed social changes are initially unacceptable, or else they would not need to be proposed . . . . Measures to stop population growth cannot be found which can be guaranteed in advance to be acceptable. They have to *win* acceptance . . . [32].

FamPlan—► A question of moral (though not intellectual) legitimacy is raised when research leads to the recommendation of actions, the cost of which are [sic] borne entirely by other people. There is something, if not illegitimate, at any rate distasteful in people from safe and comfortable positions recommending revolutions or painful reforms, or, for that matter, the maintenance of the *status quo*, to others [77]. You sit in your affluent academic armchairs and admonish others to accept the unacceptable. I seem to recall that a few years ago, when the students were prescribing university reforms and telling you to accept the unacceptable, you climbed the barricades. Now you turn the tables, and when

[37] Finnegan, p. 11. [54] McNicoll. [7] Berelson, p. 2, for an earlier listing. [45] Hardin, p. 1247. [32] Davis, p. 21; for the penalties, p. 28. [15] Boulding, p. 93. [5] Bangladesh Planning Commission, p. 537. [5] Bangladesh Planning Commission, p. 539. [30] Davis, p. 739.

[14] Blake, p. 220. [61] Ohlin, p. 158. [61] Ohlin, p. 159. [3] Bachrach and Bergman, p. 599. [32] Davis, p. 22. [77] Streeten, p. 1292.

your advice isn't taken, you sit back and say, "Well, I told them; don't blame me if they don't do as I say."

DEVDEV—All of that raises the issue of motives in providing policy prescriptions and/or policy assistance in this field. ► Many of the peoples in many countries see the expression of concern of the rich, white, northern half of the world with population increase as directed towards the not-so-rich, not-so-white, southern half of the world.... And this can certainly have undertones of racism. The word genocide occasionally is bandied about [82]. To be specific, ► political elites as well as intellectuals in most African countries question the motivations of the highly industrialized nations for actively pushing and financially supporting family planning programs in Africa [62]. ► At present, there is already political reaction against population programs in many countries because they think the advanced nations are trying to sell population control as a cheap means of achieving progress [28]. At the World Population Conference at Bucharest, ► the opponents of the Western approach were clearly in the majority [and intended] without question a repudiation of attempts to make population the culprit for poverty and underdevelopment and a backlash against the way in which imperialist countries have sought to promote birth control in the rest of the world [20]. ► That is why the "demographic approach" to the present problems of the world is so sterile: it points only to a non-solution while, at the same time, with its overdramatization about approaching disaster due to the "population explosion," it distracts the attention of the public from where real solutions may be found [75].

FAMPLAN—Inevitably, the sensitive issues involved in population get tangled up in international politics, as though the substance itself were not problem enough. Bucharest is the key example. As you have yourself said, DevDev, ► "The deep tensions in the international politico-economic system are aggravated by the world-population pressure and at the same time prevent its cure" [73].

DEVDEV—Moreover, your motives are perceived as impure in another way. ► In our opinion, the primary way of solving the population problem lies in combatting the aggression and plunder of the imperialists, colonialists and neo-colonialists, and particularly the superpowers . . . [64]. ► The most relevant and revealing fact is that a tiny minority in affluent countries is using up food, petrol and other essential commodities out of all proportion to their needs.... The threat to their life styles has led some persons to blame the growth of population in countries like India. But it is the rich who deplete resources and pollute the environment, not the poor [41]. ► It is inadmissible that those who have control of the wealth and resources of mankind should try to resolve the problem of hunger by forbidding the poor to be born.... Is it not a new form of warfare to impose a restrictive demographic policy on nations to ensure that they will not claim their just share of the earth's goods [65]?

FAMPLAN—Inadmissible? Forbid? Impose? Restrict? Such terms fit your vocabulary much better than mine. To the contrary, I'm freeing couples, chiefly women, to make a choice that history has never realistically provided them, partly thanks to you. As for the threat of resource depletion, population growth in developed countries cannot be much of a villain since there's not much of it these days—21 of 31 highly developed countries now have birth rates below replacement [27]—and don't overlook that they are the creator of resources too.

DEVDEV—Motives aside, we are dealing with a truly historic affair. ► The solution of the problems addressed . . . is in my judgment a social revolution [72]. The thrust of the conservative ideology that permeates population thinking is counterrevolutionary [72]. And on the level of politics, ► insisting on population increase as a major cause of underdevelopment can . . . serve . . . to distract attention from the

[82] Townley, p. 5. [62] Okediji, p. 17. [28] Concepción, p. 28. [20] Carder and Park, p. 19. [75] Singer, p. 13.

[73] Seers, p. 108. [64] People's Republic of China, p. 7. [41] Gandhi. [65] Pope Paul VI. [27] Coale, p. 30. [72] Ryder, p. 8. [72] Ryder, p. 8.

real political-economic issues facing the Third World [59]. ► In fact, I've got a feeling that to change the system we're going to have to get a little closer to chaos, by even a greater explosion of population in these countries . . . [55]. ► This is why population policies are opposed by revolutionaries . . . [73]. In any case, population and family planning is seen as a safety valve, a band-aid, a cop-out, that only buttresses the existing system. Moreover, ► the response of the Population Establishment to this new challenge was to concede the importance of economic and social factors but to carry on as before, arguing that each question should be dealt with separately, with separate strategies and plans for each sector [20].

FamPlan—If the population establishment or what you call its masters wanted to retard the development of the poor countries, wouldn't encouraging their population growth be a cheap way to do so? If we had gone the other way and withheld the modern technology of fertility control, what would we then be accused of? As for the demographic revolution, I am of course enlisted: the question remains, how? With regard to social revolution, that's just another term for development—women's liberation, income equalization, popular education, decent health, and so on. But make no mistake, enabling women to control their own fertility may well count as a revolutionary contribution to their liberation. As for political revolution, that isn't made for demographic reasons, but the demography can help in that it can help to produce light at the end of the tunnel, and that's when revolutionary change occurs.

AcCrit—But that poses the issue too narrowly. You always try to push the issue back to the provision of contraceptives, FamPlan, as though that has ever been really important. The two of you focus on your own interests, yet even the two together—development and family planning—aren't enough. ► To date efforts at curtailing population growth in developing countries have been bipolarized into the "economic development" approach on the one hand, and the family planning approach on the other. . . . Neither approach seems to be practical taken alone, nor do they even appear to be adequate in combination [13]. ► Modernization and birth control alone will clearly not bring family size into line with modern levels of mortality unless this reproductive institution is itself modified . . . [13].

[59] Nikolinakos et al., p. 2. [55] Maione, p. 19. [73] Seers, p. 106. [20] Carder and Park, p. 18.

DevDev—And how is that to be done, if not through economic development?

AcCrit—Through ► a significant lessening of involvement in familial roles . . . , direct manipulation of family structure itself—planned efforts at deflecting the family's socializing function, reducing the noneconomic utilities of offspring, or introducing nonfamilial distractions and opportunity costs into people's lives [13]. For example, ► offer [Egyptian] women employment as an alternative to childbearing . . . . [as in] small sewing factories [11]. Or encourage female participation in the Indian labor force [13] or institute ► rigidly compulsory education of children which would remove them as potential economic utilities . . . , all the while effectively putting intellectual barriers between them and the past generation [13]. ► Many of these policies for influencing the family do not depend on prior economic development, they can be implemented concomitantly with modernization strategies [13].

DevDev—They *are* modernization strategies, to be sure, but let's not fuss over the semantics. Do you think they can be done outside the development package, any more than fertility control can?

FamPlan—► To wonder . . . why the intensification of employment opportunities for women as a means of lowering fertility had not been attempted in India is to wonder as Marie Antoinette did, why the people did not eat cake [87]! Nor is it accidental that the sewing factories are not yet running. As for popular education, if all the funds used to support the family planning effort were shifted to education, it would add only a few days to the school year or increase the enrollment by a tiny fraction [51]. The proposals having to do with tax reforms, marriage licenses, maternity leaves, child

[13] Blake, p. 67. [13] Blake, p. 69. [13] Blake, pp. 61–62. [11] Bindary, p. 193. [13] Blake, pp. 66–67. [13] Blake, pp. 68–69. [13] Blake, p. 68. [87] Wolfers, p. 19. [51] Jones, pp. 356–357, for data.

assistance, public housing, and university fellowships [30] are simply irrelevant in most of the developing world. Such suggestions ► depend on a level of social organization in which the great majority are tax-payers and in employment. If you cannot get blood from a stone, you cannot operate schemes of this kind in the vast populous rural areas of the developing world [87].

DevDev—AcCrit and I are not saying that your effort or your budget can do much to reduce poverty or educate children or employ women but only that such things must happen before you can be even moderately successful.

FamPlan—Not so fast—*plus* community pressure *plus* minimizing insecurity [24] *plus* raised age of marriage *plus* heavy antinatalist propaganda in the name of the revered leader (hardly an unmixed blessing) *plus* a vigorous family planning effort including induced abortion. Anyway, we really don't know yet.

AcCrit—When you get right down to it, you have to face the fact that in today's world, on an issue that so sharply divides the rich countries from the poor ones, what's really lacking is the political will. And that has to be based on a stronger appreciation of what is involved. ► The effort should be directed toward generating demand for population policies through advancing the analysis of the consequences of population processes [34]. Potentially effective measures ► cannot be proposed seriously until or unless a high level of felt social need for such policies emerges [34]. When natural pressures and contraceptives fail, ► society will have to find other means to solve its demographic problems, relying on disincentives, moral suasion, or command. Such solutions must be national solutions par excellence [35].

FamPlan—Yes, but let the record show that they are still unspecified.

Last Words

The debate seems to keep circling back upon itself. The time has come for summaries and conclusions.

[30] Davis, p. 738, for data. [87] Wolfers, p. 16. [24] Chen, pp. 13–18 passim. [34] Demeny, p. 11. [34] Demeny, pp. 12–13. [35] Demeny, p. 11.

DevDev—The basic problem is not population growth but the reduction of poverty, with all that entails both as cause and as consequence. Attacking that basic problem is the best way, in efficiency as well as in morality and politics, to attack the problems of population growth. And the international community must understand this fundamental point and allocate its resources for assistance accordingly. As for "severe" measures to control population, as I said, the cure sounds worse to me than the disease. In any case, don't try to push people around with the threat of "population explosion." Family planning programs are all right, but don't expect them to do very much; anyway they are good for other than demographic reasons and can't do any harm. My last word?—Develop, and in the process, Distribute income more equitably.

AcCrit—We simply do not know how to proceed in order to reduce birth rates in traditional societies, which is why I keep calling for more research in order to find out how. Where we do know, we are unwilling to pay the price: people ► do not want runaway population growth . . . but they want to avoid it painlessly [32]. ► In short, they want a miracle [32]. Neither DevDev nor FamPlan has a viable answer: development takes too long and is itself retarded by the very growth it is meant to relieve; family planning doesn't work, except trivially where it isn't really needed. Some direct demographic measures are required; they aren't altogether clear except that they won't be easy. But the alternatives will be worse. In the longer view, one can only be pessimistic: after all, mankind has never been very good at controlling individual behavior for the common welfare. My last word is double: Research, Restructure.

FamPlan—I'm for both development and research, but both will take a long time: that's what makes basic causes and fundamental solutions so basic and fundamental. But that's not the issue, at least for me. The issue is: what if anything should the population effort now do with its small resources, in personnel and funding, that can make the most difference. I'm not sure that I have the proper answer, but I'm convinced that's the proper question. To assign to me

[32] Davis, p. 28. [32] Davis, p. 29.

poverty reduction or population education or liberation of women or any other alleged threshold of similar magnitude is ludicrous on its face. To call for more study is on the other hand too easy: one tends to remain in a Talmudic tradition where everything is very complicated and nothing can be done. At least I am doing something, however incremental, and if it could be done well it should make a nontrivial difference in softening the growth curve; anyway, it is a useful means to accompany the engine of motivation. Both DevDev and AcCrit are willing that it go on and have not yet told me what else to do that I can do. My last word, then, is: Persevere.

* * * *

A worthy yet unsatisfying debate, the needle stuck beyond science and within politics: no final guidance from the former, numerous constraints from the latter, and in between lots of room for the play of judgment.

Still, the participants seem to agree on a good deal that they still keep arguing about: the demographic facts, the absence of any panaceas, population as only a means, the need for both direct and indirect efforts, the empirical results of family planning efforts, the useful in both development and family planning, perhaps even the existence of a problem. Why then the continuing acrimony?—semantics, emphasis, point-scoring, putting down the more vulnerable extremes within the opposing camp, ideology. If nothing else, eliminating the straw men from the debate—a sophomore's game—would be a major step forward, though the dynamics of the situation make that unlikely. Given the interests imbedded in the debate, this is understandable, perhaps necessary, probably inevitable—yet at the same time it exacerbates an already difficult situation.

Perhaps the most consequential differences in the debate are not over facts or values but over the formulation of issues. DevDev and AcCrit tend to talk about theoretical analysis and basic causes and fundamental solutions, FamPlan about practical next steps and allocation of resources and incremental advances. That is where the debate seems to be least joined but most needed, on what the proper policy issue really are. And complicating the resolution is the normal sight-line of the planner and intellectual as against the operator—the long-term versus the short-term.

In reviewing another intellectual debate, the economist Marshall once observed that one was most likely to be right when promoting his own method of inquiry and most likely to be wrong when attacking the other fellow's. In this debate, the reverse seems to be the case: each debater seems most persuasive when pointing out what's wrong with the others and least persuasive when putting forward his own positive program. Taken together, that adds up to an overwhelming impression of negativism: what can be done is not "enough," what is "enough" cannot be done. As all three of the debaters made clear, proposed actions are often unadoptable for one reason or another, and if adoptable, incapable of being adequately implemented. So as a whole the debate does not lead to an optimistic conclusion, especially when put against the recalcitrance of the problem itself. It is wry comfort, as often observed, ► that the powers of the state to influence fertility or growth, at least to the extent that it has been regarded as practicable to apply them so far, are limited and marginal . . . [16].

But the modern world does not let great problems rest. ► In earlier times, problems of this character were not so readily identified and, when they were, not so readily addressed. These days the very recognition of a public problem means that something must be done about it [10]. Once recognized, they must be addressed, and readdressed.

The elementary truth is that no path into the future is likely to be painless, not least the path of demographic laissez-faire. ► It is indeed hard not to be philosophical in contemplating the most likely course of demographic-economic development in the coming decades. It holds out the promise of a sustained sense of déjà vu, continuing a developmental line that rapidly increases the gap between what man could be were he able to control his affairs and what he, in fact, is [33].

Somehow, the debate is not as it ought to be—too often repetitive, circular, untidy, pedestrian, oblique, evasive. ► It is too schematic, it assumes clear-cut and clearly formulated alternatives that do not exist. The point is that nothing works very well, and that goes for development as well as for family planning. Nor is there any substitute for

[16] Brass, p. 65. [10] Berelson, p. 133. [33] Demeny, p. 8.

local commitment, resolve, effort—including the subtleties of an international intellectual debate [48].

Still responsibility rests on these debaters and what they represent. The exchange has a valued life of its own, to generate ideas and/or the consensus to inform and improve action. The population strategy of the 1960s and early 1970s is, though still very much alive, under growing scrutiny; the population strategy from now to 1984 is struggling to be born.

References

[1] *Action Pack*. 1974. Distributed by The World Population Year Secretariat of the United Nations Fund for Population Activities.

[2] Amin, Samir. 1971. "Development strategies and population policies: Under-populated Africa." In *Population-Education-Development in Africa South of the Sahara*. Meeting of Experts, Dakar (29 November–4 December). Dakar: UNESCO Regional Office for Education in Africa.

[3] Bachrach, Peter, and Elihu Bergman. 1972. "Participation and conflict in making American population policy: A critical analysis." In *The Commission on Population Growth and the American Future, Aspects of Population Growth Policy, 6*. Edited by Robert Parke, Jr., and Charles F. Westoff. Washington, D.C.: Government Printing Office, pp. 583–607.

[4] Bahri, Ahmed, et al. 1971. "A new approach to population research in Africa: Ideologies, facts, and policies." Paper issued at the African Population Conference, Accra, (9–18 December). Mimeo.

[5] Bangladesh Planning Commission. 1973. *The First Five-Year Plan 1973–78*. Dacca: Government of the People's Republic of Bangladesh (November).

[6] Berelson, Bernard. 1961. "The great debate on cultural democracy." In *Values in America*. Edited by Donald N. Barrett. Notre Dame, Indiana: University of Notre Dame Press.

[7] Berelson, Bernard. 1969. "Beyond family planning." *Studies in Family Planning* 1, no. 38 (February): 1–16.

[8] Berelson, Bernard. 1970. "The present state of family planning programs." *Studies in Family Planning* 1, no. 57 (September): 1–11.

[9] Berelson, Bernard. 1973. "Positions on population growth." In *The Population Council Annual Report*. New York: The Population Council, pp. 19–27.

[48] Heaps.

[10] Berelson, Bernard. 1974. "An evaluation of the effects of population control programs." In *Population and Its Problems*. Edited by H. B. Parry. Oxford, England: Clarendon Press, pp. 133–168.

[11] Bindary, Aziz. 1972. "Egypt studies a new plan of action." *Studies in Family Planning* 3, no. 8 (August). 193–194.

[12] Black, Robert, and Richard Hankinson. 1974. *Population: A Progress Report*. Paris: Organization for Economic Cooperation and Development.

[13] Blake, Judith. 1965. "Demographic science and the redirection of population policy." In *Public Health and Population Change: Current Research Issues*. Edited by Mindel C. Sheps and Jeanne C. Ridley. Pittsburgh: University of Pittsburgh Press, pp. 41–69.

[14] Blake, Judith. 1971. "Reproductive motivation and population policy." *BioScience* 21, no. 5 (March): 215–220.

[15] Boulding, Kenneth E. 1973. "The shadow of the stationary state." In *The No-Growth Society*. Edited by Mancur Olson and Hans H. Landsberg. New York: W. W. Norton & Company, Inc., pp. 89–102.

[16] Brass, William. 1974. "Population size and complex communities with a consideration of world population." In *Population and Its Problems*. Edited by H. B. Parry. Oxford, England: Clarendon Press, pp. 51–71.

[17] Brown, Lester. 1974. *In the Human Interest*. New York: W. W. Norton & Company, Inc.

[18] Burch, Thomas K. 1974. "Theories of fertility decline as guides to policy." Draft of paper presented at the Annual Meeting of the Population Association of America, New York City (18–20 April). Mimeo. To be published in *Social Forces*, September 1975.

[19] Caldwell, John C. 1974. "The containment of world population growth." Paper presented at the Tribune, World Population Conference, Bucharest (August). Mimeo.

[20] Carder, Michael, and Robert Park. 1975. "Bombast in Bucharest: Report on the World Population Conference." *Science for the People* (January): 17–19.

[21] Casey, Rick (ed.). 1973. *A Frustrated Consensus*. Report on the Consultation on Population Policy, Montreal (12–13 October). Cosponsored by the Canadian Inter-Church Project on Population and the Center of Concern.

[22] Cassen, Robert H. 1974. "Economic-demographic interrelationships in developing countries." In *Population and Its Problems*. Edited by H. B. Parry. Oxford, England: Clarendon Press, pp. 216–238.

[23] Cassen, Robert H. 1974. Personal communication. (March).

[24] Chen, Pi-chao. 1974. "The 'planned birth' program

of the People's Republic of China, with a brief analysis of its transferability." As reported in "Implementing a total national program for fertility reduction." A SEADAG report on a population panel seminar, Bali, Indonesia (12–14 August).

[25] Choucri, Nazli. 1973. "Population dynamics and social inquiry: Some methodological imperatives." In *Population and Politics*. Edited by Richard L. Clinton. Lexington, Massachusetts: Lexington Books, D. C. Heath and Company, pp. 75–100.

[26] Coale, Ansley. 1969. "The decline of fertility in Europe from the French Revolution to World War II." In *Fertility and Family Planning: A World View*. Edited by S. J. Behrman, Leslie Corsa, Jr., and Ronald Freedman. Ann Arbor: The University of Michigan Press, pp. 3–24. Citing "Factors associated with the development of low fertility: An historic summary." By Ansley Coale. In United Nations, *World Population Conference, 1965, Vol. 2*, pp. 205–209.

[27] Coale, Ansley. 1974. "Too many people?" *Challenge* 17, no. 4 (September-October): 29–33.

[28] Concepción, Mercedes B. 1974. "Emerging issues on population policy and population program assistance." In *Third Bellagio Conference on Population*. New York: The Rockefeller Foundation, pp. 26–30.

[29] Davis, Kingsley. 1963. "The theory of change and response in modern demographic history." *Population Index* 20, no. 4 (October): 345–366.

[30] Davis, Kingsley. 1967. "Population policy: Will current programs succeed?" *Science* 158 (10 November): 730–739.

[31] Davis, Kingsley. 1972. "The changing balance of births and deaths." In *Are Our Descendants Doomed?* Edited by Harrison Brown and Edward Hutchings, Jr. New York: Viking Press, pp. 14–33.

[32] Davis, Kingsley. 1973. "Zero population growth: The goal and the means." In *The No-Growth Society*. Edited by Mancur Olson and Hans H. Landsberg. New York: W. W. Norton & Company, Inc., pp. 15–30.

[33] Demeny, Paul. 1973. "On the economic theory of fertility." Paper presented at the Conference on the Economic Aspects of Population Growth, Valescure, France (3 September). Mimeo.

[34] Demeny, Paul. 1974. "Population and development: An agenda for policy-oriented research." Paper prepared for the Conference on Social Science Research: Population and Development, Session 2, New York (29–30 October). Mimeo.

[35] Demeny, Paul. 1974. "Population policy: The role of national governments." Paper presented at the First Regional Population Conference, Beirut (18 February–1 March). Mimeo.

[36] Ehrlich, Paul R., and Anne H. Ehrlich. 1970. *Population, Resources, Environment: Issues in Human Ecology*. San Francisco: W. H. Freeman and Company.

[37] Finnigan, Oliver D. III. 1974. "Integrating population and development planning." As reported in "Implementing a total national program for fertility reduction." A SEADAG report on a population panel seminar, Bali, Indonesia (12–14 August).

[38] Freedman, Ronald. Circa 1964. Observation in a population meeting.

[39] Freedman, Ronald. 1974. Personal communication. (October).

[40] Freedman, Ronald, and John Y. Takeshita. 1969. *Family Planning in Taiwan: An Experiment in Social Change*. Princeton: Princeton University Press.

[41] Gandhi, Indira. 1974. Speech to a national conference on population. (December).

[42] Gray, R. H. 1974. "The decline of mortality in Ceylon and the demographic effects of malaria control." *Population Studies* 28, no. 2 (July): 205–229.

[43] Greene, Wade. 1975. "Triage: Who shall be fed? Who shall starve?" *The New York Times Magazine* (5 January): 9ff.

[44] Guzevaty, Yaropolk. 1974. Cited in "Population/family planning programs in Latin America–Problems and prospects." By Jose F. Patiño. In *Third Bellagio Conference on Population*. New York: The Rockefeller Foundation, pp. 20–25.

[45] Hardin, Garrett. 1968. "The tragedy of the Commons." *Science* 162 (13 December): 1243–1248.

[46] Hauser, Philip. 1967. "Family planning and population programs: A book review article." *Demography* 4, no. 1: 347–414.

[47] Hauser, Philip. 1969. "Population: More than family planning." *Journal of Medical Education* 44, no. 11, part 2 (November): 20–29.

[48] Heaps, David. 1975. Personal communication. (March).

[49] Interdisciplinary Communications Program. 1974. *The Policy Relevance of Recent Social Research on Fertility*. Occasional Monograph Series, no. 2. Washington, D.C.: Smithsonian Institution.

[50] Jaffe, Frederick. 1974. "Family planning and the population challenge?" Draft of paper presented at Georgetown University, Washington, D.C. (October). Mimeo.

[51] Jones, Gavin. 1971. "Effect of population change on the attainment of educational goals in developing countries." In *Rapid Population Growth: Consequences and Policy Implications*. Prepared by a National Academy of Sciences Study Committee. Baltimore: The Johns Hopkins Press, pp. 315–367.

[52] King, Timothy. 1974. "Economic research priorities for population policy." Paper prepared for the Conference on Social Science Research: Population and Development, New York (29-30 October). Mimeo.
[53] Kocher, James E. 1973. *Rural Development, Income Distribution, and Fertility Decline*. New York: The Population Council.
[54] McNicoll, Geoffrey. 1974. "Community-level population policy: An exploration." Manuscript. (Revised April 1975). To be published in *Population and Development Review*, September 1975.
[55] Maione, Romeo. 1973. Cited in *A Frustrated Consensus*. Edited by Rick Casey. Cosponsored by the Canadian Inter-Church Project on Population and the Center of Concern.
[56] Mauldin, W. Parker. 1974. "Assessment of national family planning programs." Paper presented at the Tribune, World Population Conference, Bucharest (August). Mimeo.
[57] National Academy of Sciences Study Committee. 1971. *Rapid Population Growth: Consequences and Policy Implications*. Baltimore: The Johns Hopkins Press.
[58] National Academy of Sciences et al. 1974. *In Search of Population Policy: Views from the Developing World*. Washington, D.C.: National Academy of Sciences.
[59] Nikolinakos, Marios, et al. 1974. "Population growth and social development." Statement at the occasion of World Population Year. Mimeo.
[60] Notestein, Frank W. 1973. "The quest for optimal patterns of demographic, economic and social development: Costs and benefits of population programs." Paper prepared for the Symposium on Population and Development, Cairo (4–14 June 1973) and the World Population Conference, Bucharest (August 1974). UN Economic and Social Council E/CONF .60/SYM.I/8.
[61] Ohlin, Goran. 1974. "The new breed of Malthusians." *Family Planning Perspectives* 8, no. 3 (Summer): 158–159.
[62] Okediji, Francis O. 1974. "Sociopolitical implications of family planning programs as an aspect of population policies and development planning in Africa." In *Third Bellagio Conference on Population*. New York: The Rockefeller Foundation, pp. 13–19.
[63] Oppenheimer, Valerie. 1971. "Population." *Headline Series*, no. 206. New York: Foreign Policy Association.
[64] People's Republic of China, Head of the Delegation. 1974. Speech delivered at the World Population Conference, Bucharest (August). Mimeo.
[65] Pope Paul VI. 1974. Address to the participants of the World Food Conference, Rome (9 November).
[66] Pradervand, Pierre. 1974. "The Malthusian man." *New Internationalist*, no. 15 (May): 20–24.
[67] Pradervand, Pierre. 1974. Letter of correction to Editor, regarding article in *New Internationalist*, no. 15 (May). Personal communication. (9 September).
[68] Ravenholt, R. T., and John Chao. 1974. "Availability of family planning services—The key to rapid fertility reduction." *Family Planning Perspectives* 6, no. 4 (Fall): 217–223.
[69] Ravenholt, R. T., John Chao, and James W. Brackett. 1972. "Epidemiology of world fertility." In *Clinical Proceedings of the International Planned Parenthood Federation Oceania Regional Medical and Scientific Congress*, Sydney (14–18 August), pp. 1–28.
[70] Rich, William. 1973. *Smaller Families through Social and Economic Progress*. Monograph no. 7. Washington, D.C.: Overseas Development Council. (January).
[71] Rockefeller, John D. 3d. 1974. "Population growth: The role of the developed world." Paper presented at the Tribune, World Population Conference, Bucharest (August). IUSSP Lecture Series on Population.
[72] Ryder, N. B. 1974. "Realistic pathways to fertility reduction in developing countries." Paper presented at the Annual Meeting of the Population Association of America, New York City (18–20 April). Mimeo.
[73] Seers, Dudley. 1974. "Development and population growth in poor countries." In *Population and Its Problems*. Edited by H. B. Parry. Oxford, England: Clarendon Press, pp. 101–111.
[74] Segal, Sheldon J. 1974. Memorandum. (November).
[75] Singer, Paul. 1974. "Population growth: The role of the developing world." Paper presented at the World Population Conference, Bucharest (August). IUSSP Lecture Series on Population.
[76] Singh, Karan. 1974. Statement made at the World Population Conference, Bucharest (August). Mimeo.
[77] Streeten, Paul B. 1974. "Social science research on development: Some problems in the use and transfer of intellectual technology." *Journal of Economic Literature* 12, no. 4 (December): 1290–1300.
[78] Stycos, J. Mayone. 1974. "Demographic chic at the UN." *Family Planning Perspectives* 6, no. 3 (Summer): 160–164.
[79] Tabbarah, Riad B. 1974. "Population policy issues in international instruments: With special reference to the *World Population Plan of Action*."

Unedited draft of paper for publication in *Journal of International Law and Economics*, December 1974.

[80] Teitelbaum, Michael S. 1972. "Fertility effects of the abolition of legal abortion in Romania." *Population Studies* 26, no. 3 (November): 405–417.

[81] Teitelbaum, Michael S. 1974. "Population and development: Is a consensus possible?" *Foreign Affairs* 52, no. 4 (July): 742–760.

[82] Townley, Ralph. 1973. Cited in *A Frustrated Consensus*. Edited by Rick Casey. Cosponsored by the Canadian Inter-Church Project on Population and the Center of Concern.

[83] United Nations. 1972. "Report of the Second Asian Population Conference, 1972." E/CN.11/1065 (13 December). Cited in "Population policy issues in international instruments: With special reference to the *World Population Plan of Action*." By Riad B. Tabbarah. Unedited draft of paper for publication in *Journal of International Law and Economics*, December 1974.

[84] United Nations, Senior Officer of the World Population Conference. 1974. Personal communication. (26 August).

[85] van de Walle, E., and John Knodel. 1967. "Demographic transition and fertility decline: The European case." Paper presented at the 1967 conference of the International Union for the Scientific Study of Population, Sydney, Australia. Cited in "The decline of fertility in Europe from the French Revolution to World War II." By Ansley Coale. In *Fertility and Family Planning: A World View.* Edited by S. J. Behrman, Leslie Corsa, Jr., and Ronald Freedman. 1969. Ann Arbor: The University of Michigan Press, pp. 3–24.

[86] Wallis, Allen. Circa 1955. Observation.

[87] Wolfers, David. 1974. "Non-medical factors in population change." Paper presented at the International Conference on the Physician and Population Change, Stockholm (September). Mimeo.

[88] World Bank. 1974. *Population Policies and Economic Development*. Staff Report. Baltimore: The Johns Hopkins University Press.

[89] World Population Conference. 1974. *World Population Plan of Action*. New York: United Nations Economic and Social Council. E/5585. (Also issued as E/CONF.60/19.)

3
Paths to Fertility Reduction: The 'Policy Cube'

What policy options are available to deal with the problem of rapid population growth in developing countries, and how are they to be addressed?

If a developing country seeks to improve the standard of living, health, education, human welfare . . . or quality of life of its people, one contributing measure is to reduce the rate of population growth.

If a country seeks to reduce the rate of population growth, there are in principle three ways to do so: encourage emigration, raise mortality or lower fertility. The first has occasionally been utilized in a few small island societies but clearly it is not feasible for most developing countries in today's world: The numbers are too great, the logistics are forbidding, the will is absent both on the sending and the receiving ends. The second is virtually unthinkable as a matter of public policy:* If lower mortality means higher growth, then so be it. The decision is an easy one for governments to make within the ranges currently available to them: The cure would be considered worse than the disease. That leaves lowered fertility as the means of choice.

Paths for Consideration

If a developing country seeks to reduce fertility, it may, in principle, choose from a number of reasonably specific and concrete paths—policies that are being currently employed or have been responsibly proposed. A first approximation of these paths appears in Table 3.1, which lists a number of identifiable interventions of some magnitude designed to affect either the *supply* (availability) of modern means of fertility control or the *demand* for (or motivation to use) fertility control methods. A brief reprise of these categories may be in order for descriptive clarity.

On the Supply Side

A. Access: This policy calls for the provision of information, supplies and services for voluntary fertility control in various institutionalized ways, as is now being done in family planning programs throughout the developing world (1). Most programs only provide contraceptives, but some have stressed sterilization (e.g., India), and a few add abortion (e.g., China). The systems for delivery of such services vary with local circumstances: fieldworkers and private doctors in Taiwan, paramedics in China, the commercial sector in several countries (notably, in Colombia along with local agents), 'saturation' distribution of pills and condoms in Pakistan, 'camps' for sterilization, especially vasectomy, in India, mobile clinics in Tunisia, postpartum arrangements, and various forms of 'integration' into health or development efforts.

B. Product: This policy calls for a better method of fertility control—better in the three characteristics designated in Table 3.1—to be made available for delivery. Biomedical efforts in this direction are substantial, particularly in the public sector,

---

Reprinted with permission from *Family Planning Perspectives*, 1977;9(5):214–219.

*But only "virtually"; for a serious discussion, see S.H. Preston, "Health Programs and Population Growth," *Population and Development Review*, 1:189, 1975.

TABLE 3.1. Policy paths to fertility reduction

To Affect Supply	
A. Improve access of more people to modern means of fertility control and provide better services	
1) Traditional family planning (FP) programs, in various forms and with currently available contraceptives (pill, IUD, condom)	Providing information, supplies and services for voluntary fertility control via modern contraception and various delivery systems; many examples operating today
2) . . . plus sterilization	. . . and adding sterilization, male and/or female, on an equivalent basis, as in India
3) . . . plus abortion	. . . and adding induced abortion on an equivalent basis, as in China
4) Community-based or commercial distribution of currently available contraceptives	. . . emphasizing contraceptive distribution through local agents who may profit, as in IPPF's community-based distribution (CBD) programs (e.g., in Colombia); the AID effort at saturation distribution (e.g., in Pakistan and the Philippines); and the recent efforts to stimulate commercial distribution (e.g., in India or Sri Lanka)
5) Sterilization camps	. . . concentrating communal facilities and promotion for vasectomy, as in India (first in Ernakulum district and then in Gujarat state), where highly organized and vigorous campaigns were conducted in a limited time period, with much publicity and substantial stipends
6) Postpartum arrangements	. . . systematically providing information and services in connection with institutionalized delivery, as in The Population Council program in 138 hospitals in 21 countries
7) Integration into maternal and child health (MCH) programs	. . . as in the so-called Taylor-Berelson effort in the Philippines, Turkey and Nigeria, to extend both MCH and FP services to the rural areas – a postpartum program for populations without the institutionalized delivery systems that are largely limited to the cities of the developing world; includes encouragement of breastfeeding as a spacing device in addition to its child care benefits
8) Integration into general health programs	. . . as in Narangwal (India) or Etimesgut (Turkey) – two large communities where FP has been incorporated as a normal part of the health system under experimental organization and evaluation
9) Integration into community development programs	. . . organized as part of rural improvement and community development, as in Gandhigram (India), where FP was incorporated as a normal part of a comprehensive effort at modernization in a whole range of fields
B. Improve the product, i.e., the acceptability, continuity of use and/or effectiveness of new means of fertility control	
Emphasis on development of improved contraceptives, such as a vaccine or implant, a side effect-free IUD, a safer or more convenient pill (once a month), a nonsurgical termination of pregnancy, . . . a currently unknown 'ideal' contraceptive	Research programs directed toward that end now under way in both the private and the public sectors, e.g., those conducted by drug companies, the WHO Expanded Programme of Research, Development and Research Training in Human Reproduction, and the International Committee for Contraception Research of The Population Council
To Affect Demand	
C. Promote basic socioeconomic determinants of fertility, or the most likely presumed determinants ('thresholds'), singly or together*	
1) General development: modernization, social change, sociocultural transformation . . . away from the traditional (high fertility) society	Reliance on social change, modernization, development, social-structural transformation, "New International Economic Order" to reduce fertility rates 'automatically' in the process
2) Increasing popular education: e.g., toward 6–8 years of schooling for all	. . . with special reference to extending education for girls as a necessary precondition to fertility reduction

* All of these paths work, at least in some important part, by lowering the economic value of children and thus changing family-size desires relative to other personal and social values.

TABLE 3.1. *Continued*

3) Reducing infant-child mortality: e.g., toward a rate of 50 or below	. . . as a necessary precondition for reducing birthrates
4) Increasing income: e.g., toward \$500 per capita or, better, \$800, plus perhaps more equitable income distribution	. . . with special reference to poverty reduction at the bottom of the income pyramid, or improved standard of living or social mobility or income redistribution as a necessary precondition
5) Industrialization: e.g., toward one-third or less of the labor force in agriculture	. . . with special reference to industrial development and its consequences for family, kinship, modernized attitudes, urbanization
6) Improving women's status: toward liberation from traditional childbearing and childrearing, through education and employment	. . . with special reference to emancipating women from traditional status, particularly via education and moneyed employment away from the home
7) Urbanization: toward 25 percent or more living in large cities ($\geq$ 100,000)	. . . with special reference to urban development, with implications for housing, city attitudes and behavior
D. Inform, educate, propagandize: persuade people to lower fertility through messages, arguments, appeals . . .	
1) . . . via mass media (radio, TV, newspapers, posters)	Promotion of energetic propaganda for smaller families, as in South Korea, Singapore, China
2) . . . via person-to-person communication, individually (e.g., door-to-door fieldwork) or collectively (e.g., group meetings)	. . . the same through personal contact, via residential or occupational communities, as in Isfahan (Iran) or Sialkot (Pakistan), where experimental programs were carried out along this line together with evaluation of outcome
3) . . . via formal school systems (population education)	Incorporation of population materials into primary and secondary school curricula, for long-term effect
E. Manipulate incentives/disincentives	
1) Housing and job opportunities 2) Maternity costs, leaves, etc. 3) Child allowances, educational fees, etc. 4) Social security systems 5) Money, gifts	Management of incentives/disincentives to individuals or families, in money or in kind, in antinatalist direction but without undue pressure; examples are the preferences given to small families for governmental housing in Singapore, the 1976 regulations about family size for government employees in India, the experimental schemes of educational bonds for limiting family size in Taiwan and of deferred savings accounts in certain tea estates in India, the direct stipends for vasectomy in India, and the development of obligation by the state for provision of welfare to the aged, in order to reduce the presumed need for children (sons) for that purpose, as reportedly in China
6) Communal incentives	Proposal of communal benefits (e.g., schools, roads, water supply) in return for specified fertility behavior by the collectivity
F. Manage community change and pressure to develop an antinatalist community consensus, typically guided by the political apparatus	
1) Youth corps, or equivalent work program, to change traditional behavior away from the home community	Proposals for collective employment and instruction of young people, both male and female, away from home ties, in order to delay marriage and modernize attitudes and information
2) Community pressures organized to discourage the nth child	Systematic efforts to develop community consensus in antinatalist direction, as reportedly in China, with social pressures exerted for enforcement of new norms
G. Impose legal sanctions	
1) Increase age at marriage	Increase minimum age of marriage for women to at least 18 and preferably beyond, e.g., as in China and Tunisia, and as proposed in India
2) Restriction on out-migration from villages	Limitations on mobility such that villages cannot export local unemployment to cities but must support their own 'excess' reproduction, as in China
3) Direct limitation on family size	Government imposition of a limit on number of children a couple may have

but also in the private sector via pharmaceutical companies. Reviews of such reproductive research, including appraisals of the present situation and the likely prospects, appear constantly (2).

On the Demand Side

C. Determinants: This policy calls for more or faster progress in changing the social and economic conditions associated or believed to be associated with lowered fertility—the individual or collective 'thresholds' that lead to smaller family size (3). Sometimes the call is simply for greater 'development', as in the Bucharest-related slogans "Development is the best contraceptive" and "Take care of the people and the population will take care of itself." Sometimes the focus is on those particular determinants that are or are considered to be most fertility-influencing, such as popular education or infant mortality; and there appears to be a current upsurge of interest in the potential fertility impact of concentrated efforts to improve living standards among rural populations (4). Typically, the rationale for this policy path is based on the 'causal linkage'—to affect fertility, first affect its cause(s). Those who favor this path, however, have generally given no explicit attention either to the relative allocation of interventionist resources or to the specific modes of implementation. That is, even if there were agreement (and there is not) on which factors exert how much fertility effect in what time, there has been little consideration of the costs involved: How should governments reallocate resources in order to increase the fertility effects of such large elements of the social structure? At the same time, most developing societies are actively pursuing such developmental ends by their own lights and within the limits of their resources, and seem unlikely to intensify or change their efforts very much on demographic grounds.

D. Information: This policy calls for intensive efforts to talk people into lower fertility by pointing out to them the alleged advantages of that course for individual families and/or the community at large—advantages, for example, for maternal and child health, availability of food, educational and job opportunities for the next generation, the status of women, the standard of living, the national economy and national welfare, and the natural resources, environment and ecology of the middle future. The interventions range from such instant information media as posters, leaflets and radio spots, to organized personal contacts and group discussions, to such longer range goals as population education in the schools (as in the Philippines).

E. Incentives: This policy calls for both direct and indirect manipulation of inducements to lower fertility. The most direct means is to provide money or other material rewards, as was done in India for vasectomy. A more indirect approach is represented by the 'tied' bank account used in the Tea Estate experiment in India, or by the educational bond scheme in Taiwan, in which a deferred payout is subject to certain levels of achieved parity. Still more indirect are the incentive programs affecting housing or maternity costs, as in Singapore; or the proposals to set up communal rather than individual incentives for fertility limitation (in occupational as well as residential communities) so that the community itself receives such improvements as a better school system, more roads, a cleaner water supply or preferential housing in return for the indicated fertility behavior; or the long-range effect of social security systems that are perceived as reducing the need for children (or sons) to assure welfare in old age. (This effort is really the other side of the coin of the child assistance programs adopted at least partly for pronatalist reasons in certain European nations.)

F. Community: This policy calls for systematic efforts to create and sustain a small-family norm within the community for the communal welfare. It is familiar mainly through reports of such endeavors in China, but occasionally appears by spontaneous generation elsewhere (as, reportedly, in Bangladesh). Similar efforts that have been proposed include isolated work programs for young people, both male and female, that would serve to break their communal ties with the traditional society, move them for a time outside the hold of the village, and thus expedite social change.

G. Sanctions: This policy calls for the imposition of legal sanctions and their enforcement, and takes three main forms:

- an increase in the age of marriage, as in China and as recently proposed in India;
- restrictions on migration from village to city so that the local community cannot export its excess manpower or relieve its food deficiency in this way, as in China; and
- as the last remedy, direct limits on the number of children couples may have without penalty, as was recently under consideration in India, and, in a borderline case, through community pressure to respond to politically set and supervised quotas, as in China.

There may in principle or in fact be other paths to fertility reduction for a developing society, but they are not now visible on the international scene (at least to this author) either in practice or in responsible proposal. Naturally, none of these paths need be selected in isolation; there is ample room for multiple paths to be pursued simultaneously.

There are a number of other measures that are being supported both by national governments and international assistance agencies in order to deal with the population problem. These include building construction, training programs, institution building, data collection, research and evaluation, and policy analysis. But they appear to be indirectly related to the designated task in the sense that when buildings are constructed, people trained, institutions built, data collected, research completed and policy analyzed—when all that is done, the direct paths to fertility reduction must still be identified and selected, presumably along the foregoing lines in the absence of further social invention.

Criteria for Choices

If these are the paths to fertility reduction that are available for consideration, how are they to be judged by policy makers? In any specific instance, local circumstances, not to say personalities, will rule. But one can discern general criteria by which such rulings are or can be made, standards by which the paths are appraised for the purpose of policy formulation and implementation. They are here considered as three-fold:

- *Acceptability.* Will the measure be acceptable to governmental elites and to the public—that is, in the official policy process and by general opinion ("the culture")? Is it compatible with political values and personal values?*
- *Feasibility.* If acceptable, can the program be implemented in the designated area? Is there sufficient administrative capability and resource availability to do the job? That is, can the bureaucratic infrastructure actually carry through on the measure and are there enough resources, including funds, to support the program?
- *Effectiveness.* If acceptable and feasible, will the measure reduce fertility by a worthwhile amount in a reasonable period of time—as judged, for example, against the target of reducing the crude birthrate by 10 points in 10 years—at reasonable cost? Note that this criterion is not *efficiency,* defined as effectiveness per dollar invested. It is immediately obvious that different interventions range widely in their costs. For example, industrialization or popular education is far more expensive per capita than family planning programs or, in sheer economic terms, the application of sanctions. But effectiveness here, as measured against the indicated standard, assumes that the intervention is indeed carried out, i.e., is both acceptable and feasible. The score judges the effectiveness of the intervention *if realized.*†

In short, how willing is the society to adopt the policy path? How able is it to implement the decision? How much will the path yield toward the intended result?

These criteria can be considered as a set of screens through which the policy must filter. To the

---

*The argument is sometimes heard from the outside that countries can no longer afford to consider acceptability as a criterion for action; but both those responsible for policy and those subject to policy are likely to find that injunction unacceptable.

†As for efficiency, the author and Robert Haveman of the University of Wisconsin have in process a cost-benefit analysis of resource allocation in this field that is based on these categories and that includes analyses by a number of experts of the likely effect of such interventions on fertility under a range of conditions and given the same expenditure of funds.

extent that it passes through one, it goes on to the other. Acceptability is normally gauged against some cultural and political understanding of what would be permitted in the society over the next decade or so, feasibility against some empirical knowledge of what the administrative infrastructure can carry by way of implementation, and effectiveness against what would be likely to happen to the birthrate if the policy were carried forward for a decade or so (disregarding the time lag in getting under way).

Paths Evaluated Against Criteria

Now it is immediately apparent that any particular policy path can rank quite differently across the three criteria. The path may be highly acceptable but not very feasible (for example, a sharp increase in general schooling or standard of living), or highly effective but not very acceptable or feasible (for example, some forms of sanction). Indeed, the population debate often seems to be stuck these days in dispute between a policy that is more or less acceptable and feasible but is not "sufficiently" effective (family planning) and a policy that presumably would be effective but is not "sufficiently" feasible within a reasonable time (development). In effect, the search is for a third way that scores as highly as possible on all three criteria at an affordable cost. Whatever policy choice is made, however, is in effect a trade-off among paths judged against such criteria.

By way of illustration, if nothing more, I assign values to the designated paths on a 10-point scale (10=high, 1=low) for each criterion. These rankings have only "best guess" status. They are based first on available data, then on empirical experience, and beyond these, on subjective judgment as residually required. In this respect, note, they are no different from most policy judgments. Indeed, this process illustrates the kind of policy judgment that needs to be made in this field as in others, and with these paths and criteria or with others.

Finally, the criteria must be applied in the particular national case. But these ratings may serve as prototypic approximations for developing countries in need, i.e., those with relatively disadvantaged social settings. And the scores are perhaps more revealing in their relative than in their absolute values.

How acceptable, how feasible and how effective are these paths in the typical developing country with inadequate development and a crude birthrate, say, over 35? This author's estimate for the contemporary international situation may be seen in Table 3.2.

Let me elucidate a few of these ratings, for illustrative purposes. By now, traditional family planning programs have gained a certain acceptability (7 in Table 3.2) in the developing world; but, typically, they cannot be carried out as planned in most such settings because of inadequate infrastructure (5); and, though the matter is still controversial, they appear to have had at least moderate-sized results in reducing fertility (4). Adding sterilization to the program reduces both acceptability (6) and feasibility (4)—the former because of moral and personal objections, the latter because of the need for medical personnel in numbers not now available; but sterilization increases effectiveness (5.5) because of the long-term continuity built into the method. Adding abortion reduces policy acceptability still further (4), on moral and political grounds, but increases effectiveness (6.5) in view of the empirical evidence of strong demand for legal abortion services wherever they have been made available under proper conditions—a demand which exceeds substitution for illegal abortions.

To take other examples: Popular education is highly acceptable (9) and would be highly effective (8) but is not very feasible of implementation within a reasonable time period (5). A social security system would be accepted (8) and would perhaps be somewhat effective, though with a considerable time lag (5), but it is not feasible in the absence of administrative networks (2). Sanctions on family size—for example, no more children after three—would probably be quite effective (9) but would not be acceptable (3) or feasible (4) in most societies. In general, since demand policies cover a wider range of activity than supply policies, the former have a wider range in the scoring as well.

In the real world, of course, several of these paths are being pursued simultaneously. The acceptability and the feasibility of the various paths are substantially though not wholly indepen-

TABLE 3.2. Estimated values of alternate policy paths, as measured by their acceptability (Acc), feasibility (Fea) and effectiveness (Eff), on a scale of 10–1

Paths	Acc	Fea	Eff
Supply Paths			
A. Improved access			
1) Traditional FP programs, various forms, current contraceptives	7.0	5.0	4.0
2) . . . plus sterilization	6.0	4.0	5.5
3) . . . plus abortion	4.0	4.0	6.5
4) Community-based/commercial distribution, current contraceptives	7.0	6.0	5.5
5) Sterilization camps	5.0	5.0	5.5
6) Postpartum arrangements	8.0	6.0	4.5
7) MCH integration	8.0	5.0	5.0
8) Health integration	8.0	4.0	4.5
9) Community integration	7.0	4.0	4.5
B. Improved product, appropriate delivery	8.0	3.0	6.0
Demand Paths			
C. Determinants			
1) Development	8.0	4.0	9.0
2) Education	9.0	5.0	8.0
3) Infant/child mortality	10.0	5.0	7.0
4) Income	9.0	4.0	6.0
5) Industrialization	7.0	4.0	7.0
6) Women's status	6.0	3.0	6.0
7) Urbanization	6.0	4.0	5.0
D. Information			
1) Mass media	7.0	5.0	2.5
2) Person-to-person	7.0	4.0	4.0
3) Population education	8.0	4.0	3.5
E. Incentives/disincentives			
1) Housing, jobs	6.0	2.0	3.0
2) Maternity costs	5.0	2.0	3.0
3) Child allowances	5.0	2.0	4.0
4) Social security	8.0	2.0	5.0
5) Money, gifts	6.0	5.0	6.0
6) Communal	6.0	4.0	4.0
F. Community			
1) Youth corps	5.0	3.0	6.0
2) Community pressure	3.0	4.0	8.0
G. Sanctions			
1) Age at marriage	6.0	4.0	5.5
2) Out-migration	5.0	2.0	7.0
3) Family size	3.0	4.0	9.0

TABLE 3.3. Estimated values of alternate policy paths (compressed version)

Paths	Acc	Fea	Eff
Supply Paths			
1. Public sector access: current means (A1, 5–9)	7.0	5.0	4.5
a) . . . plus sterilization (A2)	6.0	4.0	5.5
b) . . . plus abortion (A3)	4.0	4.0	6.5
c) . . . plus improved product (B)	8.0	3.0	6.0
2. Private sector distribution (A4)	7.0	6.0	5.5
Demand Paths			
1. Determinants (C)	8.0	4.0	7.0
2. Information (D)	7.0	4.0	3.0
3. Incentives (E1–4,6)	6.0	2.5	4.0
a) Money (E5)	6.0	5.0	6.0
4. Community (F)	4.0	3.5	7.0
5. Sanctions (G1–2)	5.5	3.0	6.0
a) Limits on family size (G3)	3.0	4.0	9.0

dent of one another. However, the effectiveness scores are additive; for example, if improvement of the status of women were added to the traditional family planning approach, the impact on fertility would be greater than if either were employed separately. But such scores cannot simply be added together to get a combined effectiveness measure. Moreover, as we have noted, this array does not directly take into consideration the obvious cost factors that could affect the choice of interventions—that is, how much effectiveness could be purchased for an additional or alternative expenditure of $X? This scoring attempts only to estimate what the effect on fertility would be *if* the indicated intervention were carried out, disregarding cost—though the other two criteria estimate the likelihood, on political, cultural and administrative grounds, that the policy path will be taken.

No claim is made that these are definitive scores in any sense. They are personal estimates for the prototypic developing country in need, presented as illustrations of the process of policy determination; and other serious estimates could claim equal validity. If the scores seem unduly differentiated and precise for the present state of the art, they could readily be reformulated into, say, a trichotomy of high, middle and low.

Whatever the refinements, however, something like the present array would emerge—and indeed something like it is now latent in the process of policy decision. What this exercise does, one hopes, is to specify the application of standards of appraisal to the policy paths before the house. To the extent that these are the right paths and the right criteria and the right estimates, this is where the matter now stands, and these appear to be the current trade-offs.

The array in Table 3.2 has the virtue of setting forth the proposed policy options for competitive consideration in the allocation of scarce resources. But if it is considered too extended or too unwieldy—with too many options—it can be summarized into a compressed version as in Table 3.3.

Thus, the policy decision becomes a three-dimensional selection against resources: how to allocate such resources as money, staff and facilities to such policy options as are appraised. In extenso, one can think of a 'policy space' within which such decisions are made. In principle, all decisions on public policy are made within some such space, in which possible interventions are weighed against criteria for judgment and then balanced against costs. In this case, the space is three-dimensional, and equal on all sides (though uneven or weighted sides could be readily accommodated).

In physical representation, the space becomes what I term the 'policy cube'. Each side of the cube represents a standard of appraisal—acceptability, feasibility, effectiveness—and the paths can be located within the cube by their scores, across the theoretical range from 10–10–10 to 1–1–1. The initial and the compressed arrays, with paths evaluated by criteria distributed therein, as in Tables 3.2 and 3.3, are seen in Figures 3.1 and 3.2. The physical representation does not add to the foregoing description,

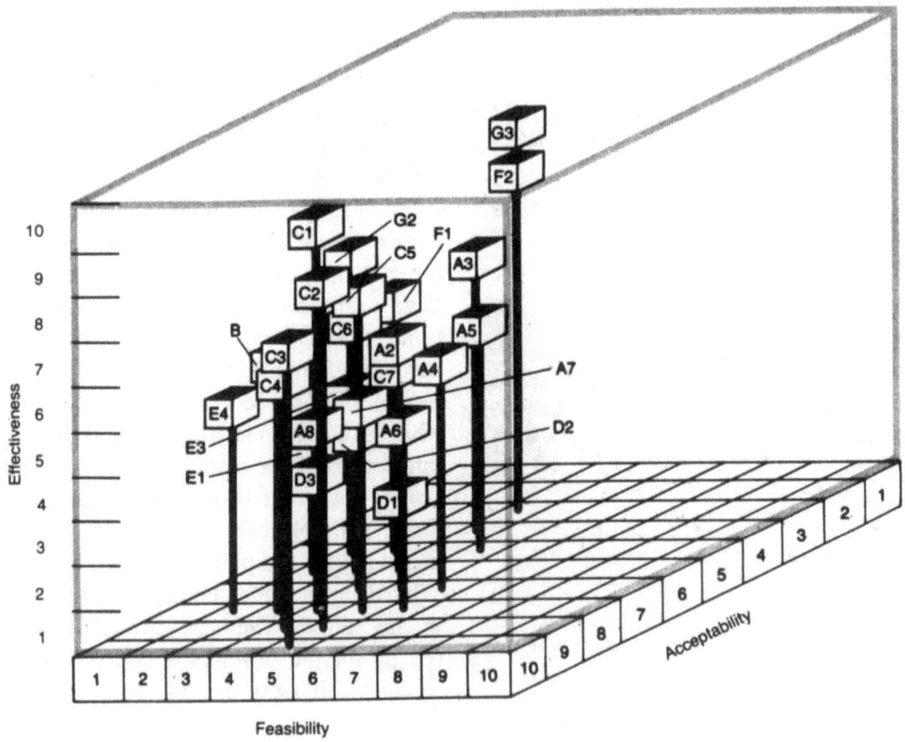

Note: Six paths hidden in illustration.

FIGURE 3.1. Schematic drawing (based on actual physical model) of the Policy Cube. Estimated values of the 31 policy paths as measured by their acceptability, feasibility and effectiveness on a scale of 10–1.

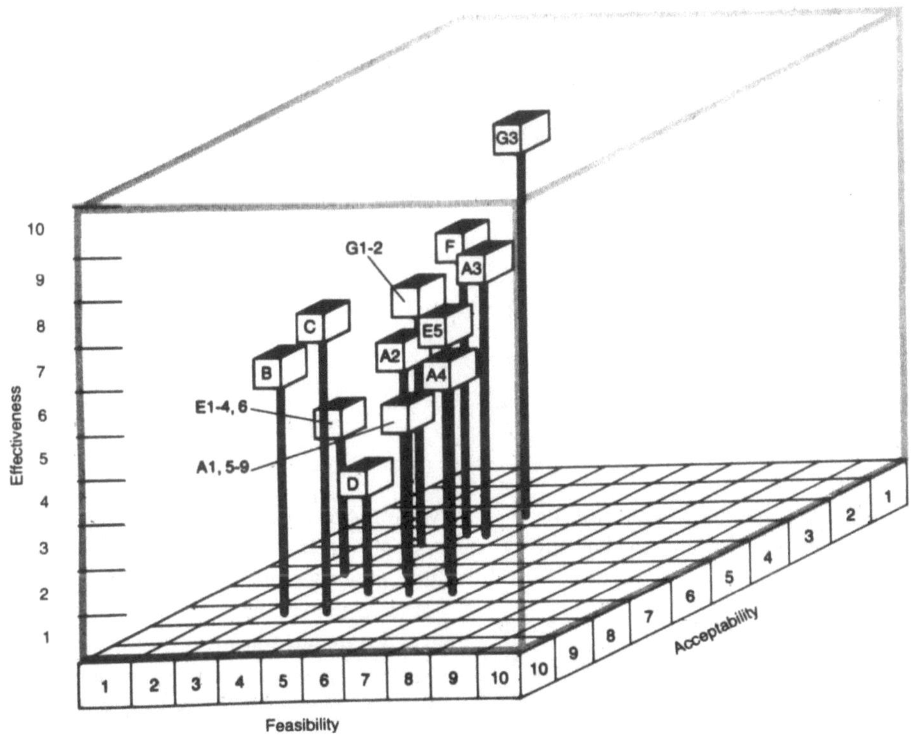

FIGURE 3.2. Schematic drawing of the compressed array (12 paths) of the Policy Cube.

but it does make clear the trade-offs involved, and hence focuses on choices and makes them more explicit.

Summary

This article has enumerated several policy paths now used or proposed for dealing with rapid population growth in developing countries; has identified three standards by which such options can be appraised; has appraised policies against standards, and has embodied that process in a 'policy cube' to represent the trade-offs involved. In a rapidly evolving field like population policy, everything is subject to change—paths, criteria and scores—but the underlying process of selection has a certain constancy. If not this set, then another—but the problem remains. It is in that spirit of continuing discourse that this effort is offered.

References

1. R. Freedman and B. Berelson, "The Record of Family Planning Programs," *Studies in Family Planning*, 7: 1, 1976. (This article contains references for most of the categories listed in Table 3.1.)
2. R.O. Greep, M.A. Koblinsky and F.S. Jaffe, *Reproduction and Human Welfare: A Challenge to Research—A Review of the Reproductive Sciences and Contraceptive Development*, The MIT Press, Cambridge, Mass., 1976; R.V. Short and D.T. Baird, eds., *Contraceptives of the Future: A Royal Society Discussion*, The Royal Society, London, 1976; S.J. Segal and O.S. Nordberg, "Fertility Regulation Technology: Status and Prospects," *Population Bulletin*, Vol. 31, No. 6, 1977.
3. N. Uphoff, "Accelerating the Movement to Smaller Families," *Development Forum*, Jan.-Feb. 1977, p. 4.
4. R. Ridker, ed., *Population and Development: The Search for Selective Interventions*, The Johns Hopkins University Press, Baltimore, 1976.

4
Beyond Family Planning

What further proposals have been made to "solve" the population problem, and how are they to be appraised?

This article rests on four propositions: (i) among the great problems on the world agenda is the population problem; (ii) that problem is most urgent in the developing countries, where rapid population growth retards social and economic development; (iii) there is a time penalty on the problem in the sense that, other things being equal, anything not done sooner may be harder to do later, due to increased numbers; and accordingly (iv) everything that can properly be done to lower population growth rates should be done, now. The question is, what is to be done? There is a certain agreement on the general objective (that is, on the desirability of lowering birth rates, though not on how far and how fast), but there is disagreement as to means.

The first response to too high growth rates deriving from too high birth rates is to introduce voluntary contraception on a mass basis, or try to. Why is family planning the first step taken on the road to population control? Probably because, from a broad political standpoint, it is the most acceptable one; since it is closely tied to maternal and child care it can be perceived as a health measure beyond dispute, and since it is voluntary it can be justified as a contribution to the effective personal freedom of individual couples. On both scores, it ties into accepted values and thus achieves political viability. Moreover, it is a gradual effort and an inexpensive one, both of which features contribute to its political acceptability.

How effective have family-planning programs been as a means toward population control? There is currently some controversy among qualified observers as to its efficacy (1), and this is not the place to review that issue. There is agreement, however, that the problem is of such magnitude and consequence that additional efforts are needed to reach a "solution," however that is responsibly defined.

For the purpose of this article, then, let us assume that today's national family-planning programs, mainly based on voluntary contraception, are not "enough"–where "enough" is defined not necessarily as achieving zero growth in some extended present but simply as lowering birth rates quickly and substantially. "Enough" begs the question of the ultimate goal and only asks that a faster decline in population growth rates be brought about than is presently being achieved or in prospect—and, within the range of the possible, the faster the better (2,3). Just to indicate roughly the order of magnitude, let us say that the proximate goal is the halving of the birth rate in the developing countries in the next decade or two—from, say, over 40 births per thousand per year to 20 to 25 (4). For obvious reasons, both emigration and increased death rates are ruled out of consideration.

What is to be done to bring that reduction about, beyond present programs of voluntary family planning? I address that question in two ways: first, by listing the programs or policies more or less

---

Reprinted with permission from *Science* 1969;163 (Feb. 7):533–543.

responsibly suggested in recent years for achieving this end; second, by reviewing the issues raised by the suggested approaches.

Proposals Beyond Family Planning

Here is a listing of the several proposals, arranged in descriptive categories. The list includes both proposals for consideration and proposals for action.

A. Extensions of voluntary fertility control.

1) Institutionalization of maternal care in rural areas of developing countries: a feasibility study of what would be required in order to bring some degree of modern medical or paramedical attention to every pregnant woman in the rural areas of five developing countries, with professional backup for difficult cases and with family-planning education and services a central component of the program, aimed particularly at women of low parity (5).

2) Liberalization of induced abortion (6; 7, p. 139; 8).

B. Establishment of involuntary fertility control.

1) Mass use of a "fertility control agent" by the government to regulate births at an acceptable level. The "fertility control agent," designed to lower fertility in the society to a level 5 to 75 percent below the present birth rate, as needed, would be a substance now unknown but believed to be available for field testing after 5 to 15 years of research work. It would be included in the water supply in urban areas and administered by "other methods" elsewhere (9). A related suggestion is the "addition of temporary sterilants to water supplies or staple food" (10).

2) "Marketable licenses to have children," given to women and perhaps men in "whatever number would ensure a reproduction rate of one" (say, 2.2 children per couple). For example, "the unit certificate might be the 'deci-child,' and accumulation of ten of these units, by purchase, inheritance or gift, would permit a woman in maturity to have one legal child" (11).

3) Temporary sterilization of all girls by means of time-capsule contraceptives, and of girls and women after each delivery, with reversibility allowed only upon governmental approval. Certificates of approval would be distributed according to national popular vote on desired population growth, and saleable on the open market (12).

4) Compulsory sterilization of men with three or more living children (13); a requirement of induced abortion for all illegitimate pregnancies (6).

C. Intensified educational campaigns.

1) Inclusion of educational materials on population in primary and secondary school systems (6,14,15).

2) Promotion of national satellite television systems for directly disseminating information on population and family planning and for indirectly promoting acceptance of modern attitudes and practices in general (7, p. 162; 16; 17, especially pp. 13–14; 18).

D. Incentive programs. As used here, the term *incentive programs* refers to payments, or their equivalent, made directly to couples who use contraceptives or to couples who do not have children for specified periods. It does *not* refer to payments to field workers, medical personnel, volunteers, and others, for securing acceptance of contraceptive practice.

1) Payment, or the equivalent (for example, the gift of a transistor radio), for accepting sterilization (6,19–21) or for the effective practice of contraception (21–24).

2) A bonus for child spacing or nonpregnancy (25–28); a savings certificate to couples for each 12-month period in which no child is born (29); a lottery scheme for preventing illegitimate births among teenagers in a small country (30); "responsibility prizes" for each 5 years of childless marriage or for vasectomy before the birth of a third child, and special lotteries, with tickets available to the childless (7, p. 138).

E. Tax and welfare benefits and penalties—that is, a system of social services that would discourage child-bearing rather than encourage it, as present systems tend to do.

1) Withdrawal of maternity benefits, perhaps after the birth of *N* (3?) children (6,21,26) or in cases where certain limiting conditions, such as adequate child spacing, knowledge of family planning, or attainment of a given level of income, have not been met (31, pp. 130–31).

2) Withdrawal of child or family allowances, perhaps after the birth of *N* children (6; 26; 31, pp. 131–36).

3) Levy of tax on births after the *N*th child (21; 26; 28, p. 30).

4) Limitation of governmentally provided medical treatment, housing, scholarships, loans, subsidies, and so on, to families with fewer than *N* children (6,26).

5) Reversal of tax benefits, to favor the unmarried and the parents of fewer rather than more children (6; 7, pp. 136–37; 21; 26; 31, p. 137; 32).

6) Provision by the state of *N* years of free schooling, at all levels, to each family, to be allocated among the children as desired (33).

7) Pensions for poor parents with fewer than *N* children, as social security for their old age (21,34,35).

F. Shifts in social and economic institutions—that is, broad changes in fundamental institutional arrangements that could have the effect of lowering fertility.

1) Raising the minimum age at marriage, through legislation or through imposition of a substantial fee for marriage licenses (6,32); through direct payment of bonuses for delayed marriage (25); through payment of marriage benefits only to parents of brides over 21 years old (31, p. 130); through government loans for wedding ceremonies when the bride is over a given age, or with the interest rate inversely related to the bride's age (36); through a "governmental 'first marriage grant' . . . awarded each couple in which the age of both [sic] partners was 25 or more" (7, p. 138); or through establishment of a domestic "national service" program for all men for the appropriate 2-year period in order to develop social services, inculcate modern attitudes toward (among other matters) family planning and population control, and delay marriage (37).

2) Measures to promote or require the participation of women in the labor force (outside the home), in order to provide roles and interests for women that are alternative or supplementary to marriage (6,32,38).

3) "Direct manipulation of family structure itself—planned efforts at deflecting the family's socializing function . . . or introducing nonfamilial distractions . . . into people's lives," specifically through employment of women outside the house (39); "selective restructuring of the family in relation to the rest of society" (6).

4) Promotion of "two types of marriage, one of them childless and readily dissolved, and the other licensed for children and designed to be stable"; marriages of the first type would have to constitute 20 to 40 percent of the total in order to allow free choice of family size for marriages of the second type (16,40).

5) Encouragement of long-range social trends leading toward lower fertility—for example, "improved and universal general education, or new roads facilitating communication, or improved agricultural methods, or a new industry that would increase productivity, or other types of innovation that may break the 'cake of custom' and produce social foment" (41); improvement in the status of women (42).

6) Efforts to lower death rates even further, particularly infant and child death rates, in the belief that lower birth rates will follow (43).

G. Political channels and organizations.

1) U.S. insistence on "population control as the price of food aid," with highly selective assistance based thereon, and exertion of political pressures on governments or religious groups that impede "solution" of the population problem (7, pp. 161–66; 44).

2) Reorganization of national and international agencies to deal with the population problem: within the United States, "coordination by a powerful governmental agency, a Federal Department of Population and Environment . . . with the power to take whatever steps are necessary to establish a reasonable population size" (7, p. 138; 45); within India, creation of "a separate Ministry of Population Control" (46, p. 96); development of an "international specialized agency larger than WHO to operate programs for extending family limitation techniques to the world . . . charged with the responsibility of effecting the transfer to population equilibrium" (16).

3) Promotion of zero growth in population as the ultimate goal, and acceptance of this goal now in order to place intermediate goals of lowered fertility in proper context (6).

H. Augmented research efforts.

1) More research on social means for achieving necessary fertility goals (6).

2) Focused research on practical methods of sex determination (47).

3) Increased research directed toward improvement of the contraceptive technology (48).

Proposals: Review of the Issues

Here are 29 proposals beyond family planning for dealing with the problem of undue population growth in the developing world. Naturally I cannot claim that these are all the proposals that have been made more or less responsibly toward that end, but my guess is that there are not many more and that these proposals are a reasonably good sample of the total list.

Since several of the proposals tend in the same direction, it seems appropriate to review them against the criteria that any such proposals might be required to meet. What are such criteria? There are at least six: (i) scientific, medical, and technological readiness; (ii) political viability; (iii) administrative feasibility; (iv) economic capability; (v) moral, ethical, and philosophical acceptability; and (vi) presumed effectiveness. In other words, the key questions are: Is the scientific, medical, technological base available or likely? Will governments approve? Can the proposal be administered? Can the society afford the proposal? Is it morally acceptable? And, finally, will it work?

Scientific, medical, technological readiness. Two questions are involved: (i) is the needed technology available? and (ii) are the medical or paramedical personnel needed in order to assure medical administration and safety available or readily trainable?

With regard to temporary contraception, sterilization, and abortion, not only is the needed technology available now, but it is being steadily improved and expanded. The intrauterine device (IUD) and the oral pill have been major contraceptive developments of the past decade, and several promising leads are now being followed up (49), though it cannot be said with much confidence that any of the efforts will produce measures suitable for mass use within the next few years (50). Improved technologies for sterilization, both male and female, are being worked on, and there has been a recent development in abortion technique, the so-called suction device.

However, neither Ehrlich's "temporary sterilants" nor Ketchel's "fertility control agent" (B-1) is now available or on the technological horizon, though that does not mean that the research task ought not to be pursued against a subsequent need, especially since any such substance could be administered to individuals on a voluntary basis as well as to the population as a whole on an involuntary basis. In the latter case, if administered through the water supply or a similar source, the substance would have to be medically safe and free of side effects for men and women, young and old, well and ill, physiologically normal and physiologically marginal, as well as for animals and perhaps plants. As some people have remarked, the proposal that such a substance be added to a water supply would face far greater difficulties of acceptance, simply on medical grounds, than the far milder proposals with regard to fluoridation to prevent tooth decay.

Though a substantial technology in fertility control does exist, that does not necessarily mean that the techniques can be applied where they are most needed; this is true partly because of limitations in the number of trained personnel. In general, the more the technology requires the services of medical or paramedical personnel (or, what is much the same, is perceived as requiring them), the more difficult it is to administer in the developing countries. In the case of sterilization and abortion, the medical requirement becomes more severe. For example, when the policy of compulsory vasectomy of men with three or more children was first being considered in India (see 13), it was estimated that the policy would affect about 40 million males: "one thousand surgeons or parasurgeons each averaging 20 operations a day for five days a week would take eight years to cope with the existing candidates, and during this time of course a constant supply of new candidates would be coming along" (51)—at present birth rates, probably some 3.5 million a year. A program of large-scale abortion (provided such a program was legal and acceptable) might additionally require hospital beds, which are in particularly short supply in most developing countries. However, the newer abortion technique might not require hospitalization— theoretically, the abortion "camp" may be feasible, as the vasectomy "camp" was, though the problems are substantially greater.

In short, the technology is available for some but not for all current proposals, and the case is similar for properly trained personnel.

Political viability. The "population problem" has been increasingly recognized by national governments and international agencies over the past decade, and policies for dealing with it have been increasingly adopted: national family-planning programs in some 20 to 25 countries; positive resolutions and actions within the United Nations family; large programs of support by such developed countries as the United States and Sweden; the so-called World Leaders' Statement, in which 30 heads of governments endorsed efforts to limit population growth. There is no reason to think that the trend toward population limitation has run its course.

At the same time, the political picture is by no means unblemished. Some favorable policies are not strong enough to support a vigorous program, even one limited to family planning on health grounds; in national politics, "population control" can become a handy issue for a determined opposition; internal ethnic balances are sometimes delicately involved, with political ramifications; national size is often equated with national power, from the standpoint of international relations and regional military balances; the motives behind the support and encouragement of population control by the developed countries are sometimes perceived as neocolonialist or neoimperialist; and on the international front, as represented by the United Nations, there is still considerable reluctance based on both religious and political considerations. In short, ambivalence on the part of the elite and recognition of the issue as a political liability are not absent even in the countries that favor population limitation.

Any social policy adopted by government rests on some minimum consensus concerning goals and means. They need not be the ultimate goals or the final means; the socioeconomic plans of developing countries are typically 5-year plans, not 20- or 40- or 100-year plans. Indeed, the ultimate goal of population policy–that is, zero growth–need not be agreed upon or even considered by officials who *can* agree upon the immediate goal of lowering growth by a specified amount or by "as much as possible" within a period of years. And since there are always goals beyond goals, one does not even need to know what the ultimate goal is–only the direction in which it will be found (which is usually more readily agreed upon). Would insistence *now* on the acknowledgment of an *ultimate* goal of zero growth advance the effort or change its direction?

To start with, the proposal of compulsory controls in India in 1967 (B–4) precipitated "a storm of questions in Parliament" (52); the proposal was withdrawn, and the issue resulted in a high-level shift of personnel within the family-planning organization. No other country has seriously entertained the idea. Other considerations aside, in many countries political instability would make implementation virtually impossible.

Social measures designed to affect the birth rate indirectly–for example, tax benefits, social security arrangements, and so on–have been proposed from time to time. In India there have been several such proposals: for example, by the United Nations mission (53, chap. 11), by the Small Family Norm Committee (26), by the Central Family Planning Council (54), and in almost every issue of such publications as *Family Planning News, Centre Calling*, and *Planned Parenthood*.

As Samuel reports, with accompanying documentation (21), "the desirability of imposing a tax on births of fourth or higher order has been afloat for some time. However, time and again, the suggestion has been rejected by the Government of India." In some cases action has been taken either by the central government [for example, income tax "deductions for dependent children are given for the first and second child only" (53, p. 87)] or by certain states ["Maharashtra and Uttar Pradesh have decided to grant educational concessions and benefits only to those children whose parents restrict the size of their families" (55)]. Indicative of political sensitivity is the fact that an order withdrawing maternity leave for nonindustrial women employees with three or more living children–at best a tiny number of educated women–was revoked before it went into effect (56). There is a special political problem in many countries, in that economic constraints on fertility often turn out in practice to be selective on class, racial, or ethnic grounds, and thus exacerbate political tensions. Moreover, the promotion of female participation in the labor force runs up against the political problem that such employment would be competitive with men in situations of already high male unemployment and underemployment.

Whether programs for eliminating population growth are or are not politically acceptable appears to depend largely upon whether they are perceived as positive or negative; where "positive" means that they are seen as promoting not only population limitation but other social benefits as well, and where "negative" means that they are seen as limited to population control. For example, family planning programs, as noted above, are often rationalized as contributing to both maternal and child health and to the effective freedom of the individual family; a pension for the elderly would have social welfare benefits as well as indirect impact upon family size, in countries where a large family has been the traditional "social security system"; contraceptive programs in Latin America are promoted by the medical community as a medical and humanitarian answer not to the population problem but to the extensive illegal and dangerous practice of abortion. On the other hand, imposing tax liabilities or withdrawing benefits after the birth of the *N*th child, not to mention involuntary measures, can be attacked as punitive means whose only purpose is that of limiting population.

It would thus require great political courage, joined to very firm demographic convictions, for a national leader to move toward an unpopular and severe prescription designed to cure his country's population ills. Indeed, it is difficult to envisage such a political move in an open society where a political opposition could present a counter view and perhaps prevail.

The governmental decisions about measures to be taken to deal with undue population growth must be made mainly by the countries directly involved; after all, it is their people and their nation whose prospects are most centrally affected. But in an interconnected world, with peace and human welfare at issue, others are properly concerned, for reasons both of self-interest and of humanitarianism—other governments from the developed world, the international community, private groups. What of the political considerations in this connection?

A recommendation (G-1) that the United States exert strong political pressures to effect population control in developing countries seems more likely to generate political opposition abroad than acceptance. It is conceivable that such measures might be adopted here, but it is hardly conceivable that they would be agreed to by the proposed recipients. Such a policy seems likely to boomerang against its own objective, quite aside from ethical or political considerations.

The proposal (G-2) to create an international superagency seems more likely of success, but is not without its difficulties. The World Health Organization, UNICEF, and UNESCO have moved some distance toward family planning, if not population control, but only slowly and in the face of considerable political restraint on the international front (57). A new international agency would find the road easier only if its efforts were restricted to the convinced countries. Certainly the international organizations now concerned with this problem would not be expected to abdicate in favor of a new agency. If it could be brought into being and given a strong charter for action, then, almost by definition, the international political climate would be such as to favor action by the present agencies, and then efficiency and not political acceptability would be the issue.

Administrative feasibility. Given technical availability and political acceptability, what can actually be done? This is where several "good ideas" run into difficulties in the developing world, in the translation of a theoretical idea into a practical program.

It is difficult to estimate the administrative feasibility of several of the proposals listed above, if for no other reason than that the proponents do not put forward the necessary organizational plans or details. How are "fertility control agents" or "sterilants" to be administered on an involuntary mass basis in the absence of a central water supply or a food-processing system? How are men with three or more children to be reliably identified in a peasant society and impelled to undergo sterilization against their will; and what is to be done if they decline, or if a fourth child is born? What is to be done with parents who evade the compulsory programs, or with the children born as a result of this evasion? How can an incentive system be honestly run in the absence of an organized network of offices positioned and staffed to carry out the regulatory activity? How can a system of social benefits and penalties, including incentives to postpone or forego marriage, be made to work in the absence of such a network?

These questions are meant only to suggest the kinds of difficulties that must be taken into account if proposals are to be translated into programs. It would seem desirable that every responsibly made proposal address itself to such administrative problems. Some proposals do move in that direction. The feasibility in administration, personnel, and costs of the plan (A-1) to institutionalize maternal care in rural areas, with family planning attached, is currently under study in several developing countries.

The plan (C-1) to include population as a subject in the school curriculum has been carried forward as far as the preparation of educational materials, and in a few cases beyond that (58). The plans for incentive programs sometimes come down to only the theoretical proposition that people will do anything for money (in this case refrain from having children), but in some cases the permissible payment is proposed on the basis of an economic analysis, and in a few cases an administrative means is also proposed (59). The plan for governmental wedding loans scaled to the bride's age recognizes that a birth-registration system might be needed to control against misreporting of age (6).

Thus the *why* of population control is easy, the *what* is not very hard, but the *how* is difficult. We may know that the extension of popular education or an increase in the number of women in the labor force or a later age at marriage would all contribute to population control in a significant way. But there remains the administrative question of how to bring those developments about. In short, several proposals assume workability of a complicated scheme in a country that cannot now collect its own vital statistics in a reliable manner. Moreover, there is a limit to how much administrative burden the typical developing country can carry: it cannot manage many large-scale developmental efforts at a time, either within the field of population or overall. After all, population is not the only effort; agriculture, industry, education, health, communications, the military—all are important claimants. And, within the field of population, a country that finds it difficult to organize and run a family-planning program will find that harder when other programs are added. So, difficult administrative choices must be made.

Economic capability. From the standpoint of economic capability there are two questions: (i) is the program worthwhile when measured against the criterion of economic return, and (ii) if worthwhile, can it be afforded from present budgets?

Most of the proposals probably pass the second screen. If a fertility-control agent suitable for mass administration becomes available and politically and administratively acceptable, such a program would probably not be prohibitively expensive; incorporation of population materials into the school curriculum is not unduly expensive; imposing of taxes or withdrawing of benefits or increasing fees for marriage licenses might even return a net gain after administrative cost.

But a few proposals are costly in absolute if not relative terms. For example, the institutionalization of maternal care (proposal A-1) might cost some $500 million for construction and $200 million for annual operation in India, or, respectively, $25 million and $10 million in a country with population of 25 million (5) (although recent estimates are substantially lower). The plan for a "youth corps" in India would cost upward of $450 million a year if the participants were paid only $50 annually. The plan for payment of pensions to elderly fathers without sons could cost from $400 million to $1 billion a year, plus administrative costs (35). The satellite television system for India would cost $50 million for capital costs only, on a restricted project (17, p. 23), with at least another $200 million needed for receiving sets, broadcast terminals, and programming costs if national coverage were to be secured. All of these proposals are intended to have beneficial consequences beyond population control and hence can be justified on multiple grounds, but they are still expensive in absolute amounts.

The broad social programs of popular education, improved methods of agriculture, and increased industrialization (F-5) already absorb even larger sums, and they could no doubt utilize even more. Here the question is a different one. At present, in such countries as India, Pakistan, South Korea, and Turkey, the funds allocated to family-planning programs constitute less than 1 percent—in most cases, much less—of the total funds devoted to economic development. Would that tiny proportion make a greater contribution to population control, over some specified period, if given over to education or industrialization or road-building than it makes when utilized directly for family planning (60)? From what we now know, the answer is certainly "No."

Beyond family planning, the situation is still less clear. On the assumption that some level of incentive or benefit would have a demographic impact, what would the level have to be to cut the birth rate by, say, 20 percent? We simply do not know: the necessary experiments on administration and effectiveness have not been carried out. Let us review what has been proposed with respect to incentives. On the ground that incentives for vasectomy are better than incentives for contraception—since vasectomy is a one-time procedure and is likely to be more effective in preventing births—Pohlman (20) proposes for India a range of money benefits depending upon parity and degree of acceptance—from $7 to a father of four or more children if half the villagers in that category enter the program up to $40 to a father of three children if 75 percent enter. If the 50-percent criterion were met in both categories throughout India, the current plan would cost on the order of $260 million in incentives alone, apart from administrative costs. The decline in the birth rate would be slightly over a fourth, perhaps a third—roughly equivalent to $35 to $40 per prevented birth (61).

Simon proposes an incentive of half the per capita income "each year to each fertile woman who does not get pregnant" (23). Here a special problem arises. In a typical developing population of 1000, about 25 to 30 percent of the married women of reproductive age give birth each year: a population of 1000 means from 145 to 165 such women, and a birth rate of, say, 40. Thus, the incentives paid to about three-fourths of the married women of reproductive age would have no effect on the birth rate, since these women would not be having a child that year in any case; thus the cost could be three to four times the amount "needed" for a desired result. Even if the incentive were fully effective and really did prevent a birth, a cut of ten points in the Indian birth rate would cost on the order of $250 million (or 5 million prevented births at $50 each). The cost would be substantially larger if the women (including the nonfecund or the semi-fecund) who would not have had a child that year in any case, could not be screened out effectively.

But these and other possibilities are only speculations: to date we simply do not know whether incentives will lower a birth rate, or, rather, we do not know how large the incentives would have to be in order to do so. These illustrations show only that an incentive program could be expensive. In any case, incentive systems would require a good amount of supervision and record-keeping; and, presumably, the higher the incentive (and hence the greater the chance of impact), the greater the risk of false reporting and the greater the need of supervision—which is not only expensive but difficult administratively.

Moral, ethical, and philosophical acceptability. Next, is the proposal not only politically acceptable but considered right and proper—by the target population, government officials, professional or intellectual elites, and the outside agencies committed to aid in its administration?

Coale states (3,62), "One reason the policy of seeking to make voluntary fertility universal is appealing—whether adequate or not—is that it is a natural extension of traditional democratic values: of providing each individual with the information he needs to make wise choices, and allowing the greatest freedom for each to work out his own destiny. The underlying rationale is that if every individual knowledgeably pursues his self-interest, the social interest will best be served." But what if "stressing the right of parents to have the number of children they want . . . evades the basic question of population policy, which is how to give societies the number of children they need?" (6). The issue rests at the center of political philosophy: how best to reconcile individual and collective interests.

Today, most observers would acknowledge that having a child is theoretically a free choice of the individual couple. However, for many couples, particularly among the poor of the world, the choice is not effectively free in the sense that the individual couple does not have the information, services, and supplies needed to implement a free wish in this regard. Such couples are restrained by ignorance, not only of contraceptive practice but of the consequences of high fertility for themselves, their children, and their country; they are restrained by religious doctrine, even though they may not accept the doctrine; they are restrained legally, as in the case of people who would choose abortion if that course were open to them; they are restrained culturally, as in the case of women subject to a tradition that reserves for them only the childbearing and childrearing roles. Hence effective freedom of choice in the matter of childbearing is by no means realized in the world today, as recent policy statements have remarked (63).

To what extent should a society be willing to compromise its ethical standards for the sake of solving a great social problem? Suppose a program for population control resulted in many more abortions in a society where abortion is morally repugnant and where, moreover, abortion by acceptable medical standards is widely unattainable; how much fertility decline would be "worth" the result? What of infanticide under the same conditions? How many innocent or unknowing men may be vasectomized for a fee (for themselves or for others who obtained their consent) before the practice calls for a moral restraint? How large an increase in the regulatory bureaucracy, or in systematic corruption through incentives, or in differential effect by social class to the disadvantage of the poor (64) is worth how much decrease in the birth rate? How much association of childbearing with monetary incentive is warranted before "bribing people not to have children" becomes contaminating, with adverse long-run effects on parental responsibility (65)? How much "immorality," locally defined as extramarital sex, outweighs the benefits of contraceptive practice (assuming that there is an association)? How much withholding of food aid is ethical, judged against degree of fertility decline? If it were possible to legislate a later age at marriage, would it be right to do so against the will of young women, in a society in which they have nothing else to do? In countries, like our own, where urbanization is a serious population problem, is it right to tell people *where* to live, or to impose heavy economic constraints that in effect "force" the desired migration? Is it right to withdraw educational benefits from children in "too large" families? Such withdrawal would not only be repressive from the standpoint of free education but in the long run would be unfortunate from the standpoint of fertility control. In the balance—and this is a question of great but neglected importance—what weight should be given the opportunities of future generations as against the ignorance, the prejudices, or the preferences of the present one?

Guidance on such ethical questions is needed. For further consideration, these propositions are put forward. (i) "An ideal policy would permit a maximum of individual freedom and diversity. It would not prescribe a precise number of children for each category of married couple, nor lay down a universal norm to which all couples should conform" (3). (ii) "An ideal program designed to affect the number of children people want would help promote other goals that are worth supporting on their own merits, or at least not conflict with such goals" (3). (iii) An ideal program would not burden the innocent in an attempt to penalize the guilty—for example, would not burden the *N*th child by denying him a free education simply because he *was* the *N*th child of irresponsible parents. (iv) An ideal program would not weigh heavily upon the already disadvantaged—for example, by withdrawing maternal or medical benefits or free education from large families, policies that would tend to further deprive the poor. (v) An ideal program would be comprehensible to those directly affected and hence subject to their response. (vi) An ideal program would respect present values concerning family and children, values which some people may not be willing to bargain away in a cost-benefit analysis. (vii) An ideal program would not rest upon the designation of population control as the final value justifying all others; "preoccupation with population growth should not serve to justify measures more dangerous or of higher social cost than population growth itself" (3).

Presumed effectiveness. If proposals are scientifically ready to be implemented, politically and morally acceptable, and administratively and financially feasible, to what extent will they actually work in bringing population growth under control? That is the final question.

To begin with, the compulsory measures would probably be quite effective in lowering fertility. Inevitably in such schemes, strongly motivated people are ingenious enough to find ways "to beat the system"; if such people were numerous enough the system could not be enforced except under conditions of severe political repression (66). Otherwise, if the scheme was workable, compulsion could have its effect.

What about the proposals for the extension of voluntary contraception? Institutionalizing maternal care in the rural areas, with family planning attached, does promise to be effective within, say, 5 to 10 years, particularly in its potential for reaching younger women and women of lower parity. The International Postpartum Program did have that effect in the urban areas (67), and presumably the impact would extend to the rural areas, though probably not to the same degree because of the somewhat greater sophistication and modernization of the cities.

A liberalized abortion system—again, if workable—could also be effective in preventing unwanted births, but it would probably have to be associated with a contraceptive effort; otherwise there might be too many abortions for the system, as well as for the individual woman (who might need three a year to remain without issue).

Free abortion in cases where contraception had failed would probably make for a decline in fertility, but how large a one would depend upon the quality of the contraceptive program. With modern contraception (the IUD and the pill) the failure rates are quite small, but women who only marginally tolerate these two methods could fall back on abortion. Free abortion has certainly lowered fertility in Japan and in certain countries of eastern Europe (68) and, where medically feasible, would do so elsewhere as well; as a colleague observes, in this field one should not underestimate the attraction of a certainty as compared to a probability.

The large question of the impact of the various incentive and benefit or liability plans (D and E) simply cannot be answered: we have too little experience to know much about the conditions under which financial factors will affect childbearing to any substantial degree. Perhaps everyone has his price for everything; if so, we do not know what would have to be paid, directly or indirectly, to make people decide not to bear children.

Such as it is, the evidence from the pro-natalist side on the effectiveness of incentives is not encouraging. All the countries of Europe have family allowance programs of one kind or another (69), most of them legislated in the 1930s and 1940s to raise the birth rate; collectively Europe has the lowest birth rate of any continent. The consensus among demographers appears to be that such programs cannot be shown to have effected an upward trend in the birth rate where tried.

As in the case of abortion for illegitimate pregnancies, several of the benefit or liability proposals would affect only a trivial fraction of people in much of the developing world. However, because the impact of incentive and benefit or liability plans is uncertain and may become important, we need to become better informed on the possibilities and limitations, and this information can come only from experimentation under realistic circumstances and at realistic levels of payment.

A higher age at marriage and a greater participation of women in the labor force are generally credited with effecting fertility declines. In a recent Indian conference on raising the age at marriage, the specialists seemed to differ only on the magnitude of the fertility decline that would result: a decline of 30 percent in the birth rate in a generation of 28 years if the minimum age of the woman at marriage were raised to 20 (70), or a decline of not more than 15 percent in 10 years (71). I say "seemed to differ" since these figures are not necessarily incompatible. In either case, the decline is a valuable one. But an increase in the age at marriage is not easy to achieve, and that must come before the fertility effect.

Similarly, an increase in the proportion of working women would have its demographic effect, but could probably come about only in conjunction with other broad social trends like education and industrialization, which themselves would powerfully affect fertility, just as a decline in fertility would assist importantly in bringing these trends about (72). Both compulsory education and restrictions on child labor would lower the economic value of children, hence tend to produce a decline in fertility. The question is, how are they to be brought about?

Finally, whether or not research would affect fertility trends depends of course upon its nature and outcome. Most observers believe that, under the typical conditions of the developing society, any improvement in contraceptive technology would lead toward the realization of present fertility goals and might help turn the spiral down. Indeed, several observers believe that this is the single most important desideratum, over the short run. Easy means of determining sex should have some effect upon the "need for sons" and thus cut family size to some extent. Research on the social-economic side would probably have to take effect through programs of the kinds discussed above.

The picture is not particularly encouraging. The measures that would work to sharply cut fertility are politically and morally unacceptable to the societies in question (as with coercion), and in any case unavailable; or they are difficult of attainment in any foreseeable future, as in the case of broad social trends or a shift in age at marriage. The measures that might possibly be tried in some settings, like some version of incentives or benefit or liability plans, give uncertain promise of results at the probable level of operation. Legalization of abortion, where the needed medical facilities are available, would almost certainly have a measurable effect, but acceptability is problematic.

Conclusion

This review leaves us with some conclusions concerning proposals that go beyond family planning.

1) There is no easy way to achieve population control. If this review has indicated nothing else, it has shown how many obstacles stand in the way of a solution to the population problem. Table 4.1 shows, by way of recapitulation, how the various proposals seem to fit the several criteria (73). That is only one observer's judgment of the present situation, but, whatever appraisal is made of specific items, it would appear that the overall picture is mixed.

2) Family-planning programs do not compare unfavorably with other specific proposals, especially when one considers that any *actual* operating program is at a disadvantage when compared with any competitive *ideal* policy. Indeed, on this showing, if family-planning programs did not exist, they would have to be invented; it appears that they would be among the first proposals to be made and the first programs to be tried, given their generally acceptable characteristics.

TABLE 4.1. Illustrative appraisal of proposals, by criteria

Proposal	Scientific readiness	Political viability	Administrative feasibility	Economic capability	Ethical acceptability	Presumed effectiveness
A. Extension of voluntary fertility control	High	High on maternal care, moderate-to-low on abortion	Uncertain in near future	Maternal care too costly for local budget, abortion feasible	High for maternal care, low for abortion	Moderately high
B. Establishment of involuntary fertility control	Low	Low	Low	High	Low	High
C. Intensified educational campaigns	High	Moderate-to-high	High	Probably high	Generally high	Moderate
D. Incentive programs	High	Moderately low	Low	Low-to-moderate	Low-to-high	Uncertain
E. Tax and welfare benefits and penalties	High	Moderately low	Low	Low-to-moderate	Low-to-moderate	Uncertain
F. Shifts in social and economic institutions	High	Generally high, but low on some specifics	Low	Generally low	Generally high, but uneven	High, over long run
G. Political channels and organizations	High	Low	Low	Moderate	Moderately low	Uncertain
H. Augmented research efforts	Moderate	High	Moderate-to-high	High	High	Uncertain
Family-planning programs	Generally high, but could use improved technology	Moderate-to-high	Moderate-to-high	High	Generally high, but uneven, on religious grounds	Moderately high

In fact, when such proposals are made, it turns out that many of them call for *more* family planning, not less, but in a somewhat different form. In the present case, at least a third of the proposals listed above put forward, in effect, simply another approach to family planning, often accepting the existing motivation as to family size. In any case, family-planning programs are established, have some momentum, and, importantly, would be useful as the direct instrument through which other proposals would take effect. So, as a major critic (74) acknowledges (6), "there is no reason to abandon family-planning programs."

What is needed is the energetic and full implementation of present experience. Much more could be done on the informational side, on encouraging commercial distribution of contraceptives, on the use of paramedical personnel, on logistics and supply, on the training and supervision of field workers, on approaches to special groups of individuals, ranging from women after childbirth to young men drafted into the armed forces. If workers in this field did well what they know how to do, that in itself would in all likelihood make a measurable difference, competitive in magnitude with the probable effects of other specific proposals—not to mention the further impetus of an improved contraceptive technology.

3) Most of the proposed ideas are not new; they have been around for some time. So, if they are not being tried, it is not because they have not been known but because they have not been accepted—presumably, for reasons like those discussed above. In India, for example, several of the social measures being proposed have been, it would seem, under almost constant review by one or another committee for the past 10 to 15 years. So it is not correct to imply that it is only new ideas that are needed; the ideas are there, but their political, economic, or administrative feasibility are problematic.

4) All of the proposers are dissatisfied to some degree with present family-planning efforts, but that does not mean that they agree with one another's schemes for doing better. Thus, Ohlin believes that "the demographic significance of such measures [maternity benefits and tax deductions for children] would be limited" (34). Ketchel eloquently opposes several "possible alternatives to fertility control agents" (9). Meier argues against the tax on children on both humanitarian and political grounds (16). The U.N. Advisory Mission to India comments (53, p. 87), "it is realised that no major demographic effects can be expected from measures of this kind [maternity benefits], particularly as only a small proportion of families are covered . . . but they could contribute, together with the family planning programme, to a general change in the social climate relating to childbearing." Earlier, in supporting a family-planning effort in India, Davis noted that "the reaction to the Sarda Act [the Child Marriage Restraint Act of 1929] prohibiting female marriage [below age 14] shows the difficulty of trying to regulate the age of marriage by direct legislation" (75). Myrdal warns against cash payments to parents in this connection and supports social awards in kind to the children (76). Kirk believes that "it might prove to be the height of folly to undermine the existing family structure, which continues to be a crucial institution for stability and socialization in an increasingly mobile and revolutionary society" (77). Finally, Ehrlich is contemptuous of the professors whose "ideas of 'action' is to form a committee or to urge 'more research.' Both courses are actually substitutes for action" (7, p. 191).

5) In a rough way, there appears to be a progression in national efforts to deal with the problem of population control. The first step is the theoretical recognition that population growth may have something to do with the prospects for economic development. Then, typically, comes an expert mission from abroad to make a survey and report to the government, as has occurred in India, Pakistan, South Korea, Turkey, Iran, Tunisia, Morocco, and Kenya, among others. The first action program is in family planning, and most of the efforts are still at that level. Beyond that, it apparently takes (i) some degree of discouragement about progress combined with (ii) some heightened awareness of the seriousness of the problem to move the effort forward. To date, those conditions have been most prominently present in India—and that is the country that has gone farthest in the use of incentives and in at least consideration of further steps along the lines mentioned above.

6) Proposals need to be specific—proposals both for action and for further research. It is perhaps too much to ask advocates to spell out all the administrative details of the way their plan is to operate in the face of obstacles and difficulties, or even to spell out how it is to get permission to operate; the

situations, settings, opportunities, and personalities are too diverse for that. But it does seem proper to ask for the fullest possible specification of actual plans, under realistic conditions, in order to test out their feasibility and likely effectiveness. Similarly, advocates of further research ought to spell out not only what would be studied, and how, but also how the results might be applied in action programs to affect fertility. Social research is not always readily translated into action, especially into administrative action; and the thrust of research is toward refinement, subtlety, precision, and qualification, whereas the administrator must act in the large. Short of such specification, the field remains confronted with potentially good ideas, such as "raise the age at marriage" or "use incentives" or "substitute pension systems for male children," without being able to move very far toward implementation.

7) Just as there is no easy way, there is no single way. Since population control will at best be difficult, it follows that every acceptable step that promises some measure of impact should be taken. The most likely prospect is that population control, to the degree it is realized, will be the result of a combination of efforts—economic, legal, social, medical—each of which has some effect but not an immediately overwhelming one (78). Accordingly, it is incumbent upon workers in the professional fields concerned to look hard at various approaches, including family planning itself, in order to screen out what is potentially useful for application. In doing so, it may be the path of wisdom to move with the "natural" progression. Some important proposals seem reasonably likely of adoption—institutionalization of maternal care, population study in the schools, the TV satellite system for disseminating information, a better contraceptive technology, perhaps even liberalization of abortion laws in some settings—and we need to know not only how effective such efforts will be but, beyond them, how large a money incentive would have to be to effect a given amount of fertility control and how effective those indirect social measures are that are morally acceptable and capable of realization. It may be that some of these measures would be both feasible and effective—many observers 15 years ago thought that family-planning programs were neither—and a genuine effort needs to be made. The "heavy" measures—involuntary measures and political pressures—may be put aside for the time being, if not forever.

8) In the last analysis, what will be scientifically available, politically acceptable, administratively feasible, economically justifiable, and morally tolerated depends upon people's perceptions of consequences. If "the population problem" is considered relatively unimportant or only moderately important, that judgment will not support much investment of effort. If it is considered urgent, much more can and will be done. The fact is that, despite the large forward strides taken in international recognition of the problem in the 1960's, there still does not exist an informed, firm, and constant conviction in high circles that this is a matter with truly great implications for human welfare (79). Such convictions must be based on sound knowledge. Here it would appear that the demographers and economists have not sufficiently made their case to the world elite—or that, if made, the case has not sufficiently commanded their attention and support. Population pressures are not sharply visible on a day-to-day or even year-to-year basis, nor, short of major famine, do they show themselves in dramatic events. Moreover, the warnings of demographers are often dismissed, albeit unfairly and wrongly, on the basis of past forecasts that were not borne out (80). After all, only a generation ago we were being warned about a decline in population in the West. Asking government leaders to take steps toward population control is asking them to take very substantial steps indeed—substantial for their people as well as for their own political careers—hence the case must be virtually incontrovertible. Accordingly, the scientific base must be carefully prepared (and perhaps with some sense of humility about the ease of predicting or urging great events, for the record is not without blemishes). Greater measures to meet the problem—measures which exclude social repression and needless limitation of human freedom—must rely on heightened awareness of what is at stake, on the part of leaders and masses alike.

What is beyond family planning? Even if most of the specific plans are not particularly new, that in itself does not mean that they are to be disregarded. The questions are: Which plans can be effected, given such criteria? How can they be implemented? What will be the outcome?

This article is an effort to promote the discourse across the professional fields concerned with this important issue. Given the recent stress on family-planning programs as the "means of choice" in dealing with the problem, it is natural and desirable that counterpositions be put forward and reviewed. But that does not in itself settle the critical questions. What can we do now to advance the matter? Beyond family planning, what?

References and Notes

1. See, for example, K. Davis, *Science* **158**, 730 (1967); R.G. Potter, R. Freedman, L.P. Chow, *ibid.* 160, 848 (1968); F.W. Notestein, "Population growth and its control," paper presented before the American Assembly on World Hunger, Fall 1968.
2. See, for example, the section on "Goals" in K. Davis, *Science* **158**, 730 (1967).
3. A.J. Coale, "Should the United States start a campaign for fewer births?", presidential address presented before the Population Association of America, 1968.
4. For current targets of some national family-planning programs, see B. Berelson, "National family planning programs: Where we stand," paper presented at the University of Michigan Sesquicentennial Celebration, November 1967; the paper concludes: "By and large, developing countries are now aiming at the birth rates of Western Europe 75 years ago or the United States 50 years ago."
5. H.C. Taylor, Jr., and B. Berelson, *Amer. J. Obstet. Gynecol.* **100**, 885 (1968).
6. K. Davis, *Science* 158, 730 (1967).
7. P.R. Ehrlich, *The Population Bomb* (Ballantine, New York, 1968).
8. S. Chandrasekhar, *Population Rev.* **10**, 17 (1966).
9. M.M. Ketchel, *Perspect. Biol. Med.* **11**, 687 (1968); see also Ketchel's article in *Med. World News* (18 Oct. 1968), p. 66.
10. Ehrlich appears to dismiss the scheme as unworkable (7, p. 136), though two pages later he advocates "ample funds" to "promote intensive investigation of new techniques of birth control, possibly leading to the development of mass sterilizing agents such as were discussed above."
11. K.E. Boulding, *The Meaning of the Twentieth Century: The Great Transition* (Harper & Row, New York, 1964), pp. 135–36.
12. W.B. Shockley, in a lecture delivered at McMaster University, Hamilton, Ontario, December 1967.
13. S. Chandrasekhar, as reported in *The New York Times*, 24 July 1967. Just as the present article was being completed, Chandrasekhar proposed (*ibid.*, 21 Oct. 1968) "that every married couple in India deny themselves sexual intercourse for a year. . . . Abstinence for a year would do enormous good to the individual and the country." The reader may wish to consider this the 30th proposal and test it against the criteria that follow.
14. S. Wayland, in *Family Planning and Population Programs*, B. Berelson, R.K. Anderson, O. Harkavy, J. Maier, W.P. Mauldin, S.J. Segal, Eds. (Univ. of Chicago Press, Chicago, 1966), pp. 353–62; ______, in "Family Planning Programs: Administration, Education, Evaluation," J. Ross and J. Friesen, Eds., in preparation; "Teaching Population Dynamics: An Instructional Unit for Secondary School Students" (Columbia University, New York, 1965); "Critical Stages in Reproduction: Instruction Materials in General Science and Biology" (Columbia University, New York, 1965). The two last-named publications are pamphlets prepared under Wayland's direction at Teachers College.
15. P. Visaria, *Economic Weekly* (8 Aug. 1964), p. 1343.
16. R.L. Meier and G. Meier, "New Directions: A Population Policy for the Future," unpublished manuscript.
17. *Preparatory Study of a Pilot Project in the Use of Satellite Communication for National Development Purposes in India* (UNESCO Expert Mission, 1968).
18. W. Schramm and L. Nelson, *Communication Satellite for Education and Development–The Case of India* (Stanford Research Institute, Stanford, Calif., 1968), pp. 63–66.
19. S. Chandrasekhar, as reported in *The New York Times*, 19 July 1967.
20. E. Pohlman (Central Family Planning Institute, India), "Incentives for 'Non-Maternity' Cannot 'Compete' with Incentives for Vasectomy," unpublished manuscript.
21. T.J. Samuel, *J. Family Welfare* **13**, 11 (1966).
22. J. Simon, "Money Incentives to Reduce Birth Rates in Low-Income Countries: A Proposal to Determine the Effect Experimentally," unpublished manuscript; "The Role of Bonuses and Persuasive Propaganda in the Reduction of Birth Rates," unpublished manuscript.
23. ______, "Family Planning Prospects in Less-Developed Countries, and a Cost-Benefit Analysis of Various Alternatives," unpublished manuscript.
24. S. Enke, *Population Rev.* **4**, 47 (1960).
25. M. Young, "The Behavioral Sciences and Family Planning Programs: Report on a Conference,"

Studies in Family Planning, No. 23 (1967), p. 10.
26. D. Bhatia, "Government of India Small Family Norm Committee Questionnaire," *Indian J. Med. Educ.* **6**, 189 (1967). As the title indicates, this is not a proposal but a questionnaire soliciting opinions on various ideas put forward to promote "the small family norm."
27. S. Enke, "The Gains to India from Population Control," *Rev. Econ. Statist.* **42**, 179, 180 (1960).
27a. J.W. Leasure, *Milbank Mem. Fund Quart.* **45**, 417 (1967).
28. J.J. Spengler, "Agricultural development is not enough," paper presented before the Conference on World Population Problems, Indiana University, May 1967.
29. M.C. Balfour, "A Scheme for Rewarding Successful Family Planners," *Population Council Mem.* (1962).
30. W.P. Mauldin, "Prevention of Illegitimate Births: A Bonus Scheme," *Population Council Mem.* (1967).
31. R.M. Titmuss and B. Abel-Smith, *Social Policies and Population Growth in Mauritius* (Methuen, London, 1960).
32. A.S. David, *National Development, Population and Family Planning in Nepal* (1968), pp. 53–54.
33. J. Fawcett, personal communication.
34. G. Ohlin, *Population Control and Economic Development* (Development Centre of the Organisation for Economic Co-operation and Development, New York, 1967), p. 104.
35. W.P. Davison, personal communication. Davison suggests a good pension (perhaps $400 a year) for men aged 60, married for at least 20 years, with no sons.
36. K. Davis, personal communication.
37. B. Berelson and A. Etzioni, brief formulations, 1962 and 1967, respectively.
38. P.M. Hauser, in "The Behavioral Sciences and Family Planning Programs: Report on a Conference," *Studies in Family Planning*, No. 23 (1967), p. 9.
39. J. Blake, in *Public Health and Population Change: Current Research Issues*, M.C. Sheps and J.C. Ridley, Eds. (Univ. of Pittsburgh Press, Pittsburgh, 1965), p. 62.
40. For the initial formulation of the proposal, see R.L. Meier, *Modern Science and the Human Fertility Problem* (Wiley, New York, 1959), chap. 7.
41. P.M. Hauser, *Demography* **4**, 412 (1967).
42. "Family Planning and the Status of Women: Interim Report of the Secretary-General" (United Nations Economic and Social Council, Commission on the Status of Women, New York, 1968), especially p. 17 ff.
43. R. Revelle, quoted by M. Viorst, *Horizon* (summer 1968), p. 35; D.M. Heer and D.O. Smith, "Mortality level and desired family size," paper presented before the Population Association of America, April 1967.
44. Ehrlich makes the same point in *New Scientist* (14 Dec. 1967, p. 655: "Refuse all foreign aid to any country with an increasing population which we believe is not making a maximum effort to limit its population.... The United States should use its power and prestige to bring extreme diplomatic and/or economic pressure on any country or organization (the Roman Catholic Church?) impeding a solution to the world's most pressing problem."
45. In an earlier article Ehrlich calls for a "Federal Population Commission with a large budget for propaganda," presumably limited to the United States.
46. S. Chandrasekhar, in *Asia's Population Problems*, S. Chandrasekhar, Ed. (Allen & Unwin, New York, 1967), p. 96; Chandrasekhar cites a suggestion made in 1961 by Julian Huxley.
47. S. Polgar, in "The Behavioral Sciences and Family Planning Programs: Report on a Conference," *Studies in Family Planning*, No. 23 (1967), p. 10.
48. *The Growth of World Population* (National Academy of Sciences, Committee on Science and Public Policy, Washington, D.C., 1963), pp. 5, 28–36. This recommendation has of course been made on several occasions by several people. For an imaginative account of the impact of biological developments, see P.C. Berry, appendix to *The Next Thirty-Four Years: A Context for Speculation* (Hudson Institute, Croton-on-Hudson, New York, 1966).
49. See, for example, S.J. Segal, "Biological aspects of fertility regulation," paper presented at the University of Michigan Sesquicentennial Celebration, November 1967.
50. It is worth noting that such expectations are not particularly reliable. For example, in 1952–53 a Working Group on Fertility Control was organized by the Conservation Foundation to review the most promising "leads to physiologic control of fertility," based on a survey conducted by Paul S. Henshaw and Kingsley Davis. This group did identify a "lead" that became the oral contraceptive (then already under investigation) but did not mention the intrauterine device. It was searching specifically for better ways to control fertility because of the population problem in the developing world, and considered the contraceptive approach essential to that end: "It thus appears imperative that an attempt be made to bring down fertility in over-

populated regions without waiting for a remote, hoped-for transformation of the entire society. . . . It seems plausible that acceptable birth control techniques might be found, and that the application of science to developing such techniques for peasant regions might yield revolutionary results" [*The Physiological Approach to Fertility Control, Report of the Working Group on Fertility Control* (Conservation Foundation, New York, 1953)].

51. A.S. Parkes, *New Scientist* **35**, 186 (1967).
52. *The New York Times* (17 Nov. 1967). The then Minister had earlier suggested a substantial bonus (100 rupees) for vasectomy, the funds to be taken from U.S. counterpart funds, "but both Governments are extremely sensitive in this area. Yet in a problem this crucial perhaps we need more action and less sensitivity" [S. Chandrasekhar (46)].
53. *Report on the Family Planning Programme in India* (United Nations Advisory Mission, New York, 1966).
54. *Implications of Raising the Female Age at Marriage in India* (Demographic Training and Research Centre, Chembur, India, 1968), p. 109; *Centre Calling* (May 1968), p. 4.
55. *Planned Parenthood* (Mar. 1968), p. 3.
56. *Ibid.* (Apr. 1968), p. 2.
57. For a review of this development see R. Symonds and M. Carder, *International Organisations and Population Control (1947–67)* (Institute of Development Studies, Univ. of Sussex, Brighton, England, 1968).
58. At present, population materials are being included in school programs in Pakistan, Iran, Taiwan, and elsewhere.
59. See, for example, Balfour (29), Mauldin (30), and Pohlman (20) and, for the economic analysis, Enke (27) and Simon (22).
60. For the negative answer, see Enke (27) and Simon (22). Data are from family-planning budgets and national development budgets contained in 5-year development plans.
61. E. Pohlman, "Incentives in birth planning," in preparation.
62. Coale, however, does point out that "it is clearly fallacious to accept as optimal a growth that continues until overcrowding makes additional births intolerably expensive."
63. See, for example, the World Leaders' Statement [*Studies in Family Planning*, No. 26 (1968)] and the Resolution of the International Conference on Human Rights on "Human Rights Aspects of Family Planning," adopted 12 May 1968, reported in *Population Newsletter*, No. 2 (issued by the Population Division, United Nations) (1968), p. 21 ff. Incidentally, the issue of population policy was apparently a live one in classical times, and resolved by the great philosophers in ways not fully consonant with modern views. Plato, in the *Republic* (Modern Library edition, pp. 412, 414), says, "the number of weddings is a matter which must be left to the discretion of the rulers, whose aim will be to preserve the average of population and to prevent the State from becoming either too large or too small"– to which end certain marriages have "strict orders to prevent any embryo which may come into being from seeing the light; and if any force a way to the birth, the parents must understand that the offspring of such a union cannot be maintained, and arrange accordingly." Aristotle, in *Politics* (Modern Library edition, p. 316) says, "on the ground of an excess in the number of children, if the established customs of the state forbid this (for in our state population has a limit), no child is to be exposed, but when couples have children in excess, let abortion be procured before sense and life have begun. . . ."
64. After noting that economic constraints have not been adopted in South Asia, though often proposed, Gunnar Myrdal continues: "The reason is not difficult to understand. Since having many children is a main cause of poverty, such measures would penalize the relatively poor and subsidize the relatively well off. Such a result would not only violate rules of equity but would be detrimental to the health of the poor families, and so of the growing generation" [*Asian Drama: An Inquiry into the Poverty of Nations* (Pantheon, New York, 1968), vol. 2, pp. 1502–03].
65. F.W. Notestein, in *Family Planning and Population Programs*, Berelson *et al.*, Eds. (Univ. of Chicago Press, Chicago, 1966), pp. 828–29: "There is a real danger that sanctions, for example through taxation, would affect adversely the welfare of the children. There is also danger than incentives through bonuses will put the whole matter of family planning in a grossly commercial light. It is quite possible that to poor and harassed people financial inducements will amount to coercion and not to an enlargement of their freedom of choice. Family planning must be, and must seem to be, an extension of personal and familial freedom of choice and thereby an enrichment of life, not coercion toward its restriction."
66. In this connection see the novel by A. Burgess, *The Wanting Seed* (Ballantine, New York, 1963). At the same time, Myrdal, a long-time observer of social affairs, remarks that "the South Asian countries . . . can, to begin with, have no other principle than that of voluntary parenthood. . . . State direction by compulsion in these personal matters

is not effective . . . " [G. Myrdal, *Asian Drama: An Inquiry into the Poverty of Nations* (Pantheon, New York, 1968), p. 1501].

67. G.I. Zatuchni, "International Postpartum Family Planning Program: Report on the First Year," *Studies in Family Planning*, No. 22 (1967), p. 14 ff.
68. For example, the repeal of the free abortion law in Rumania resulted in an increase in the birth rate from 14 in the third quarter of 1966 to 38 in the third quarter of 1967. For an early report, see R. Pressat, *Population* **22**, 1116 (1967).
69. See *Social Security Programs Throughout the World, 1964* (U.S. Department of Health, Education, and Welfare, Washington, D.C., 1964).
70. S.N. Agarwala in *Implications of Raising the Female Age at Marriage in India* (Demographic Training and Research Centre, Chembur, India, 1968), p. 21.
71. V.C. Chidambaram, *ibid.*, p. 47.
72. Actually, recent research is calling into question some of the received wisdom on the prior need of such broad institutional factors for fertility decline. If further study supports the new findings, that could have important implications for present strategy in the developing countries. See A.J. Coale, in *Proc. U.N. World Population Conf.* (1965), vol. 2, pp. 205–09, and ______, "The decline of fertility in Europe from the French Revolution to World War II," paper presented at the University of Michigan Sesquicentennial Celebration, 1967.
73. As the roughest sort of summary of Table 4.1, if one assigns values from 5 for "high" to 1 for "low," the various proposals rank as follows: family-planning programs, 25; intensified educational campaigns, 25; augmented research efforts, 24; extension of voluntary fertility control, 20; shifts in social and economic institutions, 20; incentive programs, 14; tax and welfare benefits and penalties, 14; political channels and organizations, 14; establishment of involuntary fertility control, 14.
74. Davis was a strong advocate of family planning in India, and quite optimistic about its prospects even in the pre-IUD or pre-pill era. See K. Davis, in *The Interrelations of Demographic, Economic, and Social Problems in Selected Underdeveloped Areas* (Milbank Memorial Fund, New York, 1954). Davis concludes (pp. 87–88): "Although India is already well-launched in the rapid-growth phase of the demographic transition, there is no inherent reason why she should long continue in this phase. She need not necessarily wait patiently while the forces of urbanization, class mobility, and industrial development gradually build up to the point where parents are forced to limit their offspring on their own initiative and without help, perhaps even in the face of official opposition. . . . Realistically appraising her situation, India has a chance to be the first country to achieve a major revolution in human life—the planned diffusion of fertility control in a peasant population prior to, and for the benefit of, the urban-industrial transition."
75. K. Davis, in *The Interrelations of Demographic, Economic, and Social Problems in Selected Underdeveloped Areas* (Milbank Memorial Fund, New York, 1954), p. 86.
76. G. Myrdal, *Asian Drama: An Inquiry into the Poverty of Nations* (Pantheon, New York, 1968), p. 1503.
77. D. Kirk, "Population research in relation to population policy and national family planning programs," paper presented before the American Sociological Association, August 1968.
78. It begins to appear that the prospects for fertility control may be improving over the decades. Kirk, after reviewing several factors that "favor a much more rapid [demographic] transition than occurred in the West" – changed climate of opinion, religious doctrine, decline of infant mortality, modernization, fertility differentials, grass-roots concern, and improved contraceptive technology—shows, in a remarkable tabulation, that the later a country began the reduction of its birth rate from 35 to 20 births per thousand, the shorter the time it took to achieve this reduction: from 73 years (average) for the period 1831–60, for example, to 21 years after 1951; the trend has been consistently downward for over a century [D. Kirk, "Natality in the developing countries: recent trends and prospects," paper presented at the University of Michigan Sesquicentennial Celebration, 1967].
79. Nor, often, does such a conviction exist among the general public. For example, in midsummer of 1968 a national sample of adults was asked in a Gallup poll, "What do you think is the most important problem facing this country today?" Less than 1 percent mentioned population growth (Gallup release, 3 Aug. 1968, and personal communication).
80. For an old but enlightening review, see H. Dorn, *J. Amer. Statist. Assoc.* 45, 311 (1950).

5

Romania's 1966 Anti-Abortion Decree: The Demographic Experience of the First Decade*

During the first ten post-war years the Romanian crude birth rate fluctuated around the mid-20s, averaged 24.9, and at the end of the period stood at 24.2 in 1956.[1] In September 1957 following the Soviet lead, a governmental decree made abortion on request available in Romania. From that point the crude birth rate declined continuously to 14.3 in 1966. At the same time the number of abortions per 100 live births rose steadily from 30 in 1958 to 408 in 1965,[2] or about 80 percent of all conceptions. By this time, abortion had become the major means of fertility control in Romania.

At that time, the Romanian government decided to reverse the downward trend in the birth rate. As later reported by Muresan and Copil, the targets were 'to stimulate the natality to reach 18–19 per 1,000, a rate corresponding to the economic progress of the population'; and to help realize the 'national socio-economic plan of development (which) desires a population of about 24–25 million inhabitants by 1990 . . .',[3] extended in Trebici's still later citation of the Programme of the Romanian Communist Party to 'at least 25 million' by 1900 and 'around 30 million' by 2000.[4]

Since abortion was then the main instrument of fertility control, it became the centrepiece of the new pro-natalist policy. In October 1966, another decree suddenly made abortion legally available only under certain limited conditions: danger to life, risk of deformity of the foetus, rape, mother's age over 45, and specified life situations.[5] The crude birth rate showed an historically dramatic,

---

Reprinted with permission from *Population Studies* 1979; 33(2):209–220, The Population Investigation Committee, London School of Economics, London, England.

*I am indebted to Ronald Freedman for encouraging me in this venture, and to him, Parker Mauldin, and Paul Demeny for their role as demographic mentors, in this particular case and in general; and I am grateful to my colleagues Ellen Hofstatter and Richard Monteverde for data and calculations that went into this paper, and to several readers of the draft manuscript for their helpful suggestions, many of which are incorporated in this version.

[1] Unless noted otherwise, the main data for the East European countries, including the figures, are from *Post-War Demographic Trends in Europe and the Outlook Until the Year 2000, Economic Survey of Europe in 1974*, Part II, prepared by the Secretariat of the (UN) Economic Commission for Europe, 1975, Table V.1, pp. 78–79 and V.2, pp. 81–82. Those data are augmented from J. Bourgeois-Pichat, 'Baisse de la fécondité et descendance finale', *Population* (Nov.–Dec. 1976), p. 1047, and updated for the last few years from UN sources.

[2] C. Tietze and Marjorie Cooper Murstein, 'Induced Abortion: 1975 Factbook', *Reports on Population/Family Planning*, no. 14 (2nd edn) (December 1975), p. 22; and C. Tietze, 'Induced Abortion: 1977 Supplement', *ibid.* (December 1977), p. 5. Note in the explanation on p. 6 that the data on Romania 'include women admitted to hospitals for after-care or the treatment of complications of spontaneous and illegal abortions'. Prior to the 1966 decree, 'probably 90 per cent (of reported abortions) were legal terminations'.

[3] P. Muresan and I.M. Copil, 'Romania', in Bernard Berelson (ed.), *Population Policy in Developed Countries* (McGraw-Hill, 1974), pp. 367–368.

[4] V. Trebici, *Romania's Population and Demographic Trends* (Bucharest, 1976), pp. 134–135. Whether these designations of targets were contemporaneous with the decree, either publicly or privately within the governing circles, I have not been able to determine.

[5] The Decree itself, No. 770, can be found in the *International Digest*, 18, 4 (1967), pp. 822–837, complete with 14 pages of medical instructions implementing the

perhaps unique, increase to 27.4 in 1967 (actually, to 39 between the ninth and eleventh months following the decree); and from this point again began a decline to its 1976 figure of 19.5.

Given the high abortion level just prior to the 1966 decree, it is clear that Romanians then controlled their fertility largely in that favoured way. After that, according to Muresan and Copil, 'the usual mechanical methods are available.... Pills and other contraceptive devices (IUDs), although they are not forbidden legally, are used only on medical indication and under the supervision of a gynecologist.'[6] David adds that 'the importation of pills and IUDs was discontinued, as was official propaganda advocating their use.... IUDs and pills are imported clandestinely.... A month's supply (of pills) ... costs approximately 100 lei ($5.50)'.[7] In short, although legal, such other modern means of fertility control were officially discouraged and made difficult to obtain through administrative measures, so that the decree withdrawing legal abortion suddenly left a virtual vacuum of modern methods in the country. (Sterilization is rare throughout Eastern Europe.)

At about the same time, the government introduced other policy changes of a pro-natalist character-maternity leave, divorce restrictions, a 'childbirth compensation' for a third or later child, and a change in income tax related to number of dependants,[8] but similar provisions had existed in Romania (and, indeed, in several other countries) without the post-1966 effect on fertility observed there.

That effect is well known, well documented, and well accepted in demographic circles.[9] The sudden withdrawal of access to legalized induced abortion had a sharp upward effect upon the Romanian birth rate[10] —what Berent refers to as the 'upheaval caused by the change in the abortion law'.[11] The official figures fell from about four recorded abortions per live birth in 1965 to 0.3 in 1967, and then rose again to 0.9 to 1973 and 1976.[12] As a standard UN study put it, among Eastern European countries 'Romania is the only country which experienced a substantial increase in gross reproduction rate.... This increase is considered to be attributable to the reversion to anti-abortion legislation enacted in 1966 to encourage higher fertility.'[13] The increase itself immediately started to level off as other means of fertility control were found (presumably including illegal abortion), and

decree itself. See also Muresan and Copil, *loc cit.* in footnote 3, pp. 367-368, 383-384; H.P. David, *Family Planning and Abortion in the Socialist Countries of Central and Eastern Europe*, Population Council, 1970, pp. 142-160; and I. Ceterechi *et al.*, *Romanian Legislation on the Population Growth and Its Demographic Effects*, Law and Population Books Series No. 15 (Bucharest, 1975). For demographic rationale, see also H.P. David and N.H. Wright, 'Abortion Legislation: The Romanian Experience', *Studies in Family Planning*, 2, 10 (October 1971), pp. 206-207.

[6] Muresan and Copil, *loc. cit.* in footnote 3, pp. 367-368.

[7] David, *op. cit.* in footnote 5, p. 134.

[8] Muresan and Copil, *loc. cit.* in footnote 3, and David, *op. cit.* in footnote 5.

[9] Along with much related detail having to do with age- and parity-specific rates, total fertility rates, gross and net reproduction rates, nuptiality and divorce rates, maternal and child health effects, and maternal deaths attributed to abortion. See: M.S. Teitelbaum, 'Fertility Effects of the Abolition of Legal Abortion in Romania', *Population Studies*, 26, 3 (November 1972), pp. 405-417; N.H. Wright, 'Restricting Legal Abortion: Some Maternal and Child Health Effects in Romania', *American Journal of Obstetrics and Gynecology*, 121, 2 (15 January 1975), pp. 246-256; Tietze and Murstein, *op. cit.* in footnote 2, Fig. 11, p. 65; and Muresan and Copil, *loc. cit.* in footnote 3, *passim*.

[10] In a detailed analysis of the post-1955 situation in three neighbouring countries, McIntyre notes 'the oddity of the coincidence of the alleged decline in "desired family size" with the sudden availability of legal abortion' (R.J. McIntyre, 'The Fertility Response to Abortion Reform in Eastern Europe: Demographic and Economic Implications', *American Economist*, 16 (Fall, 1972), p. 61), and concludes 'that both the timing and the total number of births are changing in response to the legalization of abortion' *(ibid.)*. His discussant, with a few more years of the Romanian experience available, remarks: 'If one was attempting an experiment to determine the effects of abortion, the Romanian experience would surely resemble what an experimenter would set up. Four countries with comparable backgrounds, similar governments, and similar growth patterns all enact a law legalizing abortion. After nine years one country changes and makes abortion illegal.... The change in the discussed countries is mainly the results of changes in the abortion laws' (J.T. Lindley, 'Comment', p. 64).

[11] J. Berent, 'Fertility Trends and Policies in Eastern Europe in the 1970's', *Conference on Social, Economic and Health Consequences of Low Fertility* (1977), p. 1.

[12] Tietze, *op. cit.* in footnote 2, Table 2, p. 5, and from text on p. 6 of 380,000 reported abortions by the Romanian definition as against about 417,000 live births.

[13] *World Population Prospects as Assessed in 1973*, Population Studies, No. 60 (UN Department of Economic and Social Affairs, 1977), p. 74.

fertility began to return toward its 'natural' level, whether pre-1967, pre-1957 or some other value.

As regards the demographic importance of the policy change expressed in the abortion decree, when the issue is raised in connection with population policy, the consensus among demographers today appears to be that the sharp increase was only temporary, that the birth rate fell quickly as alternatives were found to the previous reliance on abortion, that the demographic impact would be transitory and insignificant, and that the occasion was proving once again that availability of fertility control means has little effect.

For example, at the time *Pravda* commented that:

> ... one can hardly approve of the prohibition of abortion as the experience of many countries, including the USSR, shows that such a measure has never, no matter where, led to any real or prolonged rise in the birth rate.[14]

In 1971, David and Wright concluded that:

> ... it seems unlikely that legal restrictions on abortion, coupled with more benevolent pro-natalist welfare provisions, will result in more than a short-term increase in the birth rate ... [15]

In his well-known article on the matter Teitelbaum notes:

> ... the clear and accelerating downward trend in the crude birth rate and total fertility since 1967. In part this represents an artificial decline, since 1967 must be considered a year of exceptionally high birth rates due to the temporary effects of the rapid transition from low fertility by means of abortion to moderate-to-high fertility without legal abortion. However, the continued declines in 1969 and 1970 suggest that Romanian women must be controlling their fertility with considerable effectiveness by means other than legal abortion.... Such sharp declines in fertility since 1968 suggest that the drastic fertility increases resulting from the 1966 legal shift may be transitory.[16]

And finally, in a forthcoming book on Israel's population policy, in arguing the ineffectiveness of a prohibition of abortion for Israeli fertility, Friedlander and Goldscheider conclude:

> Most importantly, the high level of fertility (in Romania) as reflected in the birth rate increase following the abortion restrictions was not sustained and a sharp decline of almost 50 per cent followed. While some slight gain in the number of births may have been achieved in the long run, ... to date, there is no evidence anywhere, the Romanian example included, demonstrating conclusively that a *sustained* increase in fertility has been achieved as a result of regulations restricting the performance of abortions[17] (their italics).

The purpose of this paper is to assess the matter after ten years' experience in order to obtain a clearer perspective on its demographic meaning: was this merely a minor blip on the fertility curve or did it have a longer-term demographic importance? It is difficult to know what 'real', 'prolonged', 'more than short-term', "transitory', and "sustained' are supposed to mean in precise quantities—by some definitions, all the quotations could turn out to be correct—but the general impression appears to be that the decree would have only a minor and temporary impact on fertility. What has actually been the demographic impact on the decree in its first ten years? How much, if anything, has it contributed to its targets?

The crude birth rates between 1957 and 1976 (latest available year) for Romania and the average of the five other countries classified as Eastern Europe in the *Economic Survey of Europe* (Bulgaria, Czechoslovakia, German Democratic Republic, Hungary, and Poland) are presented in Figure 5.1.[18] I use that region as a plausible base for comparison here, and the most appropriate among the three explored, the others being the three nearest countries of the five, and Romania itself preceding the decree;[19] and I regard the crude

[14] Cited in Wright, *loc. cit.* in footnote 9, p. 254.
[15] David and Wright, *loc. cit.* in footnote 5, p. 210.
[16] Teitelbaum, *loc. cit.* in footnote 9, p. 416.

[17] D. Friedlander and C. Goldscheider, *Israel's Population: Policy, Growth and Implications* (Columbia University Press, 1978), p. 199–199a (MS).
[18] The statistics for Figures 5.1 and 5.2 are given in Appendix 1.
[19] Three such approximations might reasonably be considered by way of comparison–those five countries, the three nearest ones (Bulgaria, Czechoslovakia, and Hungary, thus omitting the highest and lowest crude birth rates among the five), and Romania itself for the preceding five years. The accounting for alternate consideration is given in Appendix 2. For the decade as a whole, the comparison used falls between the other two. Incidentally, if the Romanian trend line were simply extended beyond 1966, the differential would be greater than with the 1962–1966 average.

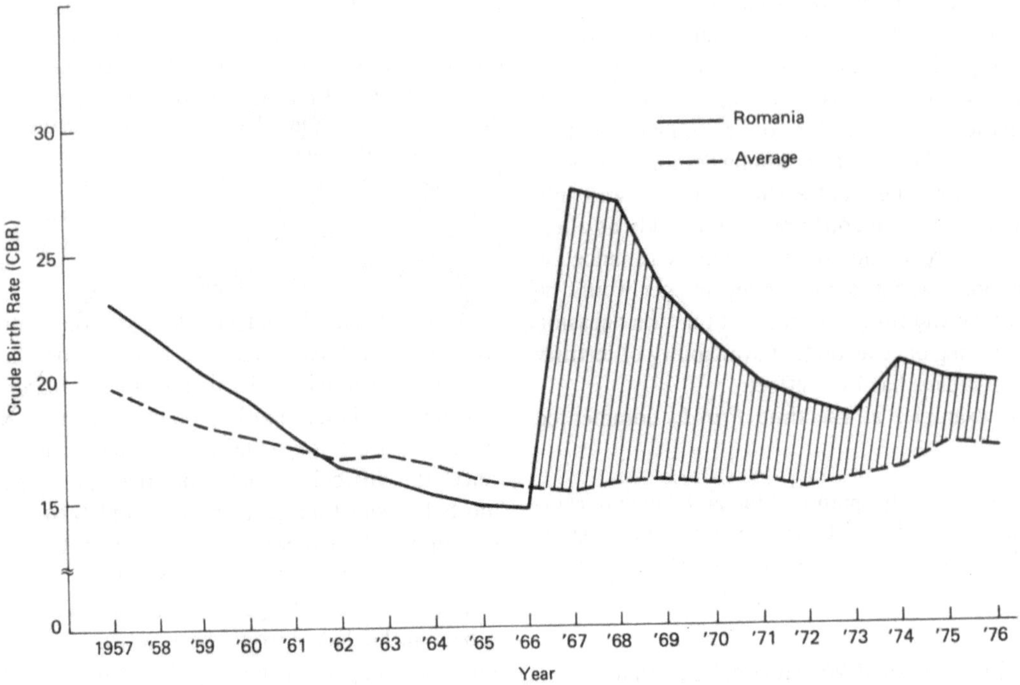

FIGURE 5.1. Trends in crude birth rate, 1957–76: Romania and average of five other Eastern European countries.

birth rate as sufficient for my purposes although some more sophisticated measures could be devised, depending upon available data. For example, the equivalent total fertility rates, as a control on possible age-structure effects, are presented in Figure 5.2, with essentially the same pattern.

For some years before the 1966 decree, the Romanian crude birth rate was actually below the average of the other five countries by nearly one point, and was following a sharper downward course since the 1957 decree which liberalized abortion. However, in 1967 a remarkable disparity became apparent, which lessened until about 1973, and has since then been maintained at an approximately even rate. The shaded area shows the difference between the Romanian rates and the average of the other five Eastern European countries, which are regarded as an appropriate approximation to Romania's fertility in the absence of the 1966 decree, if anything slightly on the high side.

Demographic Impact

How much has the 1966 decree meant to Romania demographically in its first ten years of impact? There are several ways of answering this question:

1. In the preceding five years the Romanian crude birth rate was about 0.9 points below the average of the other five Eastern European countries (or about 94 per cent of the average). From 1967 to 1971 (the major bulge) it was far above the average (52 per cent excess), and for the entire decade it was about 5.6 points above or 35 per cent in excess (averages of 21.5 and 15.9, respectively). Ten years later it is still about five points above its own 1966 value (19.5 as against 14.3) or about 35 per cent higher; and about 2.5 points, or 15 per cent above the average of the other countries. For the decade as a whole, the average excess of the crude birth rate over its 1966 level was 50 per cent. The Romanian crude birth rate has not changed much since 1971 (fluctuating within two points and essentially the same in 1971 and 1976) and the average crude birth rate of the other countries has not changed much in 15 years, except for a slight recent increase, perhaps a result of their own pronatalist policies.[20] The reported target of 18–19 was

[20] See, for examples, the chapters on Bulgaria, Hungary, Czechoslovakia, and Poland in Berelson, ed., *op. cit.* in footnote 3, and, more recently, Berent, *loc. cit.* in footnote 11, dealing with the same four countries.

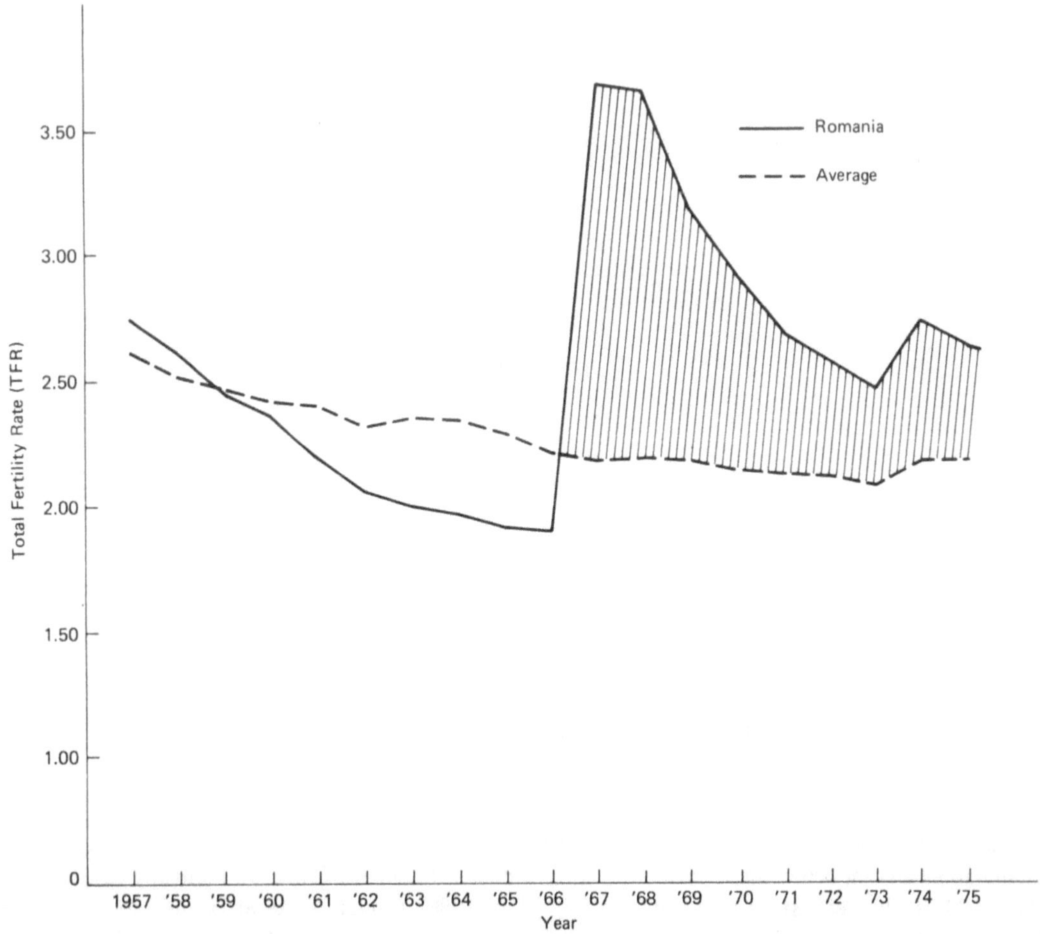

FIGURE 5.2. Trends in total fertility rate, 1957–75: Romania and average of five other East European countries.

realized after the initial rise and fall: from 1971 to 1976 an average of 19.3, with all values within one point of that figure.

The differences, taking the age structures into account, are essentially similar, as Table 5.1 shows. Since the crude birth rate is a more widely used and understood measure, because 'excess' births can be readily calculated therefrom, and since the age structure only reinforces the differences between Romania and the other East European countries, I use this measure in the following analysis.

TABLE 5.1. Total fertility rates

	Romania	Average of other five	Romania per cent of other five	Comparable percentage for crude birth rates
1957–66	2.21	2.37	93	94
1967–71	3.21	2.15	149	152
1972–75	2.57	2.13	121	119

2. The crude death rate for Romania was essentially constant during this decade (all fluctuations within one point); hence the rate of natural increase was affected in the same way as the birth rate. The average rate of natural increase with the 'excess' births was 1.14, without them 0.64 (about what it was, 0.66, in the early 1960s), or nearly double.

3. Translating crude birth rates into births, the shaded area in Figure 5.1 accounts for about 1.225 million 'excess' births—the actual figure of 4.376 million over the decade compared with about 3.151 million if Romania's birth rate had followed the average for the other five countries of

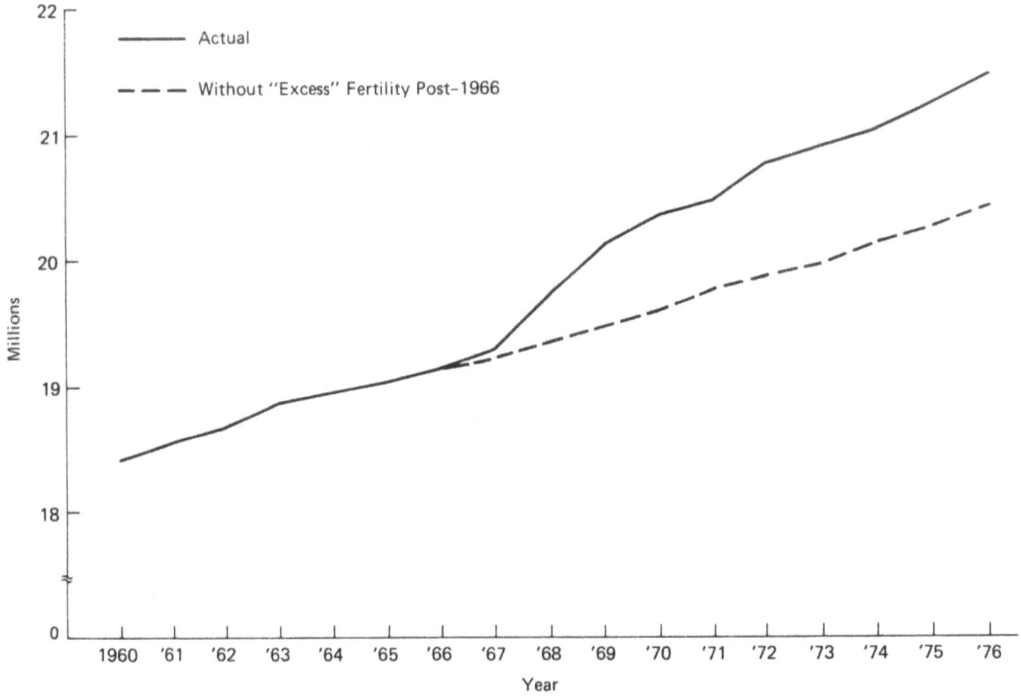

FIGURE 5.3. Population of Romania, 1960–76.

Eastern Europe (and, as noted, Romania was actually about a point below them during the early 1960s). Thus the 'excess' births that can be attributed to the non-abortion decree during this decade came to about 39 per cent more than would have been expected, had the comparative trend continued as designated.

4. The total population of Romania was 19.141 million in 1966 and 21.446 million in 1976 an increase of 2.305 million, or 12 per cent. The 'excess' births, as calculated, thus contributed about half the total increase in population for the decade (53 per cent, but if mortality up to age 5 were included, amounting to 4 per cent for this cohort, reduced to 51 per cent). In other words as noted, the actual population is now well over one million larger than would be the case if Romania had followed the average birth rate trend of the other Eastern European countries (Fig. 5.3) (several of which also took steps to increase their fertility during this period) or, indeed if its own trend had continued beyond 1967.

If these curves are simply extended to the target year of 1990, the current trend would result in a total population of 25.147 million (without consideration of the echo effect, if any, of the post-1966 births, which would in any case be small by 1990, though it could be felt soon after) as against a total of 22.316 million in 1990 under the other assumption. With these projections, the policy shift expressed in the decree will realize its target, whereas on the basis of the average Eastern European trend Romania would have missed the 25-million target by 2.7 million. As regards the target for 2000 (i.e., 30 million), extrapolation of the curves in Figure 5.3 yields 28.2 million for the actual trend since 1966, and only about 23.5 million for the other curve,[21] but without consideration of any echo effect of the baby boom. That effect might compensate for some of the approximate shortfall since there will be an increase of the order of one-third in the number of married women of reproductive age, but it could also have its own backlash in lowered fertility.

These figures may be compared with the latest traditional UN projections (Table 5.2). In both UN

[21] If the Romanian trend after 1957 is extrapolated, the comparative figures are 20.7 million for 1976, 23.1 for 1990, and 25.0 for 2000.

TABLE 5.2. Romania's population in millions

		1990	2000
From *World Population Prospects as Assessed in 1973*, Population Studies, No. 60, UN Department of Economic & Social Affairs, 1977	Low variant	23.0	24.2
	Medium variant	23.8	25.8
	High variant	25.0	27.9
From Economic Survey of Europe in 1974, Part II: *Post-War Demographic Trends in Europe and the Outlook Until the Year 2000*, UN Secretariat for the Economic Commission for Europe, 1975	Constant variant	25.0	27.9
	Moderate variant		25.6
	High variant		27.8
The projections as calculated in this paper		25.1	28.2 (without any echo effect from 1990 on)

variants, the rates of growth projected for Romania are substantially higher than for the other Eastern European countries in the same projections.[22]

The comparison between Romania without abortion (or modern contraception) and its neighbours so far presented seems firm for the 1967–71 bulge period and perhaps less so for the smaller differences of 1972–76. (The extrapolations, even without national comparisons, like any demographic projections are subject to their own uncertainties.) As regards the latter periods (and by extension the near future), there may be distinctive facets of Romanian society differing from its region that could account for some higher fertility: for example, I am advised of an extraordinarily rapid increase in gross national product accompanied by small improvements in the availability of desired consumer goods including foreign travel; or of a more youthful, optimistic, and expansionist outlook coupled with a nationalistic sentiment consequent to the country's achieving relative independence from Moscow. It is impossible to be certain how much of the trend after 1972, if any, may be attributed to these hypothetical factors supporting higher fertility, rather than to the absence of the indicated methods of fertility control.

We proceed to compare Romania's experience with a major historical landmark of a pro-natalist trend, the famous post-war 'baby boom' in the United States (which also occurred in Canada, Australia, and New Zealand). The 'baby boom' in the U.S. is estimated to have 'added about a third more people to the 1970 population . . . than hypothetically would have been added if the pre-war fertility rates had continued'.[23] Strangely, there appears to be no general agreement about the timing of 'the baby boom,' either its beginning or its end. Actually, there were two peaks in the U.S. experience (Fig. 5.4), and it is not always clear whether both or only the latter are considered to date the 'baby boom', assuming it to have occurred entirely after the war, nor when it terminated. The first immediate post-war peak occurred in 1947 and there was a fall up to 1950 when births began to increase again, and the boom is usually considered to have ended during the late 1960s. The first peak could be considered to be a direct consequence of the soldiers' return and a quick 'making-up' of births postponed during the war years, and only the large numbers between 1951 and 1968 could be considered as an aberration from the long-term trend; or the 'baby boom' could encompass both, as it is presumably in the above quotation.

Suppose, as in Figure 5.4, that the secular trend from 1945 to 1968 is represented by the dotted line between the actual crude birth rates of 20.4 and 17.5, respectively.[24] Then how many 'excess' births

[22] The UN projections are based on sophisticated techniques that take progressively evolving age structures into account. Actually, in 1970 the proportions of the female population aged 15-44 were about the same in Romania and in the average for the other five countries (44.3 per cent and 42.2 per cent, respectively). Already then, of course, the Romanian bulge showed in the 0–4 age group (9.6 per cent against 7.0 per cent) and that will increase and be carried throughout the remainder of the century.

[23] C. Westoff, 'The Populations of the Developed Countries', *Scientific American* (September 1974), p. 111.

[24] Which is roughly a continuation of the long-term secular trend, of well over a century, that was interrupted mainly by the depression and the post-war boom. For the curve, see *Population and the American Future*, The Report of the Commission on Population Growth and the American Future (GPO, 1972), Figure 2.1, p. 18. The

TABLE 5.3.

	Actual births	Estimated births at assumed average trend of crude birth rate	'Excess' births
1946–1950	18.146 million	20.0 = 14,446	3.700 or 26 per cent
1951–1968	72.105 million	18.5 = 55,674	16.431 or 30 per cent
1946–1968	90.251 million	18.7 = 70,120	20.131 or 29 per cent

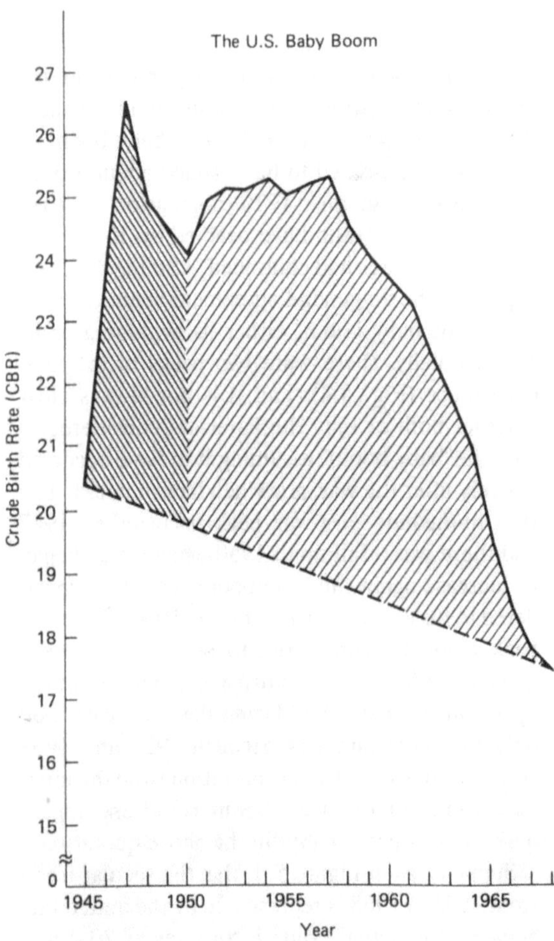

FIGURE 5.4. The U.S. 'baby boom'.

are represented above that line and below the actual curve? How does that compare with the Romanian experience and its reasonable extrapolations for an equivalent period?

We saw above that during the first ten years after the decree there were about 39 per cent more births in Romania than would have occurred if the birth rate had been equal to the Eastern European average (and still more if the Romanian trend had continued). But that included the main bulge of the 'excess' births, which were much less numerous towards the end of the period. Let us extrapolate the recent comparative plateau to the presumed length of the U.S. 'baby boom' at either 22 years (1946–68) or preferably 17 years (1951–68) (Table 5.4). Then, when these figures are put together with the actual 'excess' of 1.225 million births of 1967–76, we find that if the current Romanian experience were to continue for another seven years (to match the U.S. 1951–68 period), the 'excess' births since the decree will amount to 27 per cent; and if for another twelve years (to match the extended definition of the U.S. boom), to 24 per cent. In short, the 'transitory' effect of the Romanian policy change featuring the anti-abortion decree may well turn out to be close to the size of the U.S. 'baby boom'—which is not usually considered a minor or 'transitory' event in magnitude, duration or effect.[25]

data come from: U.S. Dept. of Health, Education, and Welfare, National Center for Health Statistics, *Vital and Health Statistics*, Series 21, No. 28, 'Trends in Fertility in the U.S.' (September 1977), Table 1, p. 26.

[25] In these calculations, the populations are extrapolated at the appropriate lowered rates of natural increase for the bottom trend and then the assumed crude birth rates applied to those figures, year by year. The rate of natural increase for Romania after 1976 was taken to be 1.0 (the average since 1971 is 0.99) and the crude birth rate as 19.5; the comparative figures for the five countries were 0.75 and 17.0 (even though the rate of natural increase since 1971 was only 0.68, it was 0.76 during the last three years of that period). For Romania between 1967 and 1976 the actual figures were, of course, used in the

TABLE 5.4.

	Extrapolated births at current Romanian crude birth rate of 19.5 (millions)	Extrapolated births at assumed Eastern European crude birth rate of 17.0 (millions)	'Excess' births (millions)
1977–1984	3.500	3.056	0.444, or 15 per cent
1985–1989	2.333	2.036	0.297, or 15 per cent

If the comparison were to extend only to the available Romanian experience of 1967–76 and compared to the equivalent decade of 1951–60 in the U.S.—which carried the 'baby boom' just across its crest—then the U.S. 'excess' is 34 per cent, below the Romanian figure of 39 per cent. In that first decade, the Romanian increase was even greater than in the U.S., and if the first decade of the 'baby boom' is considered to be 1946–55, greater still (U.S.=28 per cent 'excess').

Finally, I include two historical comparisons of an anti-natalist character for whatever they may contribute by way of criterion to the meaning of the Romanian situation: (1) The sharpest decline in the crude birth rate for a large population during the modern era, and perhaps throughout human history, appears to be the halving of the birth rate in Japan between 1947 and 1957 from 34 to 17, a level at which it has remained ever since.[26] In this case, too, a change in the legalization of induced abortion was intimately involved in the initiation, speed, and subsequent maintenance of this national decline. Abortion may not be necessary for that crude birth rate at this stage, but the legalization of oral contraceptives in Japan might well be required. In any case, induced abortion is at the centre of both the sharpest decline and the sharpest increase in crude birth rates in recent years (and in the absence of disease or compulsion, perhaps ever). (2) A decline in the crude birth rate of 30–40 per cent within a single decade in a developing country—i.e., 10–12 points—is unusually large at this time and requires favourable conditions both of social setting and programme effort.[27] So on both these inverse comparisons with anti-natalist government policy, the Romanian experience represents an impressive outcome.

Conclusion

At the Population Tribune in Bucharest in 1974, Paul Demeny said:

> The fact that Romania increased its birth rate has been widely cited here and at the Conference as a telling counterexample to so-called Malthusian policy. This is an extremely unperceptive interpretation. The Romanian policy is a classic example of a government's analyzing an existing demographic situation and concluding that a conflict exists between how individuals behave with respect to fertility and individuals' interest in their fellow citizens' behavior. One may disagree with the correctness of the outcome of the analysis but that is beside the point. Individual fertility decisions added up to a birth rate of 14 per 1,000 in 1966 in Romania. This was found socially inadequate and inconsistent with an aggregate population target identified as desirable by the end of the century. The government accordingly moved to modify individual behavior and to make it conform to the perceived public interest.[28]

one case; and in the other the actual averages of the crude birth rates of the other five countries and the difference between the rate of natural increase corresponding to this crude birth rate and the crude death rate of Romania, for a rate ranging from 0.55 to 0.77 and averaging 0.64, as noted in the text. The same procedure was used for the U.S. figures.

[26] Y. Okazaki, 'Demographic Transition in Japan', in C. Kunii and T. Katagiri (eds), *Basic Readings on Population and Family Planning in Japan* (Japanese Organization for International Cooperation in Family Planning, 1976), p. 29. The crude birth rates from 1957 to 1975 average 17.9, and all fall within the range 16.9 and 19.4 except for the Fire-Horse year of 1966 (crude birth rate 13.7). Actually, the upper figure for 1947 was probably elevated somewhat above the secular trend, as a post-war phenomenon; and in any case, Japan's record runs from peak to trough, not an arbitrarily designated decade.

[27] For the 1965–75 record, see W. Parker Mauldin and B. Berelson, 'Conditions of Fertility Decline in Developing Countries, 1965–1975', *Studies in Family Planning*, 9, 5 (May 1978).

[28] P. Demeny, 'Population on the World Agenda-1984', Comments at the Population Tribune, Bucharest (August 1974), p. 3.

This matter is naturally of direct consequence to Romania. One day in October 1966 it established a new population policy, and so far the policy seems to be meeting its two main targets. But the matter also has a larger significance for population policy beyond Romania.

In the continuing debate on the effect of family planning programmes upon fertility—where a family planning programme is defined as deliberately changed access to modern means of fertility control without direct attempt to change the so-called basic determinants or social-structural supports of fertility— the Romanian case is often dismissed from that standpoint as a transitory and insignificant event.[29]

But that by no means tells the full story. The October 1966 policy that withdrew the favoured means of fertility control (without providing for, indeed, discouraging, viable substitutes) had an important and thus far probably an enduring effect. In time, it may even turn out to be almost as large, relatively, as the U.S. 'baby boom' which certainly was and is acknowledged to be a highly significant demographic phenomenon. Over the first ten years, the decree increased fertility in Romania well beyond the going level by the order of one-half. It nearly doubled the rate of natural increase and about doubled the population increase for that decade. The effect seems to be felt a decade later, shows no certain signs of ending soon in the sense of converging to the fertility level of 1966, and could still produce its own echo effect in the 1990s. So far it is achieving the designated programme targets.

Note further that the government could establish such a policy at very little, if any, immediate, direct monetary cost. However, there are other real and serious costs to consider in consequence of the policy, e.g., the deferred social costs of dislocations in schools, housing, and jobs as the 1967–71 bulge moves through the age groups; the medico-personal costs of a six-fold increase in maternal deaths attributed to abortion;[30] and, not least, the government's deliberate interference with, if not frustration of, parental choice of family size. Whether the latter constitutes a pro-natalist equivalent of the anti-natalist 'compulsion' or 'pressure' currently deplored in developing countries is a neat question. In this connection, the Romanian case stands in sharp contrast to the U.S. 'baby boom': the latter an exercise in wanted children, the former a deliberate generation of presumably unwanted children.

The surrounding conditions need to be recalled. Here was a country that since 1957 had come to rely on abortion as its major means of fertility control; and after the 1966 decree people suddenly had to return to the discarded traditional method of withdrawal, to use with difficulty and expense the pill or the IUD which, while legal, were clearly officially discouraged and were hard to come by, or to resort to illegal abortion or otherwise find their way around the regulations (which were slightly liberalized in 1971).[31] That is the setting in which the overall effect occurred, clearly stimulated at the outset by a change in access to means—not a change in socio-economic conditions, in appraisals of the value of children, in 'population education', or in the usual manipulation of monetary incentives (e.g., child assistance). Such a country, with control over manufacture, trade, distribution and delivery of modern fertility control methods, determined to increase a 'too-low' birth rate, and did so mainly by manipulating

[29] Though not in Romania—in a kind of reversed sense. How do Romanian studies of their fertility in this period (at least, those in English) characterize the 1966 decree? The most recent, by Trebici, *op. cit.* in footnote 4, notes 'a strong straightening out of natality' that 'is a sign showing that demographic trends return to a "normal" state' (p. 21), 'the redressment of natality, from 1967 onward' (p. 28), and 'the recovery of natality' (pp. 124–125). Muresan and Copil's main reference is to 'this modified behavior . . . demonstrated also by the important increase of natality at the beginning of 1967, when the effects of the abortion law could not yet be observed,' *loc. cit.* in footnote 3, p. 361. Ceterchi *et al.*, *op. cit.* in footnote 5, call it 'a measure of natality protection, seeing that a free pregnancy interruption can greatly damage population natural growth . . . (and) was a real demographic danger. . . . So that the replacing of the free pregnancy interruption regime by a prohibitive one responded to a categorical demographic necessity, . . . especially qualitatively as it protects female fertility from the negative effects of the free abortion practice' (pp. 51–52).

[30] Tietze, *op. cit.* in footnote 2, p. 6. And as illustrated in the chart in Appendix 3.

[31] Muresan and Copil, *loc. cit.* in footnote 3, p. 367: for women over 40 or under 14, for mothers caring for four or more children, and in cases of additional diseases.

supply, and within that context, mainly through accessibility to legal abortion.

In this case, contrary to the usual interpretations, what can legitimately be termed a family planning policy and programme (i.e., a change in access to modern services of fertility control)[32] has had a major demographic impact by normal standards, albeit in a pro-natalist direction. The final irony is that the very country whose capital is symbolic of, virtually synonymous with, the relative put-down of that population policy at the World Population Conference of 1974,[33] was at the same time realizing the remarkable consequences of its own family planning intervention which today constitutes one of the world's major examples and successes.

---

[32] In this regard, abortion appears to have a special power as a means of fertility control, beyond today's contraceptives, because of its selective certainty, post-event: either when added, as in Japan and 1957–66 Romania, or withheld, as in post-1966 Romania. In general, as concluded by Tietze and Bongaarts, 'it is unlikely that any population ever attained a low level of fertility (total fertility rate=2.2 or less) without the use of induced abortion, legal or illegal'. And thus, especially in view of the recent increase in Romania under the less severe restrictions of the 1971 revision, legal abortion made easier or harder (plus control over the availability of pills, IUDs, and sterilization) may be the most effective valve available to 'fine-tune' a birth rate under the conditions prevailing in Romania, and perhaps under certain other conditions as well. (The quotation is from C. Tietze and J. Bongaarts, 'Fertility Rates and Abortion Rates: Simulations of Family Limitation', *Studies in Family Planning*, 6, 5 (May 1975), p. 119. For further material, see J.A. Ross *et al.*, 'Findings from Family Planning Research', *Studies in Family Planning*, 12 (October 1972), pp. 34ff; and C. Tietze, 'The Demographic Significance of Legal Abortion in Eastern Europe', *Demography*, 1 (1964), pp. 119–125.)

[33] B. Berelson, 'The World Population Plan of Action: Where Now?' *Population and Development Review*, 1 (September 1975), pp. 115–146.

Part III – Resource Allocation

6
On the Efficient Allocation of Resources for Fertility Reduction

Written with Robert H. Haveman

Population experts believe it would be most effective to give most population funds to countries with relatively high levels of development and strong "augmented" family planning programs. In the real world, however, the allocation priorities are reversed, with urgency of need to limit births given priority over sheer efficiency of resource allocation.

Since the early 1960s, governments throughout the developing world have adopted policies to reduce the rate of population growth. The adverse effect of rapid population growth on economic development has been the primary motivation, and the reduction of fertility has become the primary means.

In view of the importance of the objective and the large volume of resources involved, the efficiency with which resources are allocated is a significant question, often raised, but seldom explicitly addressed. Within the population field, what are the efficient strategies of intervention to secure fertility reduction? Can a superior allocation of resources be determined that would secure a larger reduction in fertility? In this article, we have combined the methods of applied welfare economics with information on the determinants of fertility reduction to shed some light on this issue. Our approach focuses on fertility reduction not as an end in itself, but as one determinant of the ultimate objectives of socioeconomic development and increased human welfare.

The estimates used here are not based on scientific empirical studies of the fertility response to various interventions under various social and political conditions. That knowledge does not now exist. This is not to say, however, that nothing is known, believed or acted upon with regard to the fertility effects of various interventions. Numerous analyses have tried to track the success of differing approaches under differing conditions, and strong convictions are held about appropriate policy interventions. Such studies, plus personal observations and experiences, do enable experts in the population field to judge the relative effectiveness of different interventions in different social and political settings. Our inquiry is based upon such judgments. Because the marginal contribution to fertility reduction from an additional dollar spent on each strategy under specified conditions is not known, we rely on informed judgment as the best available surrogate. This, of course, is what policymakers also do. The difference is that we have explicitly gathered the information and judgments pertinent to this issue, and organized them so as to bring them to bear directly on the question at issue.

The first step in our analysis is to delineate the means by which fertility reduction could be achieved through expenditures by donor agencies. By compressing a comprehensive array of 31 such means, we identify 12 strategies representing

Reprinted with permission from *International Family Planning Perspectives* 1979:5(4):133–142. This article is adapted from *On Allocating Resources for Fertility Reduction in Developing Countries* (Working Paper No. 40), published by the Council in 1979; the more detailed paper is available from the Council's Center for Policy Studies, 1 Dag Hammarskjöld Plaza, New York, NY 10017. The paper was prepared with the assistance of Myunghoon Lee, Project Assistant at the University of Wisconsin-Madison.

TABLE 6.1. Strategies for fertility reduction

Strategies involving the supply of fertility control means
(1) Improve public-sector access to current contraceptive methods, i.e., "*family planning programs*"
(2) . . . *plus sterilization*
(3) . . .*plus abortion*
(4) . . .*plus new and improved methods* with better acceptability, continuity and/or effectiveness
(5) Improve *private-sector distribution* of current means of fertility control
Strategies seeking to influence the demand for fertility control
(6) Advance *socioeconomic determinants* of fertility singly or collectively; e.g., general development, popular education, infant/child mortality, income, industrialization, women's status, urbanization
(7) Promote *information*, education, propaganda on fertility control
(8) Manipulate *incentives* and disincentives affecting fertility behavior; e.g., maternity costs, child assistance, housing, social security, social services
(9) . . . through direct payment of *money* or gifts for desired fertility performance
(10) Manage *community "pressure"* for an antinatalist consensus
(11) Impose *legal sanctions* on age at marriage, internal migration
(12) . . . *limits on family size*

major approaches to reducing fertility now being pursued or proposed in developing countries. These strategies of intervention (SI) are shown in Table 6.1.

Each of these strategies can be undertaken in a variety of circumstances. Whereas they may vary in their effectiveness in reducing fertility per dollar of expenditure, effectiveness also depends on other factors. As a second step, we identify two other factors that can determine the effectiveness of any expenditure in reducing fertility: the *social setting* (SS) in which the expenditure is made, and the strength of *program implementation* (PI) by the government. Social setting refers to those conditions of economic and social development that are or are believed to be determinants of fertility behavior—for example, infant mortality rate, percentage of school-age population in school, and per capita gross domestic product (1). Program implementation refers to a country's commitment and capacity to vigorously implement any policy intervention (2). Hence, effectiveness can vary by strategy (among the 12), by the socioeconomic characteristics of the participating society (from favorable to unfavorable), and by political commitment and administrative capacity in the public sector of that society (from strong to weak). For purposes of analysis, we establish three SS categories (high, medium, low) and three PI categories (strong, moderate, weak).

From this framework, then, we obtain a matrix of 108 cells: 12 SI categories × 3 SS categories × 3 PI categories. The question then becomes: By how much would fertility be reduced by an expenditure of $N in *each* of the 108 cells? Answering this question requires an estimate of the impact on fertility of the same level of investment in each strategy–SS-PI combination. We refer to this measure of fertility impact as an effectiveness rating.

Obtaining an effectiveness rating for each of the 108 cells is the next step. This was accomplished by obtaining a kind of judgmental distillation of knowledge based, in large part, on evaluative research. The cumulative results of such research, in conjunction with practical experience and observation, have led to judgments on the relative effectiveness of various strategies in various settings among experts and scholars in the population field. In our view, such effectiveness ratings reflect informed judgment on the matter more or less equivalent to the (largely implicit) policy evaluations made by responsible officials for their own situations.

The judgments were requested of 19 individuals. All have been long-standing and close observers of international population efforts, all have published substantially on the issues involved, and several have participated in the allocation decisions within the donor community. (None was directly involved at the time with such programs in an individual country.) Six are demographer-sociologists, four are demographer-economists, four are economists with strong interests in population issues, two are public health physicians, and the remaining three are administrators of agencies concerned with population policy. Eight are Americans, and the other 11 are citizens of nine different countries. As a whole, the group would be perceived as representing a wide range of knowledge, experience and views as to preferred population strategies. Their policy positions would probably be perceived as ranging from a strong "family planning" position through a middle or "neutral" position to a strong "developmental" position.

The basic description of our procedure was sent to each respondent along with a request for a professional judgment on the *relative effectiveness* of the 108 strategy–social setting–implementation combinations in the matrix, *given the same investment of funds*. We gave the following instructions: "Assume that the only objective is to reduce fertility. Each of the 108 options in the table represents a way in which donor agencies could allocate a given amount of money (realistically estimated) in order to achieve such reduction. Assume a scale from zero to 20, taken to express the possible range of effectiveness in fertility reduction per amount expended. The filled-in cell is given a value of seven on that scale. Using that as the anchor point, indicate the value which you believe each of the cells should be assigned."

We received 16 responses on the 108-cell matrix, and they constitute the information on which our analysis is based.

Effectiveness Ratings

The full 108-cell matrix with entries representing the mean effectiveness ratings given by the 16 respondents is presented in Table 6.2; Figures 6.1 and 6.2 present a summary of responses by strategy, SS and PI.

In the view of the panel, substantial differences in effectiveness exist among the strategies. Moreover, regardless of strategy, both social setting and program implementation are judged by the respondents to have a substantial impact on effectiveness. We note these main findings based on panel judgments:

- On average, the most effective strategies are judged to be augmented family planning programs that would include abortion (strategy 3) or a new method (4). The least effective are information campaigns (7) and incentives (8 and 9). The others are intermediate and are clustered within about three points of one another. Among the individual respondents, 11 ranked strategies 3 and 4 either first or second, and nine ranked strategy 6 (determinants) either last or next-to-last.
- The supply strategies as a whole have an average rating of about 150 percent of the demand strategies – 8.7 compared with 5.7, respectively. No respondent gave the demand interventions as a group a higher average rating than the supply interventions. However, note that the rating for strategy 1, the traditional family planning program, is only of average magnitude without the augmentation of sterilization, abortion or a new method.
- Without exception, the effectiveness ratings are positively related to strength of social setting and program implementation.* Within strategy categories, High SS and Strong PI have effectiveness ratings about double those of their low and weak counterparts. Across the entire range of strategies, the rating for the High/Strong combination is over four times greater than for the Low/Weak combination (11.7 as against 2.6). On average, each step up or down on either the SS or the PI variable means a difference in effectiveness of about 2.3.
- The two variables characterizing an intervention (SS and PI) are of approximately equal strength in contributing to effectiveness. That is, a Strong PI in a Low SS has an effectiveness rating about equal to that of a Weak PI in a High SS (6.4 vs. 6.9). Other appropriate comparisons off the diagonal convey the same result.
- We suggested to our panel that the rating was considered to be double the points off the crude birthrate (CBR) in 15–20 years. By that standard, the most effective strategy–SS-PI combination would take about eight points off the CBR, and the most effective strategy or setting or implementation, about five points. The overall average rating would take off 3.5 points, not far from what can be discerned in developing-country settings.
- With respect to the 108-cell matrix, the five most effective combinations are strategies 3 and 4 in the first two columns of Table 6.2 and strategy 2 in the first column; and the five least effective are all in the last column (strategies 7, 12, 1, 9 and 11).

---

* It is notable that there are very few reversals in the ratings by individual respondents.

TABLE 6.2. Mean effectiveness ratings, all 16 respondents (scale, 0–20)

	Social setting (SS) and program implementation (PI)									
	High SS			Middle SS			Low SS			
Intervention strategy	Strong PI	Moderate PI	Weak PI	Strong PI	Moderate PI	Weak PI	Strong PI	Moderate PI	Weak PI	Row average
Supply										
(1) Public sector, current methods	13.1	10.1	6.9	9.7	7.0	4.4	5.9	4.1	1.9	7.0
(2) ... plus sterilization	14.8	12.0	8.6	11.4	8.8	5.6	7.6	5.5	3.1	8.6
(3) ... plus abortion	16.6	13.8	10.6	13.3	10.8	7.3	9.4	7.1	4.3	10.4
(4) ... plus new method	16.4	13.9	10.7	13.4	10.8	7.4	9.4	7.0	4.3	10.4
(5) Private-sector distribution	12.1	10.0	8.2	9.2	7.1	5.1	5.4	3.9	2.3	7.0
Demand										
(6) Determinants	8.0	6.5	5.6	7.3	5.9	4.4	4.9	4.0	2.9	5.5
(7) Information	7.7	6.3	4.9	6.4	4.8	3.1	3.1	2.3	1.2	4.4
(8) Incentives	8.5	6.5	5.0	7.1	5.7	4.2	5.1	3.6	2.2	5.3
(9) ... money	8.0	5.9	4.7	6.4	5.1	3.8	4.8	3.3	1.9	4.9
(10) Community "pressure"	13.0	9.6	6.5	11.3	8.2	5.1	8.3	5.3	3.0	7.8
(11) Sanctions	11.3	7.8	5.1	10.1	6.8	4.2	6.9	3.8	2.1	6.5
(12) ... limits on family size	10.6	7.5	5.5	8.9	6.0	3.9	5.8	2.9	1.5	5.8
Column average	11.7	9.2	6.9	9.5	7.3	4.9	6.4	4.4	2.6	
SS average (all PIs)		9.2			7.0			4.8		
PI average (all settings)	9.3	7.2	4.5							

It should be noted that there is a wide disparity of views among the 16 expert respondents as to what is and is not effective in reducing fertility per unit of investment. The range of effectiveness ratings across strategies (not shown) averages 9.4, or nearly one-half of the maximum possible range of 20. On average, there is a larger variation in responses on demand strategies than on supply strategies, with mean ranges of 10.8 and 7.4, respectively. As might be expected, there is almost twice as much variation in judgment with regard to lesser tried strategies (determinants, limits and sanctions, community "pressure" and private-sector distribution) than with regard to those more fully experienced (traditional family planning programs, FP programs plus sterilization, and information efforts). The ranges within SS and PI categories do not differ substantially except perhaps at the two extremes, because of high ratings in the High/Strong and low ones in the Low/Weak column.

Profiles of Effectiveness Ratings

The pattern of effectiveness ratings can be viewed as a strategic profile. Such a profile can be displayed for an individual respondent, for subgroups of respondents, or for the group as a whole. Although substantial inconsistencies occur among individuals, there are clusters of respondents who have similar appraisals of the pattern of effectiveness. By inspecting the actual patterns of ratings of the respondents, we discerned a complex set of common clusters. The 16 respondents are grouped into five clusters on the basis of their actual patterns of response. These patterns can be described as follows:

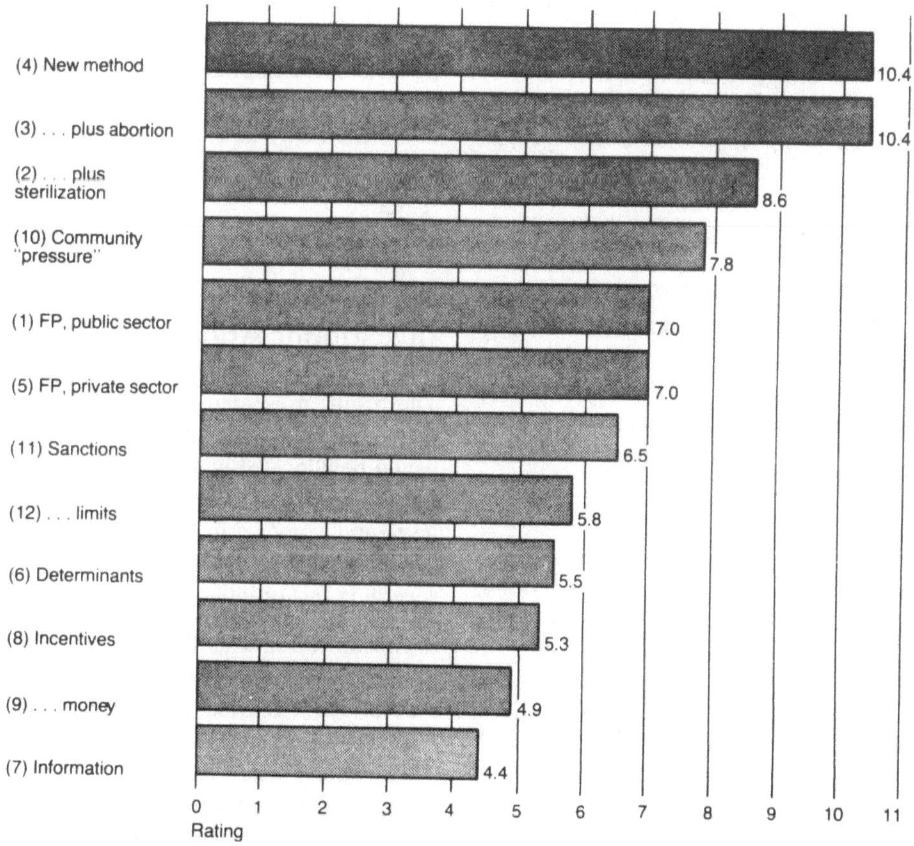

FIGURE 6.1. Average effectiveness ratings of intervention strategies (scale, 0–20).

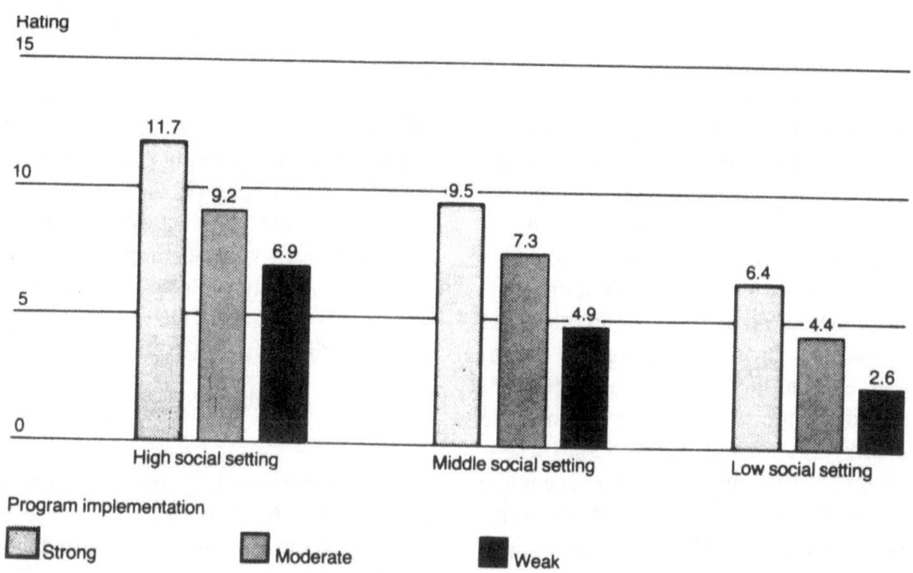

FIGURE 6.2. Average effectiveness ratings, by social setting and program implementation (scale, 0–20).

1. *Family planning/determinants (two respondents)*: This profile is strongest on determinants (6), with family planning (2–3) in second place.
2. *Primarily family planning (two respondents)*: This profile gives very high ratings to the supply strategies, especially as augmented with sterilization, abortion and new methods. Relatively low effectiveness is assigned to the other interventions.
3. *Family planning/"pressure" (five respondents)*: This profile has two main concentrations: high ratings for the augmented family planning interventions (2–3), especially abortion (3), and a smaller peak for community "pressure" (10). This profile can be seen as intermediate between profiles 2 and 4.
4. *Family planning/sanctions (three respondents)*: This profile also has two emphases: augmented family planning interventions (2–3), especially abortion, and the harder measures culminating in sanctions (11) and limits (12).
5. *Low differentiation (four respondents)*: The effectiveness ratings in this profile are relatively high for all interventions, with relatively little differentiation among them.

Toward Efficient Resource Allocation for Fertility Reduction

The data presented above provide the basis for estimating how expenditures should be allocated among the various strategy–SS-PI combinations, if fertility reduction is the objective and if the judgments of the respondents are accepted or respected as reasonable approximations to empirical fact.

The procedure, defined more precisely in the original paper, yields the optimal allocation of a fixed investment so as to secure maximum fertility reduction, based on certain assumptions of diminishing returns. In implementing this procedure, we used $200 million as the total investment to be allocated. It approximates the amount the donor community is applying (as of 1975) to activities *directly* aimed at fertility reduction, as against support for such other activities as research, training, institutional development and data collection. In recent years, according to the best available estimates, about 70 percent of "population assistance" has been applied to the former set of activities and about 30 percent to the latter set. Thus, of a total figure of $290 million in population assistance for 1975, we consider that about $200 million is now devoted directly to the goal of fertility reduction, mainly through family planning and associated support (3).

Implications of Responses for Investment Allocation

The results presented in Table 6.3 show how the $200 million of fertility reduction expenditures would be allocated when the average responses of the 16 respondents (as shown in Table 6.2) set the level and composition of the total effectiveness curves used in the analysis. These results contain several points of interest:

- The allocation would be concentrated in only 25 of the 108 cells, and the top five cells would receive $71 million, or 35 percent of the total. Whole sections of the matrix would receive no allocations whatever–including the last four columns of SS-PI categories and, with one trivial exception, strategies 6–9. *If* each of the 12 strategies could be implemented and *if* impact on fertility reduction were the only criterion, then investment based on effectiveness ratings would be limited to a relatively small number of SS-PI strategy combinations, according to the panel's judgment.
- The supply strategies would receive the bulk of the allocation–a total of $153 million. And strategies 3 and 4 (family planning plus abortion and family planning plus a new method) would receive by far the highest allocations–each would get nearly one-quarter of the total.
- The bulk of the allocations would also be assigned to High SS ($148 million) and Strong PI ($137 million) circumstances.

We calculated the allocations in certain other ways as well:

1. In the previous allocation, in which the mean ratings of the 16 respondents set the level of the effectiveness curves, the views of respondents with evaluations far from the norm tend to be submerged. Because their pattern of ratings is incorpo-

TABLE 6.3. Optimal allocation of $200 million to 12 strategies; from average ratings (allocation in millions of dollars)

Intervention strategy	High SS Strong PI	High SS Moderate PI	High SS Weak PI	Middle SS Strong PI	Middle SS Moderate PI	Middle SS Weak PI	Low SS Strong PI	Low SS Moderate PI	Low SS Weak PI	Total
Supply										
(1) Public sector, current methods	$11.2	$3.6	–	$3.6	–	–	–	–	–	$18.4
(2) ... plus sterilization	13.4	8.0	–	5.5	–	–	–	–	–	26.9
(3) ... plus abortion	16.0	11.9	5.5	10.1	5.5	–	–	–	–	49.0
(4) ... plus new method	14.8	11.9	5.5	10.1	5.5	–	–	–	–	47.8
(5) Private-sector distribution	8.0	2.6	–	–	–	–	–	–	–	10.6
Demand										
(6) Determinants	–	–	–	–	–	–	–	–	–	–
(7) Information	–	–	–	–	–	–	–	–	–	–
(8) Incentives	0.4	–	–	–	–	–	–	–	–	0.4
(9) ... money	–	–	–	–	–	–	–	–	–	–
(10) Community "pressure"	16.1	3.0	–	8.2	–	–	–	–	–	27.3
(11) Sanctions	8.2	–	–	3.0	–	–	–	–	–	11.2
(12) ... limits on family size	8.2	–	–	–	–	–	–	–	–	8.2
Total	$96.3	$41.0	$11.0	$40.5	$11.0	–	–	–	–	$199.8

rated into a set of cell averages, and because those of the 108 combinations with the lowest averages receive no allocations, the views of such respondents may be given no effective weight. To assign such minority evaluations a greater weight, a second procedure in effect grants each respondent $12.5 million ($200 million ÷ 16), which is then allocated most efficiently according to his or her *own* effectiveness ratings. Then, the resulting allocations to each of the 108 cells are summed over the respondents.

2. Two additional allocations involve selections from the 12 identified strategies: a set of seven "independent" strategies and a set of six "available" strategies. The first set recognizes that some of the original 12 strategies are close substitutes and, hence, perhaps not fully independent options. The various family planning strategies are examples. To the extent that similar options are treated as independent, and to the extent that these options receive high effectiveness ratings, the allocation results will tend to favor such choices. To adjust for this result, an alternative list of strategies is obtained by selecting the strategies that are least substitutable. The aggregation used and the resulting set (hereafter termed the seven independent strategies) are as follows:

- public-sector family planning, current methods (strategy 1);
- the most effective of the remaining supply options for each respondent (the dominant of strategies 2–5);
- determinants (strategy 6);
- information (strategy 7);
- the more effective of the two incentive options for each respondent (the dominant of strategies 8 and 9);
- community "pressure" (strategy 10); and
- the more effective of the two sanctions for each respondent (the dominant of strategies 11 and 12).

This list of strategies, with the SS-PI combinations, yields a 63-cell matrix (i.e., seven cells by nine).

The second compressed set (hereafter termed the six available strategies) includes only those strategies that are actually being used today to some substantial degree, namely:

- public-sector family planning, current methods (strategy 1);
- . . . plus sterilization (strategy 2);
- private-sector distribution (strategy 5);
- determinants (strategy 6);
- information (strategy 7); and
- incentives (the dominant of strategies 8 and 9).

This selection recognizes that abortion is not programmatically acceptable except very selectively, that the new method does not exist, and that pressures and sanctions are unacceptable in most places for a variety of reasons.

Table 6.4 summarizes the results from the allocation analyses using these two sets of strategies, and compares them with the results for the full set of 12 strategies (as in Table 6.3). In general, the allocations based on the selected strategies, as compared with the full list, indicate:

- a somewhat less concentrated allocation, though not much difference in the top five cells;
- less spent on supply strategies in the independent list, and correspondingly more spent on demand strategies, with the reverse true for the available strategies;
- essentially the same allocations to Strong PI and High SS situations;
- increased spending on traditional family planning programs, especially with the available strategies, although even there only in the 20–25 percent range;
- less allocated to augmented family planning in the independent list, though it is still a dominant category;
- trivial amounts allotted to determinants, information and incentives, except when the second allocation method is used, and even there not a large proportion; and
- more allocated to "pressure"/sanctions where available, i.e., in the independent list.

As for the two allocation methods, the relative comparisons are essentially the same for the three lists of strategies—though at different levels as indicated above—except in the case of deter-

TABLE 6.4. Comparison of allocation patterns for all 12 strategies, 7 independent strategies, and 6 available strategies; 2 allocation methods

Allocation pattern	% Allocation: From average ratings: All 12 (108 cells)	7 independent (63 cells)	6 available (54 cells)	From individual allocations: All 12 (108 cells)	7 independent (63 cells)	6 available (54 cells)
Concentration: % of cells with allocations	23	33	41	70	76	83
% of budget allocated to top 5 cells	36	46	42	28	34	36
% of budget allocated to:						
Supply strategies	77	58	83	58	44	65
Demand strategies	23	42	17	42	56	35
High SS	74	62	71	67	59	64
Strong PI	69	71	63	69	64	60
Traditional FP	9	17	25	6	11	20
Augmented FP	67	42	58	52	33	46
Determinants	0	0	8	11	14	22
Information, incentives	0	3	9	3	5	13
"Pressure," sanctions	23	38	0	29	37	0

TABLE 6.5. Percentage allocations to full and compressed lists of strategies by five clusters of respondents; from average ratings

Intervention strategy	Cluster: FP/ determinants	FP	FP/ "pressure"	FP/ sanctions	Low differentiation
Full list of strategies					
Supply (all family planning)	30	100	83	41	63
Determinants	66	0	0	0	0
Information, incentives	0	0	0	1	7
"Pressure," sanctions	4	0	17	58	30
Seven independent strategies					
Supply (all family planning)	19	98	58	32	39
Determinants	74	0	6	0	0
Information, incentives	0	2	2	2	0
"Pressure," sanctions	7	0	34	68	61
Six available strategies					
Supply (all family planning)	11	99	79	77	73
Determinants	89	0	15	0	5
Information, incentives	0	1	6	23	22
"Pressure," sanctions	0	0	0	0	0

minants and information/incentives in the last column.

However, regardless of the allocation procedure or the number of strategies, several patterns persist. In all cases, most of the investment would go to Strong PI (60–71 percent) and to High SS (59–74 percent). Among the strategies of intervention, little would go to determinants (0–22 percent), and somewhat more to traditional FP programs (6–25 percent) and "pressure"/sanctions (0–38 percent). The heaviest allocation would be concentrated on augmented family planning programs (33–67 percent). In short, in all six analyses, family planning efforts plus "pressure"/sanctions would get from 65 percent to 99 percent of the total investment of resources.

Investment Allocation by Clusters of Respondents

Earlier, we distinguished five clusters of respondents by the similarity of their patterns of strategy effectiveness ratings (see page 76). These clusters were described as: (1) family planning/determinants, (2) primarily family planning, (3) family planning/"pressure," (4) family planning/sanctions, and (5) low differentiation. Given the procedure for transforming the patterns of effectiveness ratings into an optimal allocation of a fixed expenditure, it is possible to discern the budget allocation implicit in the effectiveness ratings of each of these clusters.

In spite of the diversity of the responses, nearly all the clusters of respondents would allocate well over one-half of the resources to the High SS or the Strong PI categories. For some of the clusters, nearly 100 percent of the budget was allocated to these categories. Further, all of the clusters would allocate very little, often nothing, to the Low SS or the Weak PI categories.* Despite different preferences for strategies, the investment would always be concentrated among the haves (High SS and Strong PI) relative to the have-nots.

There are, however, clear differences in allocation among the strategies, as summarized in Table 6.5. None of the clusters would allocate more than a trivial volume of resources to information or

*Only the family planning cluster allocates any budget to the Low SS category, and only the determinants strategy allocates any budget to the Weak PI category.

TABLE 6.6. Comparison of population distribution and investment allocations; by social setting and program implementation

Category	% of Population (a)	% Allocated* (b)	Difference between (a) and (b)
SS			
High	16	59–74, or 67	+51
Middle	18	26–34, or 30	+12
Low	65	0–9, or 5	−60
PI			
Strong	4	60–71, or 66	+62
Middle	48	23–31, or 27	−21
Weak	47	6–9, or 8	−39

*The six allocation procedures are summarized in Table 6.4.

incentives (except when "pressure" and sanctions are eliminated, and, even then, not much—see bottom panel of Table 6.5); and none would allocate nearly as much to the traditional family planning programs as to the augmented ones. Moreover, virtually all of the clusters would allocate at least 20 percent of the budget to the supply options. There the agreement ends. Beyond that, those strategies on which any given cluster would tend to concentrate its allocation are by and large omitted by the other clusters.

This is seen most clearly in comparing the allocations to the determinants, "pressure" and sanctions strategies across the clusters. The compressed display reveals three basic allocation patterns: (1) all to supply; (2) most to determinants, the remainder to supply; and (3) substantial shares to supply and "pressure"/sanctions, with little in between. Again, only when this last strategy is eliminated (in the available set of options) would more than a trivial allocation go to information and incentives. Only one cluster (FP/determinants) would allocate a major share of resources to determinants.

TABLE 6.7. Range of allocation of funds to selected countries in the various SS-PI categories using three sets of strategies; from average ratings (allocation in millions of dollars)

PI	SS: High	SS: Middle	SS: Low
Strong	S. Korea $32-37		Vietnam $3–4
Moderate	Colombia $11–12	Philippines $9–10	India $25–35
Weak	Mexico* $7-9	Egypt $2	Bangladesh $0.3–0.7

*Ed. note: Mexico's program was designated as "weak" by the authors as of 1975. In 1977, a large-scale government program was introduced, one of whose goals was the reduction of the country's population growth rate to 2.5 percent by 1982—a goal which already may have been achieved. (See: U.S. Bureau of the Census, Population Division, *Country Demographic Profiles, Mexico*, U.S. Government Printing Office, Washington, D.C., 1979, Table 3.)

Investment Allocation by Population Distributions

Actually, there is a wide disparity between the estimated budget allocations by SS and PI and the actual distribution of population in countries assigned to the various categories. As Table 6.6 shows, the categories that would receive the bulk of the allocations contain countries with relatively few people.

This disparity between the distribution of population and the allocation of budget may be overstated by assigning *all* of the population in a country to the particular SS-PI cell in which the country is located. In most countries, a variety of SS and PI combinations are represented in their regions, political jurisdictions and rural-urban areas. If more complete data were available on the SS and PI characteristics of appropriate subpopulations within a country, some proportion of the population in a country classified as one SS-PI type would actually be found to belong in other neighboring classifications.

If we distribute the population symmetrically around the SS-PI classification for the entire country, the disparity between the distribution of total (developing world) population by its SS-PI classification and the allotment of optimally allocated fertility-reduction funds is significantly narrowed.* Accepting the resulting intracountry population distributions by SS and PI category, and assuming that the optimally allocated fertility-reduction expenditures by SS and PI classifications were distributed among countries so as to reflect these population distributions, we recalculated the allocation of the $200 million among the eligible countries.

By considering the dispersion of population within countries in the distribution of the $200 million, a substantial increase in support would be granted countries with low overall PI and SS ratings. For example, the distribution of funds to countries with Moderate and Weak PI classifications would increase by 32–39 percentage points, and to countries with Low SS, by 18–21 points. The per capita figures, naturally, range widely by SS and PI, but do not vary substantially over the three groupings of strategies: from about one dollar per capita in the High SS-Strong PI category to a few cents per capita in the Low SS-Weak PI category.

Table 6.7 presents the estimated allocations of the $200 million budget to selected countries in the various SS-PI categories, based on the population redistributions discussed above. It should be emphasized that these estimates are to be interpreted with care. While they do reflect the respondents' judgments concerning the effectiveness of fertility-reduction expenditures on various strategies in various social settings and under various program implementations, and while they are relatively stable in response to alternative aggregations of ratings and strategies (e.g., average vs. individual, independent vs. available), they also incorporate our own judgments on diminishing-returns patterns, on the intracountry distributions of population, and on the assignment of countries to the nine SS-PI categories. Fundamentally, of course, they rest on the panel's judgments.

Actual budget allocations can be, and are, based on considerations other than efficient fertility reduction, including political factors, expected changes in SS and (especially) in PI because of changed national leadership, appraisals of start-up needs and on-going self-sustaining efforts, and, perhaps most important, evaluations of the need for urgency of fertility reduction (e.g., Bangladesh vs. South Korea). Efficiency of outcome, in short, is one criterion for investment but not the only one.

This is readily seen in a brief comparison with the actual current distribution of donor fundings for this purpose (see Table 6.8, p. 82). The table shows a substantial disparity between population assistance and population size: somewhat more to upper SS, substantially more to the two extreme cells (the most successful in the upper left cell, the most needy in the lower right).†

Similar comparisons can be made between the actual allocations (in 1975) and the allocations based on panel judgments in this analysis. For example, there is a sharp difference in illustrative-country allocations (Table 6.9 compared to Table 6.7).

In interpreting these results in connection with donor-agency funding decisions, one point stands out—the panel's estimates of fertility-reduction effectiveness by social setting and program implementation do not closely correspond with the current allocation. Our analysis indicates that if fertility reduction was the immediate objective, funds would flow largely to the haves relative to the have-nots according to the effectiveness ratings of the respondents; whereas, in the real world, the actual funding decisions reverse this emphasis. Thus, a perception of "need" or "urgency" leads to a trade-off of some reduction in total births worldwide for a smaller reduction concentrated in nations in which, on other than sheer efficiency grounds, there is a very strong need to limit births.

Two further points seem worth mentioning in this connection: First, if we accept the reliability of the panel judgments, the analysis highlights just how far present allocations deviate from those that

*The procedure by which we made this distribution is described on p. 46 of the Working Paper from which this article is adapted.

†Actually, the disparity by strategy is not great, if only the available ones are considered (e.g., as shown in Table 6.4). According to a recent review, about three-fourths of external assistance goes to family planning efforts in one form or another (see: K. Kanagaratnam, "Approaches to the Population Problem...," World Bank, Oct. 1978).

TABLE 6.8. Percentage distribution of external population assistance (PA) to developing countries, compared to percentage distribution of population (POP); by social setting and program implementation, 1975

	SS							
	Total		High		Middle		Low	
PI	PA	POP	PA	POP	PA	POP	PA	POP
Total	100	99	26	16	21	18	53	65
Strong	11	4	11	3	0	0	0	1
Moderate	38	48	8	2	15	8	15	38
Weak	51	47	7	11	6	10	38	26

Source: Organization of Economic Cooperation and Development, Development Centre, "Aide aux Programmes Demographiques en 1975," June 1977, Table 4.

TABLE 6.9. Actual allocations to illustrative countries, 1975 (in millions of dollars)

	SS		
PI	High	Middle	Low
Strong	S. Korea $4.4		Vietnam $0.2
Moderate	Colombia $7.5	Philippines $7.7	India $14.2
Weak	Mexico $5.4	Egypt $3.1	Bangladesh $20.0

Source: See Table 6.8.

would be undertaken if efficiency in aggregate reduction of births was the sole criterion. This deviation indicates the importance actually assigned to general development goals, urgency considerations, social objectives and political pressures in the formation of budget allocations. In short, cost-benefit comparisons, although often called for, are not really wanted in their raw form. Second, if donor agencies could make concerns for urgency or need explicit and weight them relative to the fertility-reduction objective, and if such variables could be quantified, the analytic framework developed here could be used to extract efficient allocations in the face of multiple objectives.

Summary

This study has attempted to apply the principles of economic analysis to the problem of resource allocation in the population field, in particular the allocation of available fertility-reduction funds by the international donor agencies. It is based on the assumption that a primary (though not the ultimate) objective of investments in this area is fertility reduction in developing countries. Because of the unavailability of several types of data, it has had to be an exploratory exercise: arbitrary in the designated interventions and the selected experts, based on judgments in the absence of direct empirical data, using assumptions about the shape of diminishing-returns curves and population distribution, and employing available classifications of social settings and program implementations.

Nevertheless, asking and trying to answer the question of optimal resource allocation in the population field is important, particularly in the post-Bucharest period of policy debate. We believe that the analytic techniques taken over from economics are appropriate to this issue, that the panel's responses accurately reflect what is known about the birth-reduction potential of various strategies in various settings, and that the estimates based on these responses have substantive interest and validity in themselves. We would again note the exploratory nature of this effort and the potential for expanding it in several directions—number of respondents, better specification of strategies and interactions between them, better estimates of diminishing-returns patterns, incorporation of objectives other than fertility reduction, and application to specific countries where local data and close knowledge should provide better foundations for such analyses.

Nevertheless, we believe that this effort, however primitive, is a useful first step insofar as it emphasizes that the debate over the proper policies for fertility reduction must take into account *effec-*

tiveness per unit of investment along with other considerations. It is not helpful simply to assert as a policy recommendation that increased popular education or improved health or a higher standard of living or more women's liberation would reduce fertility, without appreciating the relative effectiveness per dollar of expenditure on such efforts, not to mention the programmatic means to effect them.

The following summarizes some of the main results of our analysis:

With Regard to Intervention Strategy

- The supply options receive the highest effectiveness ratings, particularly the family planning programs augmented with sterilization, abortion or a new method. Incentives and information campaigns receive the lowest ratings. Traditional family planning programs fall in between.
- Social setting and program implementation make for substantial differences in such ratings: The better the setting and the stronger the program implementation, the more effectiveness.
- There is substantial difference of opinion within the panel regarding strategic interventions (though not much with respect to SS or PI), and especially regarding the major perceived alternatives to family planning programs, i.e., determinants and "pressure"/sanctions. There is considerably more agreement on the tried than on the proposed.
- Five distinctive profiles of effectiveness ratings can be identified within this panel of respondents.

With Regard to Resource Allocation

- The better social settings and the stronger program implementations would consistently be allocated the lion's share of the resources, regardless of analytic procedures or strategic list.
- The allocation ratios to supply/demand options range from about 3:1 to 1:1 depending upon the interventions included and the analytic procedures used. Traditional family planning programs, as now commonly pursued in developing countries, would receive only a small fraction of available resources *if* the augmented versions were available, since the latter tend to be the most favored interventions. The "harder" measures of community "pressure" and official sanctions would receive a substantial share of resources, again *if* feasible; and determinants, incentives and information campaigns would be allocated relatively little. If the allocations were limited to what we term the independent and the available lists, the SS and PI allocations would remain essentially the same; traditional FP programs would receive somewhat greater and the augmented programs somewhat smaller, though still substantial, amounts; determinants would receive significantly more only in one case; and "pressure"/sanctions would remain substantial where available for choice. Finally, when we come down to what is currently available as strategic interventions in most developing countries, the FP efforts in the panel's average judgment, should get fully 83 percent of the funding.
- The allocations are sensitive to the procedure of averaging the several responses, whether through a single mean of the ratings (quite concentrated) or through a summation of the individual allocations (less concentrated).
- The different clusters of respondents ("strategic profiles") naturally favor "their own" allocations by strategy. But beyond that, family planning programs are the only intervention which would receive any substantial allocation from all schools of thought; of the remaining strategies, those on which any given cluster would tend to concentrate its allocation would receive zero or close to it from the other profiles. Essentially, there are three patterns of allocations among the clusters: to determinants and family planning; to family planning interventions and; to "pressure"/sanctions and family planning. And, although there is considerable range in the clusters' allocations to SS and PI, the higher levels would consistently receive more.
- From the respondents' ratings, allocations of funding would flow far more to the have than to the have-not countries. The relationship is affected by our process of intracountry population distributions, as a result of which increased allocations are made to low SS and lesser PI. Nevertheless, substantial disparity still remains; the range is from about one dollar per capita to one cent.

These results echo the familiar dilemma of public policy for welfare ends: What is most effective seems to be least feasible! According to the respondents, if fertility reduction is the goal, resources would be better allocated to the augmented family planning programs (including abortion, a new method, sterilization) than to the traditional; however, sterilization is not fully included in most such programs, abortion is far less so, and a new method is neither available nor soon in prospect. Beyond family planning, the stronger measures of building community "pressure" or applying sanctions would work, in the panel's judgment, but they are unacceptable in most countries: The cure is considered worse than the disease—which is only to say that, quite properly, other impacts besides fertility reduction are taken into account in policy determination. Although the respondents recognize that changing the so-called structural determinants of fertility reduction could be successful, these options are given lower ratings because of their cost per birth avoided. Finally, the greatest reduction in fertility would be obtained with heavy allocations to better settings and stronger programs (where the need is less and the populations small); and places with low social settings and weak program implementation, where most of the people are, would receive only trivial allocations if based on fertility-reduction effectiveness alone. Benefit-cost evaluation extended to cover objectives in addition to fertility reduction, or to take into account some consideration of "need," or to apply to a local situation internally, would be most helpful in this regard.

The results highlight a dilemma of public policy toward fertility reduction: Should efforts be concentrated on making acceptable policies more efficient, or on making efficient policies more acceptable? And in a sense, that raises the allocation question to a higher level, namely, the perceived value of the end which national policy must set, as against the monetary *and* the nonmonetary costs of the means. For as we have noted before, fertility reduction is neither the first priority nor the final value of the public good.

References

1. R. Freedman and B. Berelson, "The Record of Family Planning Programs," *Studies in Family Planning*, 7:1, 1976, also Chapter 11 in this volume (for an index of social setting based on a similar concept but developed for a different purpose); and W.P. Mauldin and B. Berelson, "Conditions of Fertility Decline in Developing Countries, 1965–75," *Studies in Family Planning*, 9:89, 1978, also Chapter 15 in this volume (for a more extensive analysis).
2. R. Freedman and B. Berelson, 1976, op. cit.; and R.J. Lapham and W.P. Mauldin, "National Family Planning Programs: Review and Evaluation," *Studies in Family Planning*, 3:29, 1972.
3. H. Gille, "Recent Trends in International Population Assistance," paper presented at Fourth Bellagio Population Conference, June 1977, Table 1.

Part IV – Action Strategies

7
National Family Planning Programs: A Guide

This is a personal document, not an official one. It is also preliminary, and subject to change as more experience with such programs becomes available. Hence it should be considered simply as one observer's view of the present state of things, for consideration and discussion, and as a touchstone for local circumstances. It is only fair to add that informed specialists in this complex field take different positions on several of the following matters, so the reader should think of this document only as a guide and certainly not as the guide that will eventually emerge from the gathering experience.

This is an attempt to distill present principles of "best practice" from the experience gained so far with programs designed to implement family planning in large populations in the developing countries. Naturally, there is no single "best way" to proceed—if nothing else, local situations and personalities will largely affect any program—but it may be useful to state in brief form a set of guidelines that seem to emerge from the experience to date. These observations can be put against any particular effort for comparison and guidance; certainly they should be used with flexibility and adaptiveness to local conditions, and not adopted with undue fidelity.

What follows is not all based on scientific evidence (we shall have to wait decades for that); it is rather based on a combination of evidence, critically viewed experience, and informed opinion. Moreover, it assumes that the government or other responsible agency has decided to proceed with such a program, and hence includes no rationale for that decision, e.g., on the contribution of family planning to the total scheme for development. This document deals with how to conduct a program once it is authorized.

The guide is offered in a pragmatic, empirical spirit of where-are-we-missing-out and how-can-we-do-better.

Strategy

The basic strategy at the outset should be to bring family planning to the people who want it—to give them the information, services, and supplies they need to practice birth control effectively. The primary aim, and the direct effort, should be to satisfy the existing interest in family planning, not to spread that interest: indeed, the best way to spread the interest is to satisfy the current interest. The initial strategy, then, should be primarily to change behavior, not attitudes: it is often easier to do so; peripheral attitudes will later change to conform to behavior; and, particularly in this case, it is more feasible and more consequential.

This strategy, in short, stresses action by the already motivated, rather than trying to affect attitudes of the unmotivated. It calls for information and service, not "persuasion." Naturally, as much of the latter should be attempted as possible—but not at the expense of the former. Information and services, plus generating some social support for the practice among the local elite, should be stressed at the outset—i.e., until the target population has been reached well in that way. By then, in any case, the attitudinal problem will look quite different, because of the circulation effect that

---

Reprinted with permission from *Studies in Family Planning* 1964;1(58):1–12, The Population Council, New York, NY.

spreads the idea from the satisfied users to the rest of the community as they become aware and interested. The point is to get those people who want no more children actually to begin the effective practice of family planning now—and to leave the notion of "the small family norm" for more gradual inculcation as the practice itself spreads.

In this way, to the extent successful, the program will set up a momentum in which family planning will be spread in the most efficient and least costly way, namely, from trusted person to person. In any case, few if any programs will be able to afford personal contacts by field workers with "everyone," so channels must be found for indirect effect. In addition—and this is an important point in practice—field workers will find it much more congenial to give people what they say they want than to try (usually unsuccessfully) to argue them into a new attitude. The objective, then, is to make family planning available, as nearly as possible on the same basis, to everyone in the society so that they have the opportunity to realize their own desires with regard to number and timing of children—and this is a highly desirable ethical position on which to base a program.

This strategy is based partly on the results of fertility surveys carried out in a variety of countries—i.e., studies of people's information about family planning, their attitudes, and their practices. The studies naturally vary in outcome, not to mention validity, but typically they reveal more interest in and approval of family planning than governmental and medical leaders expect or perceive. In this sense, the people are usually ahead of the leadership.

Here is a rough picture of the situation in the developing countries:

Practice family planning now	5–20%	say, 10%
Have some detailed information about reproduction and contraception	10–40%	say, 20%
Want no more children, of those with three or more	40–60%	say, 50%
Interested in learning about family planning	50–70%	say, 60%
Approve of birth control	65–80%	say, 75%

Hence there does appear to be a sizable reservoir of interest to be satisfied (even after discounting mere verbal expression). Since any program will necessarily be limited, in personnel and funds, it seems prudent at the start to allocate scarce resources where they can be most effective. What about the others? First, they will be brought along, as well as they can be in the short run, by the general informational campaign; and second, they can later be approached in the new situation that will exist when a substantial minority of their fellows have already achieved family planning practice.

Finally, it is very important not to think of the target, at a given time, as consisting of "everyone." That is an unrealistic, frustrating, and inherently deceptive position. Note, preliminarily, that not everyone needs to practice contraception completely successfully to make a difference in the birth rate. In any case, it will be all most programs can manage just to satisfy the interested, and for a good time that will be enough. Where the already interested fall below, say, 20%, then it is probably best to carry on only a general informational campaign, as well as one can, and not invest in a full effort that will not pay off, or even pass by the situation altogether for the time being (unless the 20% are quite easy to reach). It may be hard to accept, but it is probably true that in some populations, family planning simply cannot be implemented, at least with conventional methods, in a reasonable period of time, and it would be wasteful to try. In such cases, the emphasis should probably be on activities designed to interest and involve major sectors of the professional community, the formal and informal leaders, in the nature of the problem.

Moreover, it is well to think of the over-all program in phases, with flexibility to review matters and shift the course of action as experience indicates. Preparation and training come first, and then an intensive effort to get the program launched successfully in a substantial population (e.g., a few hundred thousand, or even more).

By that time, enough experience will be at hand to decide whether it is better in the local case to extend geographically or to re-till the ground already covered or to move after different groups within the target population or to concentrate on reinforcing the present users, etc., etc. Not everything needs to be done at once, or can be.

The corollary of all this is to concentrate, at the start, where the task is easier, or even easiest; it will still be hard enough there.

The two personal characteristics most favorable to acceptance of family planning are higher education and higher parity (i.e., those couples with 3–4 children or more—including one or more sons, in most developing countries). The educated people come to family planning "by themselves"; they will participate earliest, most frequently, and most successfully—but there are not many of them. The high parity group requires a program to bring them the necessary information, services, and supplies—and they are many.

However, since such couples are not residentially segregated, it is usually most economic to carry the program to the married population in the reproductive ages, but one should expect much more interest from those of higher parity and should tailor the educational materials for them. This implies that mass programs should begin with primary attention to stopping (for the high parity) rather than spacing (for the low parity). In many ways it would be better to succeed with the latter—and hence with the young couples who have most of their childbearing career ahead of them—but in the developing countries today it is much harder to bring them to family planning. Spacing can have more effect on the birth rate, but it is a more sophisticated and hence harder notion to realize. The idea of spacing should be introduced, and tried experimentally wherever feasible: whatever positive results are obtained will be that much extra; the idea of spacing will help to legitimize stopping, and is often more acceptable, as a first step; and in those developing countries with established popular education, the younger people will be congenial to social change and reasonably receptive to this innovation. Once the practice of family planning gets well-established among those couples with 3-4 children, it will filter down to be acceptable at the lower ranges too. (For this reason among others, incidentally, a program should not be limited to sterilization.)

The strategy of starting where prospects of success are best forces a difficult decision. Geographically, prospects are best in the better-educated, more modernized areas, and that means in the cities and towns. Almost certainly, everywhere in the developing world, the chances of implementing family planning are better there than in the rural areas—more medical support, better mass media, more sophisticated people, denser population, greater convenience for field workers, etc. But the cities are not representative of the countryside, and typically contain less than one-fourth of the population. Hence, in the end—and hopefully sooner than that—the program must reach out to the rural masses, and do so effectively.

At this time, perhaps the best way out of this dilemma is to try to have the best of both worlds: to start the program in cities and towns *and* in the surrounding rural areas, more or less concentrically. This will have some benefits in training personnel and in "working the bugs out of the program." More than that, it will effect most family planning at least cost most quickly, and will have a carry-over impact into the rural areas, particularly where there is a good deal of back-and-forth movement between city and country.

By the same general token, wherever one region of the country is more advanced than another, the program would do well to start there. For political reasons it may often be necessary to make the service more or less equally available everywhere at the same time, but such extension is almost never justified on substantive grounds, or indeed possible. Concentrating in the more favorable sectors and providing token service for a time in the others may be the best answer in situations where political considerations are closely involved.

Although it may not seem a part of strategy, it is very important to appreciate that the semantics of family planning are treacherous and should be carefully watched. The terms "control" and "planning" often have undesirable implications, in translation, of government intervention; to some people "birth control" and even "family planning" may mean abortion or sterility. Euphemisms may be needed—"family welfare" and "pre-pregnancy health" have been used—and translations should be done with great circumspection to be sure that people get the idea of voluntary contraception.

Design and Content

The typical family planning clinic is not enough in the developing countries (or in the developed either, for that matter); the program must be taken to the people in addition to expecting them to come to it. This means that field workers are needed, but it should not be taken to imply that the program should consist of home visits to every couple. In point of fact, it should not. It should not consist exclusively of home visits, but of other contacts as well; and when home visits are done, they need not and should not be made to every couple.

An effective program of contact to the community at large should include whatever mass media are available, group and neighborhood meetings, and mailings in addition to personal contacts. The mass media—i.e., newspapers and, especially, radio—should be used to develop support for the program and to provide actionable information, especially on the newly-developed intra-uterine devices (IUD's), i.e., where to go, when, for what. In addition, and this is perhaps more important than initially appears, the mass media should be used to promote the legitimacy of family planning: "it is done, here as well as elsewhere, by leaders of the society and by people like you; the majority agree it is a good thing." The idea is to get family planning in the air, taken for granted, accepted as normal for the social group involved. If that can be done, the media will have made a very important contribution, and program plans should be prepared with that theme in mind, expressed by the society's most respected leaders. Except perhaps for the IUD's, and even there in a limited way, the media cannot "sell" the actual practice of family planning in a low-literacy population and should not be expected to—except indirectly and in the long run.

Group meetings and mailing can be used in the same way, and the former can probably "sell" the IUD and perhaps, though not as well, some conventional methods. In any case, that should be the effort. With group meetings, the secondary objective is to get family planning talked about—to dispel the pluralistic ignorance and again legitimize the practice within the group. It is important to appreciate that there is a good deal of latent support for family planning in most societies that does not get expressed simply because the matter is not openly discussed, or even discussed between spouses, so it is essential to build up a forum, through the mass media as well as group sessions. In such meetings, every means of communication attractive to the group should be used—films, film strips, puppet shows, flash cards, etc.

As for home visits themselves, or individual personal contacts, it is normally not economic to make them to every couple, or to every wife. That scheme might get a few more acceptors than spaced visits, but almost surely not enough to be worth the cost. As has been said, it is necessary to rely on individual word-of-mouth to spread family planning, perhaps the most effective way. As a rough order of magnitude, contacts with every second or third couple may be about the right ratio to maximize cost to return—relying upon friends, neighbors, and relatives to spread the word (especially, again, of the IUD). By the time the first round of home visits has been completed, the proper distribution of repeat visits should be reasonably apparent.

How much should the husband be brought into the program? He needs to be given the same basic information as the wife, perhaps more information on the "population problem" of the country and less on methods except for male methods (particularly the condom). Almost everywhere in the developing countries the husband will be dominant in the family so he needs to be directly involved in the decision; and almost everywhere, studies show, he will be about as concerned about the matter as the wife. In most cases, though, program resources and other realities will determine the balance of effort at least as much as fine distinctions over husband/wife emphasis. For example, heavy emphasis upon the IUD (a female method) will require less attention to the men than emphasis upon the condom. In any case, the primary emphasis with men should be the same as with women—the welfare of the family.

However, there is one special group that it is important to reach, if at all possible, namely, postpartum women (or couples). It is often thought that women are more highly motivated at that time than at any other; certainly in the United States a good deal of family planning is effected at the six-week checkup. The problem in the developing countries, where few births take place in hospitals, is how to reach such women systematically. As noted later, this is where the traditional midwife becomes of critical importance. Since hospital delivery would be excellent for this purpose—the collected audience at the right psychological time—it may be useful to look carefully at costs and returns of setting up some sort of delivery system for this purpose, especially in urban centers. If post-partum women visit a health center with any frequency, that is a natural place for program effort; and so is a post-abortion service. It would appear that some imaginative experimentation with a simple centralized delivery system, with family planning built in, is called for in the developing countries; or a systematic approach to post-partum women through the midwives; or even a field program aimed at such women. The effort may well turn out to be economic in operation.

As for the informational content of the program, that follows from the central strategy. It should be direct and factual on *why* family planning and *how*. The *why* should focus on the benefits to the individual family but might also include some information on the national problem as well, especially for men. The desirable norm of the 3-child family should be reiterated, for both personal and national interests, but the material and the workers should not use "the hard sell." (An informational and educational campaign is available, in prototypic form.) It is worth stressing, since the programs are typically administered through medical offices, that the health reasons for family planning are normally not so compelling to the potential users as the economic ones, having to do with family welfare and education for the children.

It should also be mentioned that it is probably not worth looking for "deep" psychological motives for practicing contraception, or "clever" arguments to persuade people into family planning, or "gimmicks" that can spread the practice. There is none—or at least none has yet appeared, and it seems wasteful to look further. Utilizing the central and available argumentation for the individual case (e.g., economic well-being of the family and the children), providing convenient and satisfactory services and supplies, and trying to build a sense of social acceptance for the practice of family planning—that seems to be the best that can be done. If that will not do the job, it is highly unlikely that the other would.

In designing the program in the large, the principle of diffusion should be utilized. To the extent possible, the program should be organized in units of population arranged around centers that can provide service, personnel, etc.—for example, a city or large town with its satellite area, like a district. Then the service and program should be provided not to every village but to every Nth one (N will vary, probably, from 2 to 5 depending on local conditions), so that the word can spread in between. The program can be based in existing health centers of various kinds and they can be used particularly for medical contraception like the IUD and the pill. In addition, mobile teams may be needed for such a program—mobile informational teams, perhaps mobile service teams as well. (We do not yet know whether mobile IUD service into the countryside is feasible as against bringing the client to the health station or other medical site for insertion. So far the latter course has been more common.)

The stylized picture would look like the accompanying diagram, for a region of say 500,000–800,000 population (this version may be too urbanized in some developing countries, but it gives the general idea). Within large centers of population, a similar allocation of effort and resources is probably desirable. When a total area, or some large segment thereof, has been intensively covered once, the program should be repeated, with whatever modifications were suggested by the first experience. By that time, there should be a new layer of interested and motivated clients. As the layers grow in depth, the task should become progressively easier. And to repeat, if sufficient funds or personnel are not available for an intensive effort throughout the entire country or region to be covered, it is strategically better to concentrate effort in part of the field and move sequentially, rather than to spread the resources thinly throughout the area. Naturally, a sound distribution system for conventional contraceptive supplies must be established.

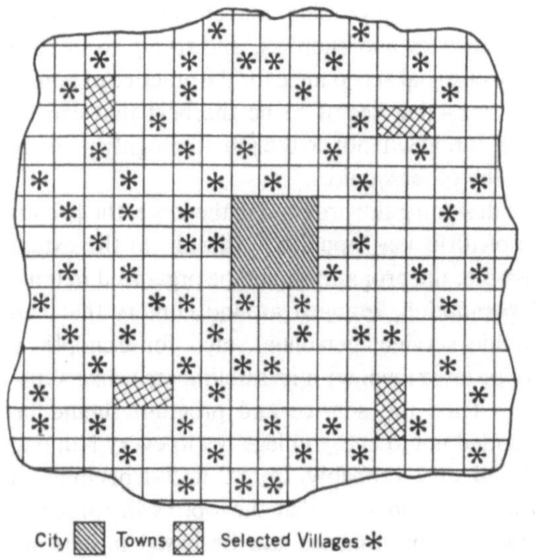

Stylized example: region of, say, 750,000 population with 1 city of 150,000, 4 towns of 25,000 each, and 250 villages of 2,000 each. Program to operate in city and towns (i.e., every Nth district within them) and in selected villages (about every 3rd).

Organization and Administration

The specific form of organization and administration of a national family planning program will depend on local conditions and, it must be noted, upon local personalities. Hence it is idle to suggest the ideal form or forms, but still a few things can be said:

1. Whatever its form, the family planning program should be set up as high in the government as possible, mainly in order to attract a strong director but also in order to enable him to call upon other agencies as needed for assistance to the program (as well as upon the highest level of government for support when necessary). Implementing family planning is at best difficult and it is made virtually impossible if it is not given a sufficiently high priority. On the administrative side this cannot be stressed too strongly.
2. The capacity of the director is naturally a key element for the success of the program. A man of unquestioned respect and prestige is needed —able, courageous, dedicated to this effort, ingenious, and administratively well-situated. It is often desirable that he be an M.D. as well, but that qualification is not so important as these others. All in all, it is probably fair to say that within reasonable limits, the person of the director is more important than the specifics of the organization—in the sense that a strong director can do more with an imperfect organization than a weak director with a good organization on paper. One strong, dedicated, able man, well located and well supported, can do a great deal in leading a national program.
3. Given the likely realities, some family planning agency with autonomous or semi-autonomous status is usually found to be necessary, as a way to get around bureaucratic restrictions of various kinds—in salary limits, subsidy restrictions, speed of action, etc. Thus there are semi-autonomous family planning institutes in some countries, a specially-created private association for maternal and child health in another (that channels medical fees for IUD insertion), a private family planning association in another to do the government's training and other services.
4. Some regional decentralization is desirable, especially in a large country, again in order to attract good people at the top and also as a way to build some healthy internal competition into the program. So far, at least, family planning programs have been carried out most successfully in units of 25 to 30 million population and below. What the local administrative unit should be will depend on local circumstances, but a unit of 250–300,000 population is not too large; indeed, for an intensive IUD program it may be somewhat too small to keep the necessary clinical team fully occupied.

Beyond these points, it appears that any of a number of possible organizations will do as well as any other. In general, it might be said that too much attention is usually given to formal administrative arrangements as against other, more central matters discussed in this memorandum.

Field Workers

They are usually needed to bring the program directly to the potential users, with the probable exceptions of the better-educated people in the cities, who will find their own way to contraceptive practice; and of post-partum women who are reachable through a clinic or health center or hospital. Some field workers need to be devoted to this task full-time, partly because of the magnitude of the job and hence the time required to do it, but also so that this receives their undivided attention and hence becomes their full responsibility. It is good to bring family planning into other programs as a residual or additional matter—e.g., community development or village education—but that way the responsibility often becomes so diffuse that no one really has it. There is no substitute for a full-time staff of field workers if the program needs to be taken to the people.

Who should they be? That depends upon who is available locally. Trained nurse-midwives are probably best as a type, provided that they have not been so highly trained that they would perceive such work as beneath them or that their potential clients would not perceive them as "one of us." Untrained but able women with some education can also be used. Being unmarried or quite young is a handicap for the obvious reasons, but not an absolute disqualification if the workers are genuinely impressed with the importance of the job and genuinely sympathetic to the women to be served. Acceptability to the public concerned is a requirement, particularly on such a delicate subject as contraception, and so is the worker's informed dedication to the task. A superior or patronizing attitude, in short, is bad and in general a lesser-trained but more humane person is to be preferred to a better-trained but unsympathetic one. In those countries where women workers cannot readily speak to men about family planning matters, male workers will naturally be required and the same goes for them—which automatically means lesser training in their background. Since sufficient numbers of trained personnel will probably not be available, field workers should be recruited with this personality factor given attention along with educational background.

All such workers, regardless of background and prior training, will need some special training to fit them for field efforts in family planning. Just what that should be will vary with local circumstances, but in general about three weeks of training at the outset might suffice, plus refresher and "feedback" work for two to three days every six to twelve months thereafter—perhaps oftener at the start, less often later on. The refresher sessions, held regionally in the field and close to their home bases, should deal with (a) recent developments in family planning, e.g., introduction of a new contraceptive method or a new set of informational materials and (b) the workers' own problems and questions as encountered in the field. The initial training session of about three weeks might best be conducted centrally or regionally—in part, simply to give the workers a sense of their importance—and should consist roughly of the following subjects:

*Introduction (by high level officers)	½ day
*The population situation	1½ days
*The population program	1 day
*Physiology of reproduction	1½ days
*Contraceptive methods	2 days
Field work operations	2 days
*Informational and educational materials and their use	2 days
Survey work and record-keeping	1½ days
Actual field work (as apprentices under supervision)	4–5 days
Review and summary	1–2 days
TOTAL	17–19 days

On the appropriate topics the workers should be trained with the same materials they will use in the field, plus some more detailed materials to be used for elaborating, answering questions, etc. It is important to emphasize that the "human relations" aspects of the task need conscious attention, in the training and apprenticeship period as well as in supervision on the job.

In addition, the regular staff of all public health centers should receive some background instruction so that they can be knowledgeable about the program and serve as referral agents. Two to three days may be all that is feasible, but that is much better than nothing; the training should include something on the items starred above. This training should be given to all health station personnel, not simply the lower levels; and the indicated material should be known by the staff at central headquarters as well.

How many field workers? That too will be dictated by local capacities but again as a rough order of magnitude, here are some guidelines. One full-time field worker can make up to 40 home visits a week in the urban areas and about 25 in the rural. This means that to cover a population of 1,000,000 in one year, with an initial visit to every second married woman in the reproductive ages and a follow-up visit to every fourth would require about 65 field workers in the cities and about 100 in the country.

Roughly, one supervisor is needed for every 20 field workers; one for 10–15 would be much better. Supervision is a critical matter, more important probably than the refresher courses. The day-to-day administration of the program is actually run by the intermediate level personnel, and they can mean the difference between success and failure. The supervisors should be carefully selected for industry, leadership, flexibility, and dedication to the effort.

One key suggestion with regard to field workers: it is likely that such workers, under most circumstances prevailing in the developing countries, will respond favorably and well to an incentive system in which they would receive a small fee for every successful acceptor of family planning (e.g., one who persists for six months or so). Perhaps such fees could be paid from the funds taken in payment of contraceptive supplies, and perhaps on a group basis, including supervisors. If some such incentive arrangement can be worked out, politically and financially, it will probably make a substantial difference in the success of the program.

One should not overlook the importance of the traditional midwives for such programs. They exist almost everywhere in the developing countries, they have the ear and usually the trust of the village women, they know who is pregnant and who has just been delivered, they are a natural channel of information and perhaps supplies—and they will normally perceive a family planning program as a threat to their livelihood, as indeed it will be. Accordingly, wherever they are even moderately important, it is critical to get them on the side of the program early and firmly—e.g., by making field workers out of them, for pay. The same goes, though in the nature of the case less strongly, for traditional medical personnel.

Special Publics

Taking family planning to married couples in their communities is central to the whole enterprise but it is not enough in itself. The key principle is to bring family planning to people's attention through as many windows of the society as possible, and particularly through the windows of special interest to them. The more sources carry the message, and especially the more trusted they are, the better. Hence, it is important to look in all directions for ways to bring the message home. Here are some important ways—there may be others in local situations:

The Military

Most countries interested in family planning have large numbers of young men under arms—young men at the start of their own marital careers who will return to all areas and all segments of the society. Here is a "captive audience" for instruction in family planning—in the *why* as well as the *how*—who can serve as agents of change back in their home communities. Wherever possible an intensive informational program should be instituted in the armed forces, especially just before the men's release from service. It is hard to over-estimate the potential importance of such a program. (Prototypic materials are available for such an informational program within the armed forces.)

The Schools

In the longer run, there is a good opportunity in the educational system—to bring the basic facts about reproductive physiology and about the country's population situation to the attention of students in the secondary and elementary schools. Soon enough they will be marrying; moreover, they will bring the information home with them now. In addition, the teachers themselves will become better aware of the problem through having to teach it, and as respected local leaders they can be influential supporters of the program. Note that such educational efforts should be proper academic work on population, not "family planning." (Again, materials and course units are now being prepared.)

Industry

Wherever possible, individual firms should be enlisted to include family planning as part of their own health programs. This has been successfully done in Japan and is thus far under-utilized in the efforts of the developing countries. The industrial employees are a kind of urban elite so there is an indirect advantage as well. Family planning can be covered not only by industry's doctors and nurses, but also in informational materials distributed under industrial sponsorship. The same goes for farmers' associations and labor unions.

Women's Organizations

Where they exist, it is only natural to involve the women's associations. They will tend to be upper class, but they can do an important job of supporting the program—not least by influencing husbands, fathers, other relatives, and friends in positions of power within the society—even though they are not normally ready to do much by way of direct service.

In addition, it is sometimes possible to attach a family planning message to community development or agricultural innovation or public health. Whenever that can be done it is almost certainly worth doing, simply to get another reinforcing influence into the picture. But one should not think that such indirect efforts will normally do the job. They will not; full-time family planning workers are typically needed.

The Medical Community

The medical community is central for two reasons: its support is highly desirable, even necessary, for the successful introduction and spread of family planning; and its participation in servicing the program is indispensable. In virtually every case so far, national programs are organized within the Ministry of Health, and family planning is usually seen as part of the maternal and child health services of the government. This brings the medical profession into immediate and lasting contact with the program. It would be virtually impossible to carry on a program against the opposition of the medical profession, so every effort must be made to develop a strongly favorable attitude early on. Moreover, the IUD is now being inserted only by physicians so that doctors are needed as direct collaborators in the program as well.

At the outset this means that special attention is needed to secure medical support—the more prestigious, the better. The medical community will naturally be involved in determining which contraceptive methods will be used in the program. Specifically, a highly-placed medical advisory committee should be organized at once to review the IUD and to gather direct experience with it in order to approve it for extensive use as soon as possible. This is all the more important when one recognizes, as experience has confirmed, that women's attitude toward the device directly reflects the doctor's attitude: if he is confident and secure, there is a good chance that they will be too. For continuity, special training materials need to be prepared for the medical curriculum, as refresher sources for practitioners, and for paramedical courses—mainly on medical aspects of reproduction and contraception but also containing some information on "the population problem." It is perhaps not too much to say that the medical profession, a large part of it, must be supportive before a successful program can be carried out, and especially the obstetricians-gynecologists.

Contraceptive Methods

The contraceptive technology is of critical importance in spreading family planning. Methods that require sustained motivation, repetitive action, and (usually) a strong supply system are one thing, especially if they are relatively ineffective; methods that require a single act of motivation, that last, and that do not require a supply system are quite another, especially if they are relatively effective. It is not too much to say that program plans depend largely on the contraceptive methods to be used or stressed.

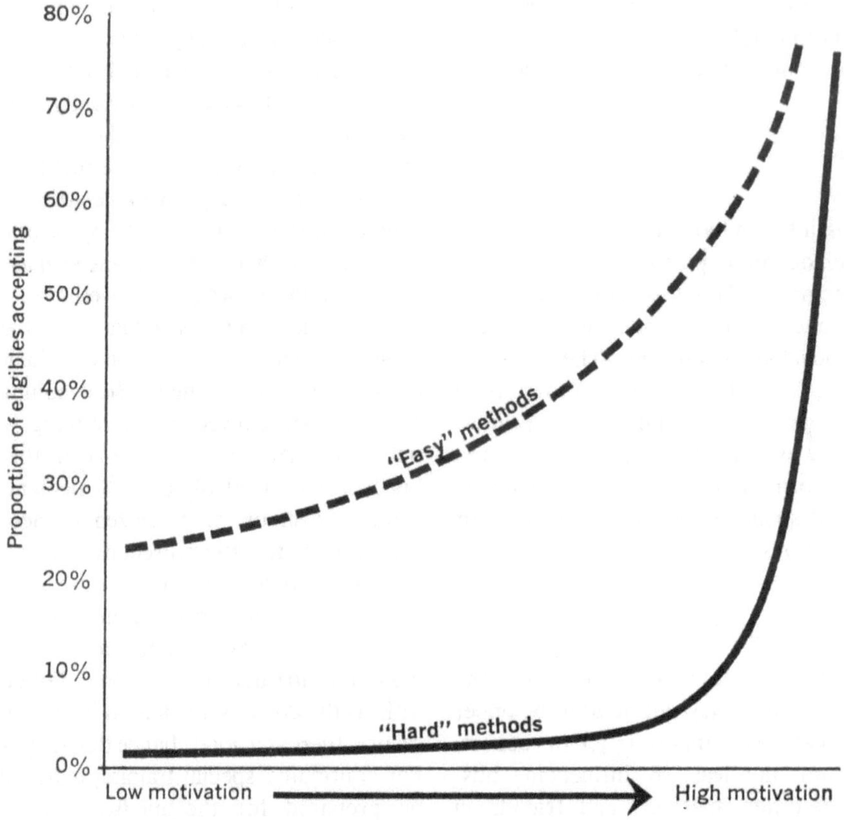

Schematic representation of relation between motivation and contraceptive technology

In general, there is an important relationship within a society between the degree of motivation required to practice family planning successfully and the ease, convenience, and effectiveness of the contraceptive method used: highly motivated people will make do with anything, weakly motivated people will need an easy method. Certainly, acceptability of the method, in this respect, is more important to a program's success than, say, the detailed informational aspects of the program itself.

At the same time, no one method will do for everyone, nor need it. At present, the IUD is a highly favorable contraceptive method for mass programs and should be utilized as fully as local circumstances permit. Beyond that, the upper classes may use the diaphragm, but that method does not appear to be worth including in a mass offering. Neither is the foam tablet: it is not highly effective, it is unattractive for many women, and it presents difficult supply problems; the contraceptive foam is better if it does not violate local notions of feminine privacy. Rhythm and withdrawal are hard to teach, and the former takes a good deal of motivation and attention to do well. The condom is definitely worth including as the best available male method (not counting vasectomy); the experience is that it gains in use even in areas where it is supposed to be unacceptable on cultural grounds (e.g., the method associated with prostitutes). The oral pill is still expensive and rather difficult for some women to use consistently, but it is probably fair to say that it has not had a full trial under low-cost conditions; it may turn out to be a useful adjunct but not the central method for mass efforts in developing countries. Thus far, at least, its cost has been a prohibitive factor in mass application, and would continue to be even at a substantially reduced rate.

From several standpoints, it may be best to provide a cafeteria choice–"here are all the recommended methods, select the one most suitable to you"–but at the same time to stress the desirability of the IUD. Actually, it would probably be more economic and no less effective to base a program on IUD and condom alone, with aerosol foam and the pill perhaps offered to women who cannot tolerate or do not wish the IUD. Both the IUD and the condom are economically feasible in almost any situation where the government is seriously interested and can provide some slight subsidy, and limiting the program to the two methods has some advantages in supply, training, informational and educational programs, etc.

Wherever possible, and to the extent possible, provision should be made in the program for sterilization operations. Typically there is a local preference for either the male or the female version, and that preference should be respected. Whether such operations can make a substantial impact on the birth rate is still an open question: the difficulties are the unavailability of medical personnel and the prevalence of the operation among those of very high parity already. Local medical circumstances and local feelings about such operations now appear to be the determining factors.

An intensive program of family planning may temporarily increase the incidence of induced abortion, by activating people's motivation to limit size of family, but it will almost certainly reduce the practice over any reasonable period of time. The proper authorities might do well to consider what their policy will be in the short run.

Supplies

There are two basic decisions that must be made here: (1) import and/or manufacture of which supplies, in what amounts; and (2) distribution of supplies, in what proportions through public and/or private channels, and at what prices.

First, in order to get at a rough order of magnitude, it is worth doing the following arithmetic: (1) to get from total population to married women in the reproductive ages, divide by six or seven; that is usually accurate enough to use as a preliminary baseline for supplies; (2) estimate that not more than 10–15% of the married women will take up family planning in the first year of the program (and they will be 30–45% of the currently eligible women–i.e., those not pregnant, lactating, or sterile, and not wanting more children now); (3) estimate that from two-thirds to three-fourths of the acceptors will choose the IUD and most of the rest the condom (which will be needed in the amount of about 100 a year per user, on the average). For a million population per annum, this works out to, say, 14,000 IUD's (perhaps of different sizes, though the modal size should do for 80% or so of the women) and 600,000 condoms. Other supplies, like diaphragms or pills or aerosol foam, will be needed in far smaller numbers. The condoms, pills, and foam will of course have to be supplied anew each year for continuing users; the IUD and diaphragms will be needed only in replacement amounts. Now, how should such supplies be secured and distributed?

It appears to be economic to manufacture both IUD's and condoms locally (assuming the prior presence of good plastics and rubber factories) only if the supplies are needed in the amounts of at least 100,000 for IUD's and about 5,000,000 annually for condoms. Such materials can be secured for about US$.15 for the IUD (probably less in large numbers) and US$.01 per condom (ditto). The decision in a particular case will of course be made in view of local circumstances but it should be made as nearly as possible on economic grounds, not political. If local manufacture is decided upon rather than import, then additional time will be required to get into good quality production; if the decision goes the other way, questions of import duty arise that need to be handled within the government.

That leads to the second question: how are the supplies to be distributed and at what prices? Naturally, a large amount will be distributed through government channels as part of the national program. Since that is normal under most circumstances, it is important to stress here that supplies should be put into private channels as early and as fully as possible–IUD's to private obstetricians and other physicians, condoms and other conventional methods into commercial enterprise. In both cases, public and private, the supplies might be offered at a subsidized cost, or even, if the government can afford it, free (at least to the indigent). Many people will be able to pay some part of their own contraceptive costs, and that is one way to support the program. However, it is usually a mistake to develop a substantial bookkeeping system on this matter; it is often cheaper to distribute the supplies gratis, and certainly less restrictive to the action effort itself, since extensive filling out of records itself repels people.

Private channels should be enabled to make a good-to-better fee or profit by extending family planning. Subsidization of private distribution is worth it to the government in that it fosters the development of an indirect network of information and service that would otherwise have to be set up on its own, and at higher cost. So it is very important to appreciate that private incentives to promote family planning should be built into the national program at every opportunity, for both effectiveness and economy, and specifically that private medicine and commercial channels should not be neglected.

Budget and Costs

Family planning cannot be spread at no cost to the government, at least not within many years, but it can be spread economically. Just as a guidepost, analyses seem to show that on economic grounds alone it would be proper to pay one to two times the annual per capita income for each prevented birth. Where it can be done at all, family planning can be spread for well below that figure—otherwise, of course, it simply would not be worth it from the economic standpoint.

Countries now engaged in national family planning programs have budgets ranging from about \$.01 to \$.05 per capita per annum. The former figure is probably inadequate to make a measurable impact on the national birth rate. Naturally, budgetary considerations will vary from country to country, from program to program, and from time-scale to time-scale, but again as a rough index of what is involved consider the following data:

For a population of one million at \$.05 per capita, the budget will total \$50,000 a year.

A program for a population of that size would require, say, 80–85 field workers (averaging urban and rural areas) who, at \$250 a year, come to \$20–22,000; plus 5–7 local supervisors at \$350 a year, or \$2,000–2,400; plus contraceptive supplies in the amount indicated above, or \$6–7,000; plus medical and midwife services as required (e.g., for IUD insertion), or \$3,500–5,000. That leaves, say, only about \$15,000 for transport and equipment plus this unit's share of central costs for top supervision, planning, evaluation, educational materials, etc. So this per capita figure is by no means on the high side.

The return should be the extension of effective family planning per year to, say, 12,000 women in the reproductive ages who in the absence of the program would give birth (at a crude birth rate of 40) to about 3,000 children. Since there will inevitably be some failures among new users, the cost might approximate \$15–20 per prevented birth the first year—well worth it economically, not to mention socially, educationally, politically, and personally. If effective family planning persists, and the acceptors have from, say, 1.5 to 2 fewer children on the average as a result, then each prevented birth might cost only about \$10 (or, considering some indirect and longer-run effects on others, even less).

The economic position of family planning is indicated in these figures. Even if the costs per prevented birth are double or triple these rough estimates, they are still well within acceptable economic limits when one considers the costs of supporting and educating children. There are other values in family planning besides the economic one, of course, but that condition does seem capable of being met.

Records

Every program needs to keep sound records and know where it is going—i.e., to evaluate itself. Such record-keeping should be kept to a reasonable minimum, partly in order not to burden the administrative staff with unduly complicated analyses of far too much data. What one really wants to know is: how well are we doing, with whom, at what cost, and (to some extent) why.

To begin with, someone in the central professional office should be given the responsibility of keeping a brief chronology of major events: when certain training started and ended, when the action program began in a certain area, what educational materials were used where and when, etc. This may seem an overly simple prescription but it often appears that such chronologies of what actually went on cannot be reconstructed from memories or available records. Into this diary, too, should go enlightened, informed, and responsible impressions of what is going well and badly, from whatever source. (The field workers themselves are usually a very good source of information on what is really going on, and why). Such a record can be of great utility in subsequent review of the program. Beyond that, there are some data that need to be kept systematically.

With an eye to the program's overall success, it is important to recognize that at any given time, a substantial proportion of married women in the reproductive ages are not eligible for family planning:

Currently pregnant or lactating	20–30%
Sterile or sterilized	5–15%
Currently practicing satisfactorily	5–20%
Miscellaneous reasons	5%

So something like 55% ± 15% are simply not in the market at any particular time—though the pregnant and lactating will be soon, and the currently practicing may well wish to shift from a poorer to a better method.

But even fewer are "currently eligible," because a good proportion of the eligible actively want another child now—normally, from one-third to one-half of them. So the 100% of married women in the reproductive ages quickly shrinks to a potential, short-run target of, say, around 30–35%. Thus if a program can get an additional 10% of the married women to become effective contraceptors in the first year, that represents about a third of the "currently eligible" and is an achievement of note. (An "acceptor," incidentally, should be defined not as someone who expresses interest or intention, or even someone who takes supplies, but rather as someone who is consistently practicing contraception six or 12 months later.)

Along this line, there is another important figure to keep in mind, though no one really knows just what its value is in different societies. That is the proportion of effective and satisfied family planners needed within a coherent society, or a major segment thereof, to sustain and spread the practice without the external impetus of a planned program. What is the "take-off point"? To repeat an earlier observation in this context, the program does not need to aim at everyone; on the other hand, 15–20% may be too few to generate a self-maintaining and -spreading system. Is a third enough? a half? are two-thirds needed? We really do not know—though as a rough guess two-thirds seems too high and one-third perhaps a little low. In any case, there probably is such a point, within a large but interacting population, and one should be on the watch for it, for all the obvious reasons of economy and efficiency.

As for the records themselves, in order to gauge success, one needs a numerator and a denominator: the number of effective practitioners (*not* simply acceptors of supplies or intenders) and the number of married women in the reproductive ages from they came—the target population. Neither is easy to get, but with care they can be collected with reasonable accuracy. The former figure, for practitioners, can come directly from the reports of field workers and health centers, together with source of referral but it needs follow-up to assess continuity of use. The experience is that not more than two-thirds to three-fourths of those accepting at the outset will still be practicing contraception a year later—and more often the figure is less; so the follow-up, while difficult, is necessary. (Many acceptors in any area program will come from outside the area, and hence the numerator need adjusting.)

The population figure can come from the register, wherever it exists—usually, however, with some corrections. The corrections can come only from a sample survey of the area, to be checked against the register. That survey is also needed in order to make the distinctions in eligibility discussed above—i.e., how many women are now pregnant, sterile, currently wanting another child, etc.; and in order to collect some evaluational data and personal characteristics. Here are the basics to be secured in the survey:

Name and address
Age of husband and wife
How long married
Formal education of husband and wife
Literacy of husband and wife
Occupation of husband
Rural/urban background
Modern household possessions (as index of modernization)
Number of known pregnancies
Number of live children born, by sex
Number of living children today, by sex and age
Pregnant or lactating now
Presumed sterile or sterilized (husband or wife)
Use of some contraceptive method ever, sometimes, or regularly now
Incidence of induced abortion
Knowledge of family planning methods
Attitude toward birth control
Current desire for children

Not all of these items are easy to interview for, but survey instruments available that have been successfully used elsewhere and hence provide comparison as well as guidance. In general, the tendency is to collect more rather than less information, so it is well to be explicit about how data will be used to guide the program, as a criterion for its collection.

It is almost automatic in some circles to say that any action experiment requires a control area with equivalent measurements. But that seems too general and uncritical a viewpoint. Controls are difficult to do well; they are costly; and in the absence of any additional stimulus, control areas normally can be safely assumed to be constant or slightly down in their birth rates, depending upon local circumstances. If the experimental area is not down rather sharply, then it has not been a highly successful effort anyway; small differences will not be measurable in most feasible sample sizes, and in any case they will not be important. So while controls are intellectually attractive, they should be carefully considered and not automatically applied.

Those observations have to do with evaluating a large-scale demonstration. The same kind of survey, somewhat expanded, can be done for an entire country, or region, in order to provide a baseline against which progress in information, attitude, and practice can be measured—as well as effect upon the birth rate itself. Such a survey should probably be done at the outset of any national program—partly for its evaluational use (since governmental records alone will not tell the full story, once the program takes hold), but also for its political use, in demonstrating to the elite that the people themselves strongly support the program and in demonstrating to the society at large that family planning is generally approved. Within not too large limits, the major results of such surveys can now be pretty well predicted, but they are still highly useful for their persuasive and informational impact. (Such surveys are not easy to do well, in sampling or questionnaire construction or field supervision, so some expert assistance is usually needed). As a baseline device for evaluational purposes, the survey should be repeated—the key items—every 2–3 years or so, to gauge over-all effect and with whom.

Pilot projects—i.e., small, carefully-controlled, research-monitored studies—are typically not now needed as prerequisites for a large program, in view of the accumulated experience. That is, they are not needed for substantive reasons, though they may be for political, strategic, or nationalistic reasons. Such projects normally take so long that the situation changes before they are finished, and in the nature of the case they are often both too elaborate and too inconclusive to provide major guidance for the larger program. Typically, progress will be made faster, and at least as efficiently, if the program is entered upon directly, evaluated informally as it goes along, and changed accordingly. Occasionally it will be useful to pre-test a specific idea within the context of the larger program, but it should be so planned that it can merge into the over-all operation within a matter of months. And any pilot effort should be planned with the administrative realities of the larger program in mind—i.e., it does not help much to learn how to do something that cannot then be afforded, in money or in personnel.

In short, the customary notion that small pilot projects have guided large national programs is more often wrong than right. But beyond that, to stress an important point, it is essential to recognize the economy of scale involved in implementing family planning—in developing informational materials, in training field workers, in any mass media effort, in securing the benefits of word-of-mouth diffusion, etc. In the end, of course, the program will have to be conducted "in the large"—and in most cases, given official support, it can start there too (or at least closer than is generally appreciated).

Finally, how much over-all effect is "enough"? How successful must a program be to be a "success"? Let us review some figures mentioned above:

> In a population of 1,000,000 in the developing countries, there will be approximately 145–165,000 married women in the reproductive ages.
>
> Of them about half will not be available for family planning at any given time—because of pregnancy, lactation, presumed or actual sterility, current practice, etc.
>
> And perhaps another fifth actively want another child now.

So only about a third of all married women in the reproductive ages are "currently eligible" in any six-month period, or about 40% in any year. If a program results in effective practice of family planning by a quarter or a third of this group—i.e., by 10% of the total number—that is good. So is a cost of $15 per effective acceptor, or even more.

The final criterion, wherever it can be correctly measured, is of course the birth rate itself. Lowering it by 3–4 points in a year is a major achievement; lowering it by 10 points in 5 years is a useful target, and has not yet been done. But then, nowhere in the world has there yet been a maximum effort on a large scale.

Time-Table

Such a program takes time—a lot of time. How much, will depend upon local circumstances: what priority is given to this program by the government? how large are the economic and human resources at hand? how committed are the key persons? how well organized are the available channels? how well trained are the available personnel? etc., etc., etc.

Accordingly, it is not possible to give more than a rough indication of the time-table involved. Here are some guideposts:

> It will take a year from the authorizing decision until a field team is recruited, trained, organized, supplied, and ready for work on any substantial scale.
>
> It will take another year before the major problems are worked out of the program and it settles into effective and efficient operation.
>
> It will take five years of action to make a major impact on the birth rate.

Summary

Here is a shorthand reminder, in 25 points, of what has been dealt with in some detail above:

1. Aim at the already-motivated couples, and leave the others for later
2. Start where the job is easiest: in the cities and large towns, with the better-educated and the high parity (where possible), and work out from them as soon as possible
3. Move into large-scale programs quickly, without waiting on pilot projects except for political reasons
4. Watch the semantics—make it clear that family planning is both voluntary and contraceptive
5. Use the mass media and the society's leaders to legitimize the idea of family planning
6. Space out home visits, for efficiency; and space out the areas covered, for the same reason
7. Go after post-partum women wherever possible—in rural areas through the traditional midwives, in urban centers through maternity hospitals and clinics
8. Provide information, not "persuasion"
9. Settle for any reasonable organization—if it is highly located enough to draw a first-class man as director
10. Provide family planning training to full-time field workers on the ground (as well as to part-time supporting personnel)—one for every 10–15,000 population
11. Provide incentive payments to field workers where practicable
12. Build the traditional midwives into the program
13. Pursue special publics—the military, the schools, industrial employees, etc.

14. Make the medical community informed supporters of the program, as early and as strongly as possible
15. Appreciate the importance of the contraceptive technology, in overcoming the need for sustained motivation and repeated action; and perhaps deal mainly with the IUD and the condom, at present the best female and male methods
16. Consider how much effect a sterilization effort can make, in view of local feelings and medical resources
17. Settle supply questions, as fully as possible, on economic grounds
18. Subsidize the distribution of supplies to provide a better-than-average return (including doctors inserting the IUD), and develop the commercial channels of distribution as fully and as quickly as possible
19. Aim at a budget of at least $.05 per capita per year for the normal program
20. Consider drastic changes in program if fewer than 5% of the target population become effective practitioners of family planning in a year
21. Keep careful and sound records of how you are doing, plus an informed diary of major events and judgments
22. Do a solid baseline survey, and repeat it every 2–3 years
23. Remember that you need not get at "everyone" all at once—take it in stages, for best efficiency
24. Consider that 10% of the target the first year is success
25. Finally, recognize that a major program cannot be developed quickly, allow a few years to get to peak performance, and hope that in five years or so you can reach the take-off point.

Remember that this is a preliminary set of observations on "best practice," based on experience to date. Accordingly, this document should not be taken for more than it purports to be—one observer's pragmatic effort to put the pieces together at an early stage of development.

8
Maternity Care and Family Planning as a World Program

Written with Howard C. Taylor, Jr.

The reasons for believing that family planning programs may be very effective when developed in association with maternity services are first discussed on a theoretical basis. Reference is then made to the demonstrated success of the "postpartum programs" developed in relation to organized hospital maternity services, notably in those of the group reported in this issue of the JOURNAL by Dr. Gerald Zatuchni. A preliminary survey of conditions in twenty-nine countries indicates that roughly a third of the women in those developing countries are now delivered in hospitals or under hospital supervision. They are the women to whom postpartum family planning programs might rather readily be extended. The further expansion of this means of giving birth control instruction, however, would require the simultaneous development of maternity and family planning services. The problems, including costs, of setting up such a system on a world-wide basis are considered.

The effectiveness of providing family planning instruction in association with other aspects of maternity care has received increasing recognition in the last 2 or 3 years. The results of a collaborative trial of the postpartum approach to family planning in 25 hospitals in 19 cities in 14 countries throughout the world are reported by Dr. Gerald Zatuchni in the section on "Current Developments" which appears in this issue of the JOURNAL (*American Journal of Obstetrics and Gynecology* 1968;100[7]:1028–1041).

The first results of this trial, organized by The Population Council, appear so favorable that it is necessary now to consider how far this promising instrument may be extended. In this article we shall first review the predictable advantages of a combination of maternity and family planning services, particularly as they seem to apply in the developing countries. We then proceed with a consideration of the problems that would have to be faced in the expansion of such combined services to the urban and rural sectors of the world, where maternity care itself is incomplete or lacking.

Background Considerations

Some of the special and compelling advantages of the association of family planning with maternity services are outlined in Table 8.1 and may be briefly described as follows:

Physiologic

The use of the event of childbirth to identify the physiologically most fertile women, those chiefly "at risk," is especially important in countries where facilities are limited and efforts must be concentrated at points where they will have the most effect. Ideally, for example, the effort in India should be directed not to the 500 million people or to the 250 million females or even to the 90 million women in the childbearing age, but rather to the approximately 20 million who each year demonstrate their current fertility, or even more, to the relatively small group of women, perhaps 4 million, who bear their first child in a given year and

Reprinted with permission from *American Journal of Obstetrics and Gynecology* 1968;100(7):885–893, C.V. Mosby Company, St. Louis, MO.

TABLE 8.1. Special advantages of a maternity-based family planning program in developing countries

1. *Physiologic*
   - Identification of the fertile woman: concentration of effort on the "high-risk" group
   - Lactation providing time and continuing contacts through child health clinics
2. *Educational*
   - The alternative to a lacking school system
   - An acutely favorable situation with respect to motivation
   - Susceptibility to advice from those to whom trust has been given for safe deliverance
3. *Accessibility*
   - Universality of contact after first pregnancy
   - Birth registration and dissemination of information
   - The special opportunity for beginning with women of low parity
   - Special means of reaching the indifferent or apathetic
4. *Acceptability*
   - Virtue by association
   - Effects of a lowered perinatal mortality
   - Development of a medical infrastructure
   - Availability of foreign aid

have the greatest residual potential for adding to the population.

In the absence of the needed information for delaying a second pregnancy, conception is likely to occur again soon after the first ovulation, possibly only a few weeks after delivery when the child is not nursed, or after a somewhat longer but undependable time in the presence of lactation. In any case, there may be little time to spare for delayed decisions.

The effects of concentrating on the pregnant or just delivered woman may of course be enhanced in the developing countries where the practice of nursing provides a somewhat longer "breathing spell" and the association of maternal with child care in the MCH clinics allows for continuing occasions for contact and repeated instruction in family planning techniques.

Educational

The educational impact of a supervised obstetric experience will be relatively greater where school systems are lacking and illiteracy widespread. It is clear that birth rates are difficult to influence where literacy is low, and the solution of the population problem cannot be delayed until systems of universal education are established. It appears to be a quicker and cheaper undertaking first to establish a system of education limited to the key problem of reproduction and to set this within the framework of supervised maternity.

Two circumstances make the woman at this time especially ready to listen and to be instructed in matters of family planning. The subject of the next child is clearly of great relevance to her and she will be at the peak of a fluctuating "motivational curve" toward family planning. Besides this temporarily heightened interest she will be receiving advice from the individual or the staff to whom her confidence for her safe delivery has already been given. The psychological circumstances for the reception of family planning instruction at these times are thus ideal.

Accessibility

A national program of family planning based on maternity can, in theory at least, reach every eligible woman. Antimalarial programs have to no small extent depended on the detection of cases of "fever" by door-to-door inspections by health workers. How much easier it will be to detect cases of pregnancy and to see to it that all puerperal women are provided with information about family planning. A program of supervised maternity care seems to promise an eventual organization for universal, systematized family planning instruction. As a demographic by-product of great importance, it would provide the means for setting up, for the first time in most developing countries, a valid system of birth registration.

A system that provides for contact with all women in their first pregnancy promises the special advantage of reaching two groups of women who are apt to be least likely to respond to general appeals. One is the primigravida or woman of low parity, whose early adoption of the principle of child-spacing would have the greatest demographic impact. The other is the woman who, from prejudice, indifference, or apathy, remains unresponsive to public appeals to take the step of visiting a birth control clinic.

Acceptability

The "public image" of population control will be enhanced by its association with such generally revered objectives as a lowered perinatal and infant mortality and with maternal welfare. From a more remote standpoint, a system of maternal

TABLE 8.2. Supervision of births in selected countries

Country	Approximate no. of annual births (column 1)	Births in hospitals or supervised domiciliary No. (column 2)	% (column 3)	Percentage of all supervised births that occur in hospitals (column 4)	Percentage of all supervised births occurring in hospitals with over 3,000 cases annually (column 5)
Africa					
Ghana	325,000	108,200	33	41	24 (2)*
Kenya	486,000	97,000	20	NA*	11 (2)
Liberia	56,000	6,000	11	NA	
Mauritius	28,000	16,100	58	41	30 (2)
Morocco	600,000	58,000	10	98	50 (4)
Nigeria (Federal District of Lagos only)	30,000	28,000	93	91	90 (1)
Tanzania	600,000	132,000	22	96	19 (3)
Tunisia	210,000	50,000	24	NA	66 (5)
United Arab Republic	1,280,000	447,500	35	29	25 (4)
Uganda	315,000	98,000	31	NA	28 (5)
Total	3,930,000	1,040,800	26		
Asia					
Afghanistan	580,000	9,000†	NA	NA	NA (1)
Ceylon	375,000	374,000	99	65	20 (14)
Hong Kong	93,000	88,000	95	98	35 (3)
Korea	1,015,000	10,000†	NA	NA	
Malaysia	300,000	83,000	28	NA	68 (11)
Nepal	400,000	12,000	3	33	
Singapore	55,000	54,500	99	76	80 (1)
Taiwan	401,000	300,000	75	34	1 (1)
Thailand	1,120,000	180,000	16	56	42 (6)
Turkey	1,400,000	64,000†	NA	NA	40 (5)
Total	5,739,000	1,174,500	21		
Latin America					
Barbados	6,500	3,500	54	100	
Chile	276,000	204,000	74	98	33 (4)
Colombia	780,000	255,000	33	92	60 (11)
Costa Rica	64,000	41,000	64	93	37 (2)
El Salvador	135,000	21,000	16	95	85 (1)
Honduras	100,000	20,000	20	100	50 (2)
Jamaica	67,000	47,000	70	55	35 (1)
Peru	450,000	127,000	28	74	42 (4)
Venezuela	376,500	230,000	61	95	45 (14)
Total	2,255,000	948,500	42		

*Figures in parentheses indicate number of hospitals. NA, not available.
†Includes only known hospital births; an unknown number of births also occur under supervised domiciliary services.

and infant care will build the medical infrastructure and lower child mortality—both useful for subsequent work in family planning—and aid may come more freely from international agencies and foreign countries when associated with other humanitarian purposes.

These theoretical constructions, along with practical experience, seem to provide fairly convincing evidence that an organized maternity service would be a successful vehicle for providing education and service in family planning to the uninformed people. The questions that now present themselves are those of cost and means of implementation.

TABLE 8.3. Thirteen hospitals in the cities of the developing world each with over 18,000 annual deliveries

Country	Hospital	No. of deliveries
Singapore	Kandang Kerbau Hospital	39,117
Mexico	Hospital de Gineco Obstetrica, No. 1, Mexico City	37,116*
Venezuela	Maternidad Concepcion Palacios, Caracas	35,355
Iran	Farah Maternity Hospital, Teheran	35,000 (est.)†
South Vietnam	Tu Du Maternity Hospital, Saigon	35,000 (est.)
Peru	Hospital de Maternidad, Lima	31,883
Mexico	Hospital de Gineco Obstetrica, No. 3, Mexico City	25,241*
Philippines	Municipal Hospital, Manila	25,000 (est.)
Nigeria	Island Maternity Hospital, Lagos	22,314
Mexico	Hospital de Gineco Obstetrica, No. 2, Mexico City	22,300*
Thailand	Women's Hospital, Bangkok	20,619
Colombia	Instituto Materno-Infantil Concepcion, Bogota	19,074
Colombia	ICCS (social security) Hospital, Bogota	18,313

*Includes some abortions. The other hospitals also treat some thousands of abortion cases as well, with a median of 3,500 to 4,000.
†Of which about 15,000 are cared for on an outpatient basis.

Present Distribution of Institutionalized Maternity Care

Against that brief background of the theoretical case for developing a joint Maternal Child Health–Family Planning Service (MCH-FPS), we turn to a review of what now appears to be available.

For the purpose of developing such a system for family planning, the conditions under which women in various parts of the world are now delivered must be analyzed. Although it is evident that one category passes gradually into another, one can perhaps recognize three major stages of development of maternity services. They may be listed as follows: (1) hospitalized delivery; (2) home delivery by qualified and/or supervised personnel; and (3) pregnancy and delivery with no qualified supervision.

On the basis of this classification, the means by which a maternity service can be adapted to a family planning purpose may be regarded as characterizing the phases of a continuous program, of which the first phase, that demonstrated in the postpartum program for the hospitalized case, has been so successfully begun.

The Population Council is currently in the process of expanding its postpartum program to include a number of additional hospitals,* and in connection with that expansion it has had the occasion to collect information on the current extent of institutionalized maternity care in several developing countries. The Council sent its inquiry to qualified informants in 50 countries and at this writing has received responses from 29 of them.

It is immediately evident from Table 8.2 that the proportion of all births that are professionally supervised is substantial in the indicated countries. Far from being negligible, the proportions across the three developing continents are perhaps surprisingly high: from over a fifth to under a half for this group of countries, with the median for all reporting countries at 33 per cent. Since most of the institutionalized maternity service is located in the cities and most of the population in the countryside, it follows that a much larger proportion—probably a sizable majority—of urban births in these countries is included within a hospital system.

A good start on the institutionalization of maternal care has clearly been made, particularly in the cities. At the same time, there is evidence of a wide range in the degree of development among the listed countries—indeed, almost the maximum possible range—from 3 per cent in Nepal to 99 percent in Ceylon and Singapore.

Of all the supervised births managed by or through hospitals in these countries, most are

* The Council's expansion is in two forms: (1) addition of large hospitals in "new" countries and (2) the spread of the postpartum program to a whole network of delivery hospitals within countries, covering 15 to 20 hospitals in each one, or even more.

TABLE 8.4. Distribution of maternity hospitals according to number of annual deliveries in the indicated countries of Africa, Asia, and Latin America* with a United States comparison

	Other countries				
No. of cases	Africa (10 countries)	Asia (10 countries)	Latin America (9 countries)	Total (29 countries)	United States
Over 10,000	4	8	12	24	3†
5,000–10,000	12	14	9	35	20
3,000–5,000	12	20	14	46	116
1,000–3,000	107	92	59	258	986
Total	135	134	94	363	1,125

*Includes cases of both labor and abortion. The latter amount to about 14 per cent of the total in Africa, 9 per cent in Asia, and 20 per cent in Latin America. In other words, about 1 out of 7 cases in these hospitals is an abortion case.
† Includes one university center with several hospitals.

handled with the woman actually in the hospital. In some countries, however, there are substantial proportions of supervised domiciliary births—that is, births in the home but attended by trained personnel under the direction of the hospital (column 4 of Table 8.2). In almost all of the countries of Latin America the births occur mainly in the hospital, but there are large proportions of supervised domiciliary births in the United Arab Republic, Nepal, Taiwan, Ghana, and Mauritius. In all other countries for which data are available, a majority, usually a large majority, of all "supervised" births are hospital births.

Furthermore, of all the professionally supervised births in these countries, a large proportion occur in, or under the direction of a relatively small number of hospitals (column 5 of Table 8.2). As medians, about 42 per cent of all supervised births are managed by only four hospitals in these countries. In Table 8.3 are some examples of hospitals in the developing world with large numbers of annual deliveries. Each of these handled more cases of labor and delivery than the largest United States maternity service, that of the Cook County Hospital, Chicago, with 18,003 cases. Besides these thirteen hospitals with large obstetric loads, there are many others in the developing world with very substantial numbers of annual deliveries. Most of these are institutions that specialize in Obstetrics and Gynecology.

In the 29 countries from which replies have been received, there are at least 363 with over 1,000 deliveries a year, and 24 with over 10,000 annual births (see Table 8.4). These institutions now offer a partly organized base for family planning services. For comparative purposes, we have included recent (1965) figures for the United States in Table 8.4. The contrast is sharp indeed: with a population of 200 million and annual births of 4.2 million, the United States has 1,125 institutions handling over 1,000 cases annually as against only 363 in these 29 countries with over 300 million population and 11.9 million births. In addition, the United States has 4,200 institutions handling fewer than 1,000 cases annually, with an average of about 300.

Projected Requirements

Not inconsiderable obstetric services are evidently available in the developing world, but they are largely limited to the cities and closely surrounding areas. What would be involved in extending some form of institutionalized care to the much larger population living in rural villages? As we have suggested, the theoretical case for providing family planning service in association with maternity care seems clear. The questions are the practical ones of costs and means of implementation.

In order to realize the essential but minimal requirements of a joint MCH-FPS system, what is needed? What are the necessary elements for the dual purposes of providing supervised maternity care and associating with it an effective, systematic organization for family planning? With due hesitation, in view of the great regional differences, it appears to us that there are only four.

1. An attendant should be present for all deliveries, however slight her training may be, but this

TABLE 8.5. Assumptions on the annual obstetric work load in a province of 100,000 people

Province	
Total population	100,000
Birth rate	40
Total births	4,000
District (four per province)	
Population	25,000
Annual births	1,000
Substations (four per district)	
Population	6,250
Annual births	250
First births	50
Emergencies and complications	12

attendant must be under the supervision of some regional health officer. From the family planning standpoint, such an attendant is the essential agent for instructing the woman in contraception or assuring her attendance at a birth control clinic.

2. A maternity health center for the area is needed for administrative purposes, as a station where expert medical attention is available and for hospitalization of the perhaps 5 per cent of women who develop major complications. Such a center is essential for the objective of a lowered maternal and perinatal mortality and, less directly, to elicit the respect and affection of the people so necessary if family planning advice is to be acceptable.
3. Any system of detecting, recording, and reporting pregnancy and birth must probably begin with a trained birth attendant. Such record-keeping is a step toward better obstetrics, for it is well known that the statistical reports of the early thirties guided the American obstetrician to a better system of maternity care. Beyond its contribution to maternal welfare, however, a system of reporting pregnancies and births would be critically important for assuring that information is given and for the follow-up activities of a family planning program.
4. Within the maternity center there must also be a clinic for ante- and postpartum examinations and for family planning instruction. Alternately or additionally, the center might serve as a station from which mobile units could carry maternal health and family planning services to the periphery.

The question now is whether the development of such an organization for the rural areas of the developing world is within the range of possibility.

As an exploratory exercise, we have attempted to calculate the costs of providing a system with such minimal functions for providing maternity and family planning services. We have undertaken several estimates, and the sample figures to be presented are clearly not universally applicable and do not pertain to any particular country. The data should perhaps be regarded only as illustrating a mode of thinking, but they may give some idea of the order of magnitude of the sums that would be required.

Let us first consider the probable annual burden of obstetrical care of a fairly typical rural "province" of a developing country. Assume that the "province" has 100,000 people and annual births of about 4,000. By dividing the province into four health districts and each district into four substations, we arrive at the annual load for those working "at the front" (Table 8.5). They will have about 5 deliveries a week to attend and advise, one primigravida a week to whose education special attention must be given, and one complicated case or emergency a month to refer to the district health center.

The division of functions of the provincial maternity service may be variously arranged. One plan would be the following:

The provincial general hospital would be the center for the supervision of the work of the districts. It would provide medical consultation, maintain hospital beds with surgical and nursing care for the seriously ill, and watch over the record-keeping activities of the districts. As staff it would require a full-time physician with some specialization in obstetrics and gynecology, two nurse-midwives or their equivalents, two clerks, and an ambulance driver.

The functions of the district health center would be the more immediate personal direction of the midwives in the substations and the provision of medical consultations or hospitalization for obstetric emergencies. It would receive reports of all pregnancies or recent deliveries occurring in the villages and would be responsible for seeing to it that all such "detected cases" received family planning instruction. The staffing of the district health center, with respect to maternity and family planning services, would require part of the time of a physician, who would not necessarily be a specialist in obstetrics, two midwives or health educators, one clerk, and one driver.

The substations would constitute the "front line" units providing service to the 95 per cent of the relatively uncomplicated pregnancies and deliveries. The duties of its staff would be the identification of pregnant, parturient, or puerperal women, attendance on women during labor, a postpartum follow-up visit, the reporting of births, the actual instruction of women in family planning, or her reference to the family planning clinic of the district or to a visiting mobile unit. An adequate staff to cover the estimated five deliveries per week would be one trained nurse-midwife with one minimally trained assistant.

The cost of construction for the various units needed for maternity and family planning services in a typical province of 100,000 will obviously vary widely from country to country. Construction would be simple in style and since the need for hospital beds is small, it should not be great. One estimate, arrived at not wholly without some knowledgeable advice, would be $100,000 for the construction of all units in the provincial system: the maternity section of a provincial hospital (10 beds) at $20,000; four district maternity health centers (4 beds each) at $10,000 each, and sixteen substations at $2,500 each.

Obtaining the needed personnel for such a service presents a twofold problem: recruitment and training on the one hand, costs on the other. Salaries, at least to American eyes, will be low; perhaps about $30,000 a year for all the provincial services in maternity-family planning care: one physician and a fraction of the time of four others at an annual cost of $4,000; 22 midwives at $500 each; 16 assistant midwives at $300 each; 6 clerks at $500 each; and drivers, maintenance personnel, and others at a total of $5,700. To this annual amount for salaries, one must add another item, taken here to be $10,000, for consumable medical supplies, food, and other commodities for maintenance and replacement. According to these assumptions the annual cost of running a provincial maternity-family planning program of this type, serving a population of 100,000, would be of the order of $40,000 or $10 for each woman delivered.

It is appropriate again to caution that these calculations are only rough estimates, striving only for an order of magnitude, and will no doubt vary greatly from place to place. But it is also proper to recognize that, as these estimates are applied to national programs, a cost-diminishing factor will come into play, based on existing facilities that do not need to be constructed and existing staff whose salaries do not need to be added as part of a new budget.

Having arrived at approximate figures for costs of construction and of annual operation for maternal health and associated family planning facilities in a typical unit of 100,000 people involving 4,000 annual deliveries, we can simply multiply to make estimates of what it would cost to set up and serve larger units. As examples, for India, the estimated bill would be $500 million for construction at most and $200 million for annual operation; for all of Latin America, perhaps $250 million and $100 million, respectively. The program of a country of 5 million population would cost $2 million a year for operating (not including construction); a country of 25 million would cost $10 million. For the entire developing world, a population of, say 2.2 billion, the operating cost would be $880 million annually. Because the figures used are related to the total population of these areas and in many countries substantial facilities for maternity care already exist, these estimates of additional financial costs may well be excessive.

For comparative purposes, the food supplied to these countries in recent years is of interest. The value of food shipments by the United States under Public Law 480 alone over the past 5 years has been relatively stable at about $1.5 billion annually (3). A more comprehensive estimate appears in Volume II of the report of the President's Science Advisory Committee Panel on World Food Supply (3) in the statement, "Under Food for Peace $2.5 billion of United States agricultural commodities have been distributed annually to less developed areas."

Again we stress the figures we are offering as the cost for setting up and operating maternity-family planning services in the developing world are only tentative. What we may have arrived at is not a "world budget" but an indication of an order of magnitude of what the cost might be to set up a system that could perhaps be in position in 10 years and which, on the basis of theoretical reasoning and some practical experience, might be expected to contribute greatly to the solution of two great problems—maternal welfare and population growth. What is now needed is a detailed study of several regions where maternity services are in various stages of development. We need to know actual costs of construction, problems of transportation, availability of personnel, training facilities, political obstacles. The beginning of such an investigation, in several more or less typical areas, is now being made under the joint supervision of the International Institute for the Study of Human Reproduction and The Population Council.

This study, we hope, may produce a blueprint for action. Such a plan need not be exclusive, but could provide at least a central guiding line of direction. The development of family planning programs through the simultaneous establishment of maternity services would then be the strategic basis for a general plan, supplementing present efforts.

The allocation of funds for population control has not paralleled the superlative statements made by responsible persons on the importance of the problem. We are accustomed to hearing that modern man lives under the two great threats of nuclear war and population growth. Predictions are freely made as to when various regions will be facing mass starvation.

Perhaps one of the reasons for under-expenditure, in the face of the high assessment of the urgency of the situation, is the lack of understanding as to how money may be spent. In a program for associating maternity service with family planning we may have in our hands the basic framework, "a grand plan," for a coordinated world effort. If after some further study a consensus can be reached that this is in fact a highly promising way in which to proceed, the needed financial support can hardly fail to be given.

References

1. The Population Council: International Postpartum Family Planning Program. Report on the First Year, Studies in Family Planning No. 22, August, 1967.
2. Taylor, Howard C., Jr.: Am. J. Obst. & Gynec. 95: 726, 1966; *and in* Family Planning and Population Programs, Chicago, 1966, University of Chicago Press, pp. 433–441.
3. Report of the President's Science Advisory Committee: The World Food Problem. Report of the Panel on the World Food Supply, Washington, D.C., 1967, United States Government Printing Office, vol. II, pp. 82 and 144.

9
18–35 in Place of 15–45?

At any point in history, the task for mankind is to manage human reproduction in a rational manner—that is, to make the reproductive means fit the valued ends in an acceptable way. The management will be exercised or defaulted in the individual event by the partners involved, but they will be strongly guided by expectations, norms, customs, pressures, laws—by social judgments, that is, of what is right in this place and time.

Such judgments vary over the world today as they have varied over the centuries. In the long view, there can be discerned two truly historic trends. The first is the trend from the large family to the small family that accompanies the long-range trends from agriculture to industry, from farm to city, from subsistence to prosperity, from illiteracy to education, from woman's subordination to equal status, from infant and child mortality to survival. The second is the trend to make reproductive decisions on the basis of the child's welfare rather than on such traditional considerations as maternal gratification or paternal *machismo* or family lineage or economic asset or ethnic prestige or military strength or political power. The first trend is still unfulfilled in most of the world; the second is barely visible.

Because of the increased interest in population problems during recent years, there has been a growing discourse about the social and philosophical issues involved in the matter. That is all to the good, especially as it tends to make reproductive behavior more conscious, more deliberate, on balance more rational. This little essay seeks to contribute to the discourse by exploring a hypothetical situation that would voluntarily cut the natural period of childbearing in half.

The period of reproductive capacity for the normal woman is, say, the thirty years from age 15 to age 45. Suppose that by common agreement children were born only to women between ages 18 and 35—or, in the developed world, between 20 and 35: in short, suppose a socially defined period of childbearing of 15–17 years in place of the biologically natural period of about 30 years. Consider the potential benefits for mothers, for children, and for the community at large if no children were born to women below 18 or 20 or above 35.

If motherhood were confined to such an age band, that would in itself lower maternal mortality by a substantial amount—maybe as much as 20 percent.* Regardless of the absolute levels, mater-

Reprinted with permission from *The Population Council Annual Report 1971*, pp. 19-27, The Population Council, New York, NY.

*The reader will appreciate that the data here and elsewhere are by no means firm, but they are to my knowledge the best available approximations and are probably correct by order of magnitude, if not in every detail or value. A technical review of the literature is now being prepared by my colleague Dorothy Nortman for subsequent publication by the Council, and this statement is partly based on that material. Her review will suitably document, elaborate, and qualify, including where possible the relationship of mother's age to such other factors as parity, socioeconomic status, and father's age. I also acknowledge the contribution of a

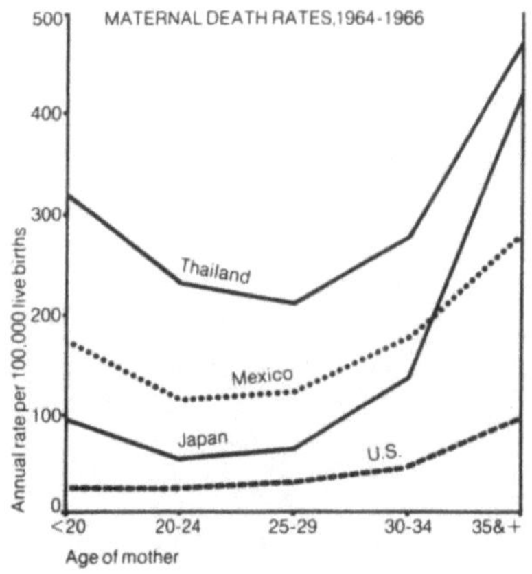

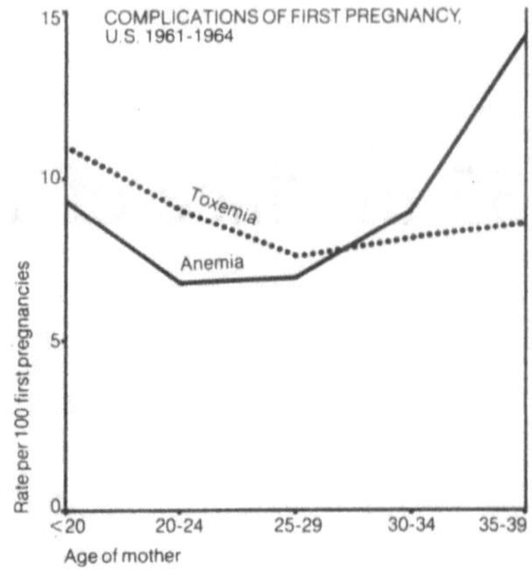

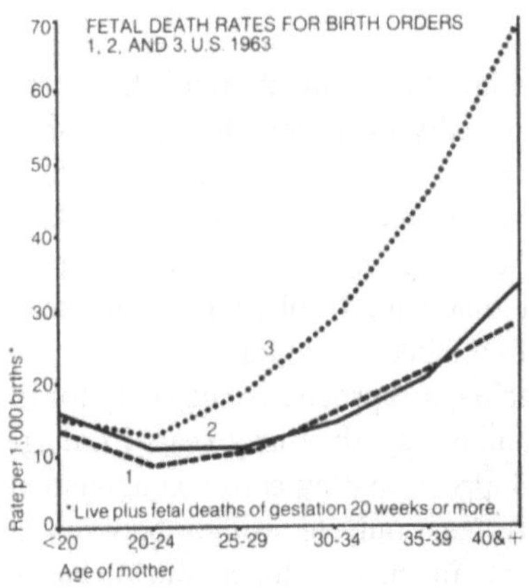

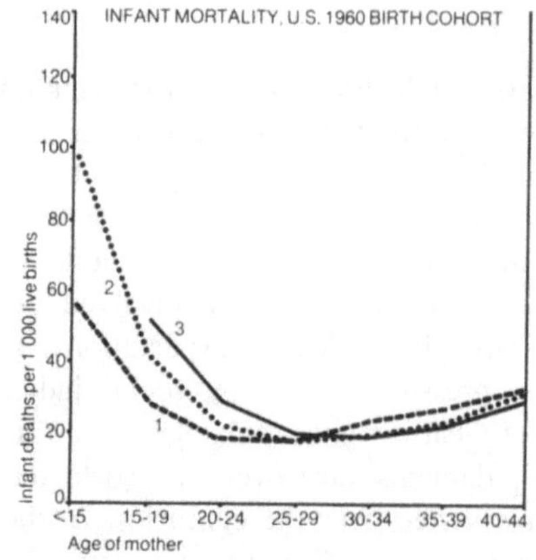

nal mortality is typically somewhat higher at the lower age, minimal in the middle years, and substantially higher at the upper ages—in some developed countries as much as four to seven times higher above age 35 as at ages 20–29, in developing countries (where the rates are higher) only two to three times as much.

A similar picture emerges with regard to certain medical complications of pregnancy. For example, in the developed countries anemia is higher among younger mothers and toxemia higher among older mothers; and in a few developing countries where data are available, the rate of complicated deliveries is higher below age 20 and much higher above age 35.

In general, then, maternity is somewhat more difficult at the younger ages, simply on medical grounds, and substantially more difficult at the older ages. What about the child, or more precisely, the potential child? What does mother's age mean for him? Here too the prospects are rather better for children born to mothers in the middle years: the children are more likely to be born alive and to be born normal.

From the beginning of pregnancy through the first year, the new life is more likely to survive with mothers in the middle age band. Again the familiar curves appear:

- for fetal death, or the spontaneous abortion of pregnancy

paper prepared for the Commission on Population Growth and the American Future by Jane A. Menken, Office of Population Research, Princeton University, on "Teenage Childbearing: Its Medical Aspects and Implications for the U.S. Population." Most studies, incidentally, break the age groups at five-year intervals so that the youngest group is typically "under 20"; presumably the under-18 group would on the average deviate even more on most factors.

- for perinatal mortality, or death from the 28th week of pregnancy through the first week of life (including still-births)
- for neonatal mortality, or death in the first month
- for infant mortality, or death in the first year.

In these cases there are complementary tendencies: a larger risk to fetal life at the older ages of motherhood and a larger risk to infant life at the younger ages, with a correspondingly smaller risk in the middle years in both cases. Indeed, postponing first births from the teens into the early 20s would have a most pronounced effect on infant mortality in the United States.

Normality of the child is also affected by mother's age. Prematurity and low birth weights—with such attendant disabilities as epilepsy, cerebral palsy, mental retardation, deafness, and blindness—are particularly high at the younger ages; and congenital abnormalities are more frequent among children of older mothers. In general, then, with regard to both mothers and children, biological nature does seem to indicate a "preferred" age-range for childbearing—roughly speaking, the first birth in the early 20s, the second and third births in the later 20s and early 30s.*

All of those are medical and biological consequences. What of the psychological implications of the mother's age? Here the data are not strong; despite the obvious importance of learning what characterizes a good parent, including age, we know very little on a scientific basis. There are some indications that IQ deficiency is related to low birth weight, which itself correlates with mother's age, but on the whole evidence is lacking.

But that does not end the matter, since experience and judgment must also be relied upon in social decisions. If there is one unmistakable sign of unwanted pregnancy, it surely must be induced abortion. Under the liberalized New York State law in the first months, about 19 percent of all legal abortions to state residents were performed on women under 20 and another 10–11 percent on

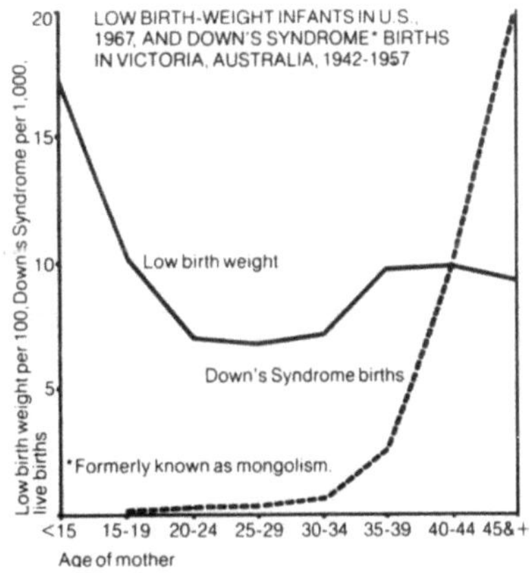

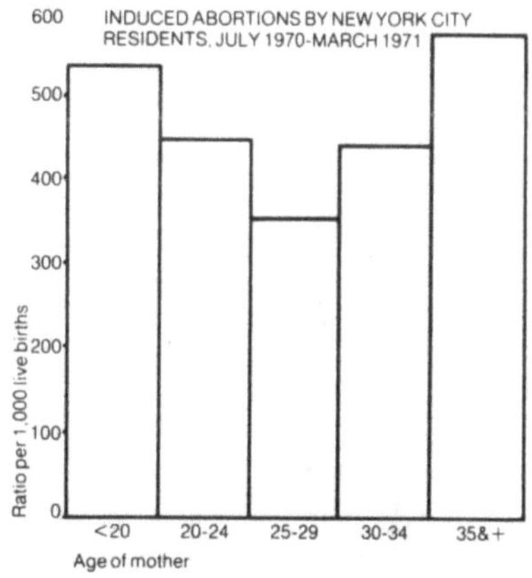

women 35 and over. Actually, the ratio of abortions to live births is highest for just these groups—in itself testimony to social pressure against childbearing at those ages. Along the same line, and with poignant consequences for the innocent children, about 25 percent of all illegitimate births in the United States occur to women under 18 and nearly 50 percent to women under 20. As someone has observed, "the girl who has an illegitimate child at the age of 16 suddenly has 90 percent of her life's script written for her. . . . Her choices are few, and most of them are bad." The whole life may be restricted, with no period of independence between reliance on the parental family and responsibility for one's own, not to mention the limited opportunities for education and employment.

Such considerations suggest the psychological burdens and sequelae of childbearing. Are American girls of 16 or 17—or, for that matter, 18 or 19—really ready to become mothers, with all the

*An on-the-scene report from some Chinese cities in early 1972 by Dr. Anibal Faundes of the University of Chile notes that "pathologies of pregnancy appear very infrequently. The most evident explanation is that most pregnancies occur in the most favorable age groups. It is unusual to find a primipara less than 23 years old or over 30, or a multipara more than 32–33 years old."

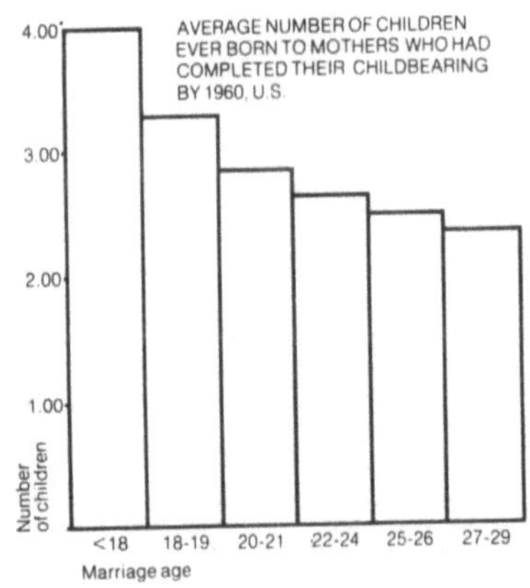

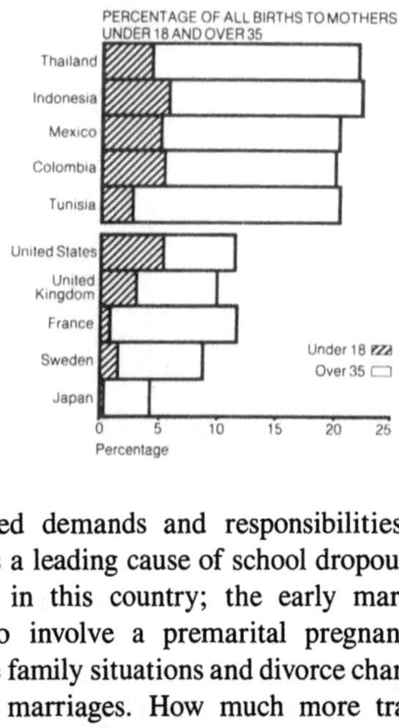

associated demands and responsibilities? Pregnancy is a leading cause of school dropout among females in this country; the early marriage is likely to involve a premarital pregnancy, and unstable family situations and divorce characterize teenage marriages. How much more tragic the outcome if based upon a casual sexual encounter leading to pregnancy and then to a premature, legitimating marriage, with burdens on the child still ahead. In many cultures around the world, is it right to expect the child of 15 to become a wife at 16 and a mother at 17? Do most women of 36 and over, allowing for compassionate exceptions, have the patience and energy to raise a child who then will not become independent until they are in the mid-50s and beyond? For many poor women throughout the world, surely 20 years of producing tissue, milk, and children should be enough–20 years of the "maternal depletion syndrome" that leaves them old before their time. At both the lower and the upper range, the lives of the mothers are particularly ruled by the fact of birth for a long period of years, with alternatives closed off or at best deferred–especially because such mothers tend to be disadvantaged on other scores as well.

So there do seem to be important benefits for those most closely at issue, the mothers and the children. The differences may not always be great, in absolute terms, but neither are they trivial, particularly for those involved. As for the community at large, it benefits not only from their improved physical and mental health, but also from the reduction of birth and growth rates.

In the United States today, 12 percent of all births occur to mothers under 18 and over 35–about half to each group:

	Percent of U.S. births			
Age	White	Black	Other	Total
Under 18	4.3	14.3	3.9	5.8
Over 35	6.2	6.1	6.1	6.2
Both	10.5	20.4	10.0	12.0

The over-35 contribution is remarkably similar across racial categories; the under-18 births are unduly concentrated in the black community where they constitute a genuine burden to the efforts at improving the quality of life, for both the mothers and the children. If the cut-off age is raised to under 20, a considerably larger portion of the births is included: a total of over 23 percent, with about 17 percent of all U.S. births occurring to mothers under 20. Actually, the proportion of all births occurring to women below 20 and above 34 has been essentially constant in the United States for the past 50 years–around 25 percent. But the two age classes have changed their contributions: the below-20 group has increased from 9 percent in 1920 to 17 percent in 1968, probably reflecting increases in both fecundity and sexual activity; and the older group has decreased, from 16 percent in 1920 to 8 percent in 1968. Thus the balance has shifted toward the young. In recent years, one out of every four women in this country had given birth by her 20th birthday, and nearly one out of ten by her 18th birthday. And the earlier childbearing begins, the shorter the birth intervals and the larger the total number of births.

In other developed countries, similar proportions of all births occur to mothers at the extreme age ranges—say, 10 percent plus or minus a few percentage points. But in the developing countries, the fraction is much larger, of the order of 20 percent. In both cases, more births are accounted for by the older group, and substantially more in the developing countries: somewhat more reproduction occurs there in the earlier ages but much more beyond age 35.

In the world as a whole, then, about one in every seven births occurs to mothers under 18 and above 35, or about 18–19 million a year. The figures become one in five, or 25–26 million births, if the lower age is under 20. Those births would not necessarily be eliminated if mankind were to follow the indicated pattern, because some births would alternately be encompassed within the 18–35 age range. Many births, in other words, would simply be transferred to a "legitimate" age, either delayed or anticipated. There is no sure way to calculate the outcome; the issue is highly complicated by the counter-effects of lengthening the duration of the generation at one end while shortening it at the other, the counter-effects of later childbearing against health benefits that could improve fecundity.

But, on balance, there would probably be a decline in total fertility if the 18–35 range were observed. It is hazardous to estimate the amount, but as an order of magnitude it would appear to be a significant decline that might in itself lower the birth rate of the typical developing country by five to eight points off a birth rate in the 40s per thousand population per year, lower the birth rate of the typical developed country by half what is needed to achieve a replacement fertility, and bring the world's birth rate from its present level of about 35 per thousand down to about 30.* The outcome will not "solve the population problem" but it will help, and in the process it will contribute to human welfare.

Any such idea cannot be fully realized in the short run: human reproduction is too closely tied to a whole set of cultural prescriptions to change easily or quickly. But in all probability a good deal of reproduction at the young and old ages is not really wanted—is the product of indifference, fatalism, tradition, ignorance, inaccessibility of means. To the extent that is the case, an effective alternative in behavior is needed more than a new consensus in attitude.

For the rest, however, the question is whether the idea deserves consideration and discussion, as a contribution to the future. *Some* social norms are going to guide voluntary reproduction; which are they to be, community by community?

The issue is by no means a simple one, bound up as it is with such profound and delicate matters as the place of women within a society or the legitimacy of sexual behavior outside marriage. If women in traditional societies may not marry at 16 and start their own families, what are they to do instead? If religious and moral doctrine forbids sexual expression except in marriage, or even except in the service of reproduction, what impact would the deferral of even a few years have upon the structure of such beliefs or upon their observance?

These are not easy matters. But these are not easy decades for mankind either. In earlier times, high fertility was required for human survival in view of high mortality rates. Today that has changed in much of the world, soon in most of the world, and perhaps irrevocably so. Today a new ethic toward childbearing is needed, a new rationale to suit the new conditions, a new effort to expedite the going trends.

The idea of concentrating human reproduction in the "best years" for childbearing may have

---

*According to Menken's calculations for the United States, "if, at the 1968 level of population and age-specific birth and death rates, no births occurred to teenagers under 18 and we assumed this reduced the birth rate among 15–19 year-olds by 30 percent, the population in 50 years would be 5 percent smaller than if the teenage birth rates remained constant. If all births to teenage mothers were postponed, 75 percent until ages 20–24 and the remainder until 25–29, the population would be 6.6 percent smaller. If all teenage births were eliminated, the result would be a population 15.1 percent below the size projected with unchanged rates. The net reproduction rate would be reduced from 1.16 to just over the zero population growth target of 1.00. It seems reasonable to speculate that if postponing of first births also reduces the rapidity with which successive ones occur, birth rates at older ages might also be reduced by postponing a large proportion of teenage births."

much to recommend it. If no children were voluntarily born to women below 18 or 20 or above 35, the benefits to mankind, and especially to womankind, would appear to be considerable. The idea promises an amelioration of both individual and societal concerns at minimal costs in personal freedom. It is certainly good for both mother and child on medical grounds and it is probably good for both of them on psychological grounds as well. It would tend to reduce the number of large families, with their attendant disabilities to the children. It would contribute to the broad goals of economic development and women's status. It would be based on an informed guide to reproductive behavior in place of tradition and sometimes ignorance. Finally, it would help, in a humane way, to meet the problems of population growth throughout the world. In a situation of great personal investment and great social consequence, the idea may have merit as a rational response to the new demographic situation in which man now finds himself.

Part V – Contraceptive Technology

10
The Impact of New Technology

Under what conditions can an addition to the present technology of fertility control have a measurable demographic impact and what are the central characteristics of the required technology?

This paper tries to examine fertility control requirements into the foreseeable future, with regard to the characteristics of the methods themselves, the delivery systems, and the target populations. There is some discussion of the magnitudes involved, the three broad means by which fertility control can be pursued, the three key ways in which the technology can be improved and their relative merits, and the time frame within which tomorrow's contraceptives must optimally be sought.

In short, the paper tries to answer the question: how much better must the system be for given effects of fertility reduction in developing societies, in what ways, and when?

In this review of contraceptives of the future, it is up to the other speakers to say what is biomedically possible, likely, safe, and effective for the individual user. And as a social scientist, it is up to me to say what is demographically needed by society. I do not propose to deal with what specific methods of fertility control we need to produce, but I will try to identify the required characteristics of a fertility control system that will have demographic impact under field conditions in developing countries. How can a new technology of fertility control contribute to fertility reduction, in what magnitudes, in what ways, in what time?

Reprinted with permission from *Proceedings of the Royal Society of London, Series B* 1976;195(1118):25–35, The Royal Society, London, England.

In the developed world, today's technology readily achieves a low fertility outcome. Thus modern man can achieve close to demographic stabilization under conditions of low mortality with the present technology of fertility control. In this sense, no additional contraceptives for the future may be needed on demographic grounds. But this 'modern man' exists in only 30% of the world, and it is the other 70% that is my primary concern here.

The other 70% of the world's population has 85% of the total births. In order to lower the birth rate of the developing world by 10 points (i.e. 10 per 1000), from around 40 to around 30, would require averting over 25 million births a year. Not that a crude birth rate of about 30 is the end of the line; after all, the developed world's crude birth rate (c.b.r.) is now about 17 and that is still 13% above replacement. But lowering a high birth rate by 10 points within, say, a decade, would be a notable achievement under current conditions; moreover, that would be a reasonable signal that the fertility transition is on. Empirically, the practice of fertility control is associated with the crude birth rate within the following range: 5–10% current contraceptive practice is associated with a c.b.r. of 40–50, as in Morocco, Ghana or Ecuador; and 60–70% practice is associated with a c.b.r. of well under 20 as in the United States and Western Europe. On that scale a 30% level of current practice is associated with a c.b.r. around 30, and 2 points of additional use means 1 point off the birth rate. I take that '30/30 rule' as my touchstone for the following exercise.

The question now becomes: how can a typical developing country move to (or beyond) the 30/30 state and where do contraceptives of the future fit into that prospect?

Three Ways to Increase Fertility Control

What can a developing society do to reach or better 30/30? For our purposes here, it is convenient to reply that there are three channels by which to extend and/or improve the practice of fertility control in such a society: (1) increase or intensify the motivation for fertility control; (2) enlarge or improve the delivery systems of fertility control, typically the national family planning programs; and (3) enlarge or improve the technology of fertility control. The first works on the demand side of the equation, the other two on the supply side.

Increasing the demand is at once the most effective yet the most difficult. We know that modernization itself will in all likelihood bring a fertility decline, but that makes the end the solution of the means and basically begs the question of how fertility reduction can be brought about in the absence of and in order to facilitate modernization. Short of full modernization, some few components in combination may do the trick—infant mortality below 50, two-thirds of the children in primary and secondary schools, less than 30% of the labor force in agriculture, per capita income of $500 a year, 30% of women of reproductive age in salaried employment outside the home. But we do not know just what the thresholds of determinants are in particular cultural regions and even if we did we could not achieve them readily or quickly or cheaply. And short of affecting the fundamental determinants, how can the demand for fertility control be increased? There are not many ways: currently under experiment is the short cut of incentives in money or in kind, with at best indeterminate results so far; propaganda is uncertain; legal remedies through age at marriage or social security are extremely difficult to organize and administer; community pressure or even governmental imposition may be the only means in the short run but that has it own costs, perhaps prohibitive in nonrepressive societies.

Improving delivery systems is easier, though not easy. There is a long way to go. According to a recent compilation, in only two or three developing countries are all five means of supplied fertility control generally available, and that availability falls off quite rapidly (Mauldin 1975). These supplied methods are the pill, the intra-uterine device, the condom, sterilization and abortion, in contrast to other methods that require no drug, device or service, like the rhythm method or withdrawal. Across the world a variety of delivery systems are being used: the private sector, the commercial sector, fixed and mobile clinics, combined public/private coupon systems, professional field agents, village-based field workers, nonmedical distribution systems, post-partum programs, maternal and child health or nutrition or community development programs with family planning 'integrated' within them, and perhaps a few others. Their effectiveness depends not only on the latent demand in the particular setting but on governmental regulations and requirements, administrative and infrastructural capacities, funding, logistics, personnel, and personalities. Such delivery systems can be substantially improved but as my mentor used to say, if we learned this afternoon that prayer was an effective contraceptive, we still would not be able to deliver the message where it counts the most.

The third channel is to improve the methods of fertility control to be delivered, in order to overcome deficiencies in demand and in program. If both the latter were 'adequate' no further improvements in fertility control technology would be needed demographically in order to achieve a low birth rate. As we have noted, the present technology of fertility control is more than satisfactory for that job, given appropriate demand and delivery, though 'it is unlikely that any population has ever attained a low level of fertility without the use of induced abortion' (Tietze & Bongaarts 1975). But neither demand nor delivery exists sufficiently in many developing countries at need. In the developed world, demand and delivery take care of whatever may be the current deficiencies in technology; in the developing world, can technology take care of some of the deficiencies in demand and delivery, in motivation and in program?

Three Ways to Improve the Contraceptive Technology

Just as there are three channels by which to extend the practice of fertility control, so there are three ways in which the technology itself can be improved: (1) improved effectiveness, (2) improved continuation, and (3) improved acceptance. Thus the overall impact would be heightened (1) if those who practiced did so with greater success and fewer failures, (2) if those who practiced did so for longer durations and with fewer dropouts or discontinuations for method reasons, and (3) if the methods had more intrinsic attraction for more people to whom they were available, or as a special case of importance, if they were so distinctively attractive as to stimulate the extension of the delivery system itself (on the ground that 'we now have something we can sell'). Naturally, these three are interwoven in real life, but they can be conceptually differentiated for our purposes here.

First, *effectiveness*: we already have quite high effectiveness rates for at least four of the five modern methods listed above; moreover, if induced abortion is available, effectiveness need not be especially high. Even under field conditions the major methods do not fail very often while being used properly (Ryder 1973), and a recent analysis (see Table 10.1) showed that improved contraceptive effectiveness from 90% (the level of the condom) to 98% (the level of the IUD) would make only a small demographic difference in societies which practice below the 30% level—only 3 or 4% points in its effect on the total fertility rate, at best. Effectiveness counts for more in high-use populations, but even then it only amounts to about 15 points at the extreme. And in family size (limiting after 2 children), at 30% use the difference between 90% effectiveness and 100% is only about one-third of a birth in the total fertility rate (t.f.r.); it takes about 85% use to make a 1-birth difference. Accordingly, in the societies at issue, I conclude that improving the effectiveness of contraceptives beyond present levels would have little demographic impact, and hence from that standpoint is not worth much.

TABLE 10.1. Percentage of total fertility rate per woman when couples use contraception only, by level of family limitation (after two live births) and by contraceptive effectiveness (adapted from Tietze & Bongaarts 1975)

Proportion limiting	Contraceptive effectiveness 90%	95%	98%
0	100	100	100
20	89	87	86
30	83	81	79
70	60	54	50
80	55	48	43
100	43	35	29

Continuation is a different story. In developing societies, continuation of present methods varies quite widely by social setting, by programmatic effort, and by age-parity of acceptors as well as by method. These ranges cover most of the major cases: for new acceptors of oral pills, from 35–70% continuation per year, or say 55% as a benchmark figure; for new acceptors of IUD from 55–80%, or say 70%; and for sterilization, only 95% (not because of surgical inefficiency but because, given their age level, about 5% of sterilants move out of their fecund period each year). Figures for condoms are not generally collected because of the system of distribution; and figures for repeated abortions (would that unduly extend the notion of continuity?) are not readily available.

Unlike effectiveness, marked improvement in continuation, as measured by method, would make a significant difference to fertility. In one analysis, a hypothetically improved contraceptive was compared to the present mix of contraceptive methods in the developing countries (roughly one-third pill, one-third sterilized, one-sixth IUD and one-sixth others; no abortion) as measured by the impact on fertility over five years as against no contraception. The improved contraceptive was defined as 100% effective with 5% discontinuing for side effects or personal idiosyncrasy and another 5% for wanted pregnancy, or a continuation rate of 90%. In that analysis the present mix results in 29% as much fertility as no contraception and this improved contraceptive in its place results in 21%, not an

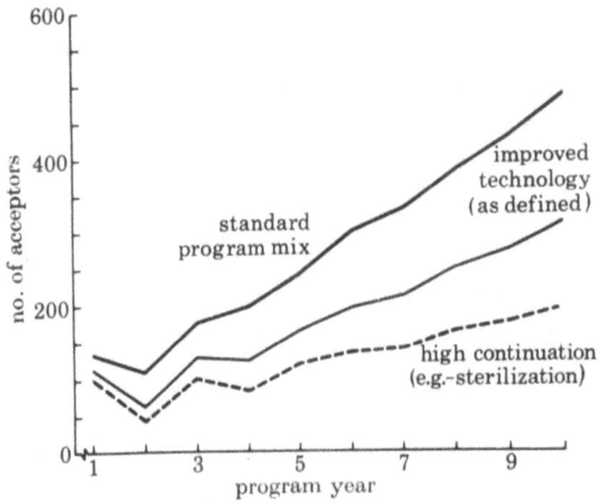

FIGURE 10.1. Annual number of contraceptive acceptors to reduce crude birth rate linearly from 45 to 35 in 10 years; illustrated for three contraceptive mixes, standard age pattern for acceptors (initial population of 2500 married women). (Adapted and extended from Nortman & Bongaarts 1975.)

overwhelming difference because the improved substitutes for sterilization and thus loses some continuation in the process. If it substitutes only for the pill, IUD, and others, in other words, if the continuation is 90% in place of 55–70%, then fertility is only 14% or about half the standard mix, which is a substantial improvement (Nortman & Sivin 1973).

Similarly, a current simulation model compares a hypothetically improved technology with sterilization on the one hand and a standard mix on the other. In this case, the improved contraceptive has a complex definition but essentially represents an increase in continuation to 75% per year in the youngest ages and 95% in the older. As measured against the acceptors required for 10 points off the c.b.r. in 10 years (Figure 10.1), that technology does not do as well as sterilization but does substantially better than the current standard. Specifically, by year 10 the improved technology would require only two-thirds as many acceptors as the standard mix in order to achieve the same target (Nortman & Bongaarts 1975).

As for *acceptance*, obviously the more of that the better, other things being equal. The other things include not only effectiveness and continuation and user characteristics, but substitution: if a new method of fertility control simply substitutes for an

TABLE 10.2. Equilibrium in use, with different combinations of acceptance and continuation (%) (calculations courtesy of Anrudh Jain and Harold Nash)

Continuation rate per year	Acceptance rate per year: 15%	10%	5%	3%
95	75	67	50	38
70	33	25	14	9
55	25	18	10	6

old one (including abortion or withdrawal), the demographic impact is nil. As new methods have been introduced into family planning programs they have tended to attract another layer of users, but often on the basis of programmatic change as well as a method innovation (Freedman & Berelson 1976). However, the latter has stimulated the former, as perhaps demonstrated most dramatically in the way the loop stimulated the early Taiwan and Korean efforts.

Trade-Offs

At the high levels of effectiveness that characterize the pill and the IUD, upwards of 95%, the main gains have come not in improved effectiveness but in extended use, through continuation and/or acceptance. What is the nature of that trade-off?

As method continuation increases, it lowers the need for acceptors in order to meet a given target; as acceptance increases, it takes the pressure off continuation. Together, the two move toward an equilibrium of use at some point (Table 10.2). The range is great, from a plateau of 75% to one of 6%; there is a sharp fall-off from very high continuation and a moderately sharp one below 10% acceptance; and the equivalences are reasonably clear (e.g. 10% acceptance with 70% continuation as against 15% acceptance with 55% continuation to achieve the level of 25% use; and so on). At the crucial level of 30% use (here in a constant population), 10 points of continuation is the equivalent of about 4.5 points of new acceptance; at 20% use, the trade-off is 10 points of continuation for 2.5 points of acceptance, and at 40% for 6.5 points of acceptance (Figure 10.2).

Or, looked at another way, how long would it take to reach 30% use (in a constant population) at

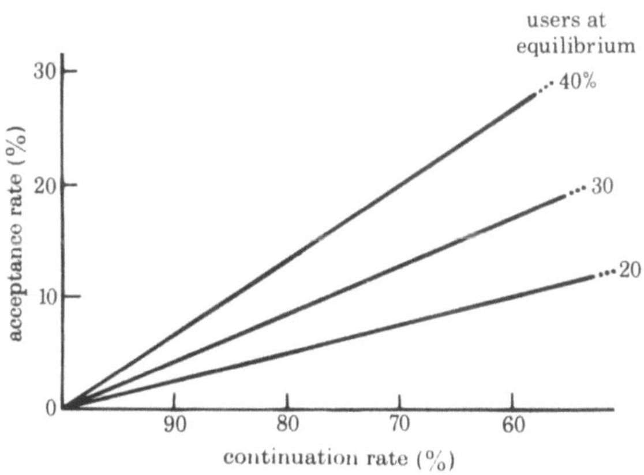

FIGURE 10.2. Acceptance rates and continuation rates corresponding to different percentages of users at equilibrium. (Calculations courtesy of Harold Nash.)

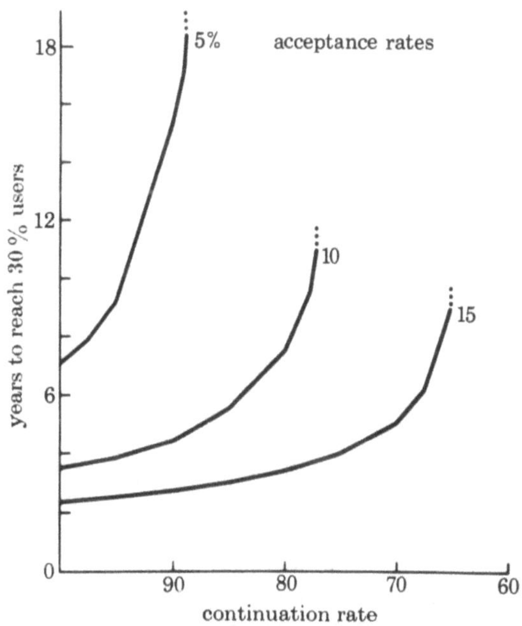

FIGURE 10.3. Time in years to reach 30% users. (Calculations courtesy of Harold Nash.)

different acceptance and continuation rates (Figure 10.3)? A low acceptance rate (5%) would never make it with less than 88% continuation (which only sterilization can now achieve); a high acceptance rate (15%) will make it in a reasonable time with any continuation rate above 65% or so.

Moreover, to extend the analysis one step further, Table 10.4 is an approximation of the joint effect on the crude birth rate after 10 years, from a simulation model with realistic assumptions for developing countries (including standard age structure of acceptors, 5% constant non-program use, 2.5% increase in target population per year). Again the importance of acceptance (among non-users) as compared with continuation is clear under these conditions. Note that it takes high acceptance combined with high continuation to take 10 points off the birth rate. At 5% acceptance and 70% continuation the effect on birth rate is, by the normal standards in such settings, barely measurable. Moreover, the effect plateaus at about those levels. That is, continued performance at those rates just holds its own, for as acceptance builds up so does discontinuance, not to mention the load of new entrants into the system.

Thus, given the normal range of performance and a reasonable time period, improved effectiveness beyond present levels does not matter much demographically; improved continuation does matter, especially as it approaches 100%; and improved acceptance matters most.

Now let us confront these hypothetical numbers about what is required for the 30/30 state with actual figures of performance in national family planning programs. Table 10.3 shows the current range in the official efforts of 36 developing countries by developmental status (demand) and by strength of program (supply); that is, our first two channels for affecting the practice of fertility control.

Note these few points: the range in absolute values of acceptance, from 2 to 15% with an average per country of under 7% (which if weighted by population size falls to 4%); the 7:1 ratio between the doubly-favored and the doubly-deprived corners of the tabulation; the lack of a strong program in a low or even a moderate setting.

We begin to appreciate our predicament anew when we consider Tables 10.3 and 10.4 together: the top figure in the 3% column (Table 10.4) approximates India today and the bottom figures Egypt, Kenya, Pakistan, Bangladesh, Mexico and Nigeria; the 70–55% continuation and 10% acceptance represent Thailand, the Philippines, Sri Lanka and Colombia; 70–55% continuation and 15% acceptance, Taiwan and South Korea. It will take decades for the major low-setting countries to

TABLE 10.3. Acceptors (1973) as percentage of estimated non-users: Country means, by social setting and program effort (adapted from Freedman & Berelson 1976)

Program effort	Social setting: High	Middle	Low	Total
Strong	14.8	–	–	14.8
Moderate	8.5	7.0	6.6	7.1
Weak	6.5	3.1	1.8	2.5
Total	12.7	5.6	3.0	6.7

TABLE 10.4. Points off a crude birth rate of 40 in ten years, with different combinations of acceptance and continuation (%) (calculations based on converse model, courtesy of Dorothy Nortman)

Continuation rate per year	Acceptance rate per year: 15%	10%	5%	3%
95	18	13	7	5
70	9	6	3	2
55	7	5	2	1

move to high social setting and consequent increase in demand; and it would take a monumental effort for the needy countries to strengthen their programs in the absence of the kinds of infrastructural improvements inherent in that higher setting. And if they could, what would the yield in acceptance be likely to be? An extrapolation to the upper right-hand corner of Table 10.3 yields, say, 8% at most, yet at that acceptance a year it would require 84% continuation to reach the 30% level of use in about a decade. At 5% acceptance, not yet attained and perhaps the most these critical countries can expect in sustained performance over the next years (compulsion absent), continuation would have to be nearly 90%. In short, if continuation is at roughly the IUD-pill level, then acceptance must be at the highest level that the most favored countries have achieved to date, around 15% per year, in order to reach the 30% level of use. Such numbers underline the importance of the single-act-plus-high-continuation of sterilization in India, where the logistical and motivational problems of continuation are severe: wherever acceptance is that low, continuation had better be very high.

As presented, this analysis is limited to method-continuation though fertility control depends on person-continuation; the same analysis would apply as well there, and the amount of switching of methods points to the need for redundancy in the system. Nevertheless, it does begin to elucidate how the contraceptives of the future are to be judged by demographic standards. Demographically, improving continuation of a method by 10 points within the current range is worth more than the entire acceptance level today in the largest, most needy countries. From their standpoint, which is easier: to get twice as many acceptors or to improve continuation by 5–10 points? If a new method could do either one, that would double the demographic impact where it is most needed.

Continuation is of course not solely the function of the technology: far from it. Increasing demand or intensifying motivation would surely make for better continuation, and improving programmatic administration might do it (e.g. better follow-up for pill users, approximating the kind of support provided by private physicians in the developed world). Ironically, however, the harder a program is pushed, the less continuation it tends to achieve since on average it reaches more marginal users. But acceptance and continuation depend on the desire to control one's fertility as well as on the character of the method. At the same time, as a colleague of mine suggests, continuation rests in part on when the user can first decide to discontinue: with sterilization, never; with an injectable 1–3 months or more; with the IUD, say a few weeks; with the pill, a day. That is why the potential implant or vaccine may be able to show a major advantage over pill and IUD: greater continuation with the same effectiveness and acceptance.

As a way of thinking about the matter demographically, then, will the contraceptives of the future attract at least 5% new acceptors a year (non-substitutional) and/or yield an additional 10 points in continuation over the present methods? This is not to mention the possibility of a new method losing ground by not attracting enough additional users to compensate for lower continuation, precisely the concern of Taiwan and Korea in introducing the pill into an IUD program, necessitating careful preliminary trials and limited offers (e.g.

under 30's, IUD dropouts). If not, its demographic utility is dubious. And if so, how many such methods a less-than-strong program can administratively absorb remains a question, though since not many are likely, perhaps only an academic one. In the next 5 years, are we more likely to gain a method or lose one?

Resources and Time

In conclusion, let us add to our consideration two key factors, both limited: resources and time.

All three channels are now moving in the right direction. Modernization is occurring throughout the developing world, but slowly: do we wait for that to 'solve' the problem of population growth through fertility reduction? If so, we need improvements in neither program nor technology. Programs are improving too, but slowly and unevenly: should we wait for them to carry the existing technology in a more effective manner, limited only by the socio-economic threshold? And the technology is improving, but that too is slow: nothing really new in 10–15 years and probably not for another 5–10 years. The easy answer, and the correct one as far as it goes, is to work on all three simultaneously, as we now do. As rough orders of magnitude so far as external assistance is concerned, it is customary to say that 98% of the resources now go into the developmental setting and 2% into 'population'. And of that 2% about half goes into family planning programs and a tenth into biomedical work. That is how the resources have come to be allocated over the years, but is that the rational allocation of resources?

That judgment needs to be made against our conception of the time required. If by these standards the contraceptive of the future were to be ready for program use tomorrow, it would be worth a great deal; if it were ready only 50 years from tomorrow, it is worth far less of today's resources. In principle, the longer it takes to produce the new, the less value it has (assuming we do not lose methods in the interim).

So there is a large trade-off in process among our initial three channels: if by the time the contraceptive of the future arrives, the social setting has sharply increased the motivation for fertility control or the programs become much more efficient, then it will have correspondingly less demographic effect and hence be less needed. In that case, the present technology will suffice. Thus there is an important discount rate that needs to be calculated. At what time, between now and the decades ahead, are the contraceptives of the future worth how much, from a demographic standpoint?

Acknowledgments. I have been engaged in exploring this matter in an informal committee of The Population Council and am much indebted for their instruction and assistance to John Bongaarts, Anrudh Jain, Harold Nash, Dorothy Nortman, John Ross, Bruce Schearer, Christopher Tietze and Walter Watson. This is in some respects a collective product, though I am fully responsible for this particular manifestation.

References

Freedman, R. & Berelson, B. 1976 The record of family planning programs. *Studies in Family Planning* 7, no. 1.

Mauldin, W.P. 1975 Assessment of national family planning programs in developing countries. *Studies in Family Planning* 6, 30–36.

Nortman, D. & Sivin, I. 1973 Fertility effect of improved ('perfect') contraceptive technology. Memorandum.

Nortman, D. & Bongaarts, J. 1975 Contraceptive practice required to meet a prescribed crude birth rate target: a proposed macromodel (TABRAP) and hypothetical illustrations. *Demography* 12, 471–489.

Ryder, N.B. 1973 Contraceptive failure in the United States. *Perspectives* 5, 133–142.

Tietze, C. & Bongaarts, J. 1975 Fertility rates and abortion rates: simulations of family limitation. *Studies in Family Planning* 6, 114–120.

Part VI – Assessment of National Family Planning Programs

11
The Record of Family Planning Programs

Written with Ronald Freedman

Preface

In the past 15 years or so, increasing numbers of developing countries, assisted by the international community at interest, have adopted policies to reduce rapid population growth. That effort has included a wide range of activities, but the major direct action has consisted of family planning programs intended to lower fertility rates. In recent years, such programs have come under more and more questioning, if not criticism; and that trend may have culminated in the World Population Conference at Bucharest, August 1974, which refrained from a strong endorsement of such programs although family planning was included within the "Recommendations for Action" of the World Population Plan of Action.

The value of family planning programs may currently be under debate on the international scene but at the same time both developing countries and donor agencies continue to allocate significant resources and funding to such programs. So while family planning programs are under some attack, they still occupy the center of the stage of population action. As such they warrant another look at the record at this time—which also happens to be precisely a decade after the first, and historic, International Conference on Family Planning Programs (the "Geneva meeting" of August 1965, reported in *Family Planning and Population Programs: A Review of World Developments*, University of Chicago Press, 1966).

As we point out several times in the text itself, neither data nor research techniques are fully adequate to this task: the former are incomplete and often questionable, the latter are insufficient for many critical issues. Still, many determinations on population policy now in controversy rest on the appraisal of such programs, so the attempt must be made—aiming for the best answers currently possible, not the definitive ones.

This report is based on the available scientific literature plus some original analysis for the purpose. As close participants in some of the history and close observers of the whole, we undertake this account of the facts of the matter and the policy conclusions to which they speak. We have both attempted such appraisals in the past, and we have both been closely identified with such efforts; nonetheless, we attempt here a comprehensive and objective and fair evaluation. At this stage of the matter, hardly any qualified observer would be completely free of the charge of prior bias. In any case, the report will stand on its merits.

Introduction

As countries have sought to deal with the "population problem" of rapid growth, they have focused on reducing fertility. As countries have sought to reduce fertility, they have focused, in large measure, on providing easier access to modern means of

Reprinted with permission in an abridged form from *Studies in Family Planning* 1976; 7(1):1–40, The Population Council, New York, NY.

fertility control through family planning programs. How if at all have such programs affected fertility?[1] What have they done and not done to change demographic trends in the participating areas? We deal primarily with the period 1960–1975, within which most family planning activity has been carried out in the sense used here.

In what sense? What is meant here by family planning programs? We refer to organized programs – mainly governmental in sponsorship, support, and administration, but often involving private efforts (family planning associations) and occasionally commercial ones – designed to provide the information, supplies, and services of (modern) means of fertility control to those interested. Such programs frequently have a persuasional component as well, advocating the small-family norm, but that element is not strong. Usually the programs more or less accept existing levels of motivation and seek to meet the existing "need" by minimizing the cost of fertility control not only monetarily but personally, by legitimizing the idea and by providing services through trusted sources.

The family planning program takes a variety of forms in the real world: (1) it can include all or only a few of the five major supplied or programmed[2] means of fertility control (oral contraceptive, IUD, condom, sterilization, abortion); (2) it can give more or less attention to the "creation of demand" in addition to facilitating supply, typically through informational efforts; (3) it can encourage or not encourage supplementary efforts through private and/or commercial channels; (4) it can provide or not provide special inducements in the form of incentives and disincentives, monetary or in kind; and (5) it can be administered via a variety of delivery systems (fixed or mobile clinics, postpartum, local agents, full- or part-time field workers, private doctors, camps for sterilization, incorporation in broader systems of maternal and child health, and a few others). And in scope, it can cover, or intend to cover, the whole of a country, as in a national family planning program, or only a limited sub-area thereof, as in a pilot, experimental, or demonstration program. So it is well to remember the variety that exists around the world: different programs, different forms.

The distinguishing key is that family planning programs work primarily on the supply side of the behavioral equation. As for demand, the family planning rationale (1) takes that as more or less given at a particular time, and/or (2) considers that the most realistic way to extend motivation is to satisfy existing motivation, and/or (3) addresses motivation through symbolic appeals ("education" or "propaganda") rather than through basic social and economic changes in the society, and/or (4) believes that legitimizing family planning in this manner will tend to make latent demand manifest, and/or (5) considers that motivation will build with the process of historical modernization now being sought in the developing world and that minimizing supply problems will significantly facilitate the total process.

The supply/demand equation is close to the heart of the controversy over family planning programs. Is there "enough" existing motivation (demand) to make for a significant fertility decline if it were met (supply)? Can something worthwhile be achieved by reducing the number of "unwanted" pregnancies or must the "wanted" be dealt with as well? How much effect can the easing of supply make in the demand situations that characterize traditional as against modernizing societies? It is such questions that are addressed here, along with some attention to possible alternatives. We do not deal with other questions involved in the full controversy: for example, family planning policy as "a substitute for population policy," or the political motives for international assistance to family planning programs, or the symbolic importance of family planning programs as "neocolonialism," or the rationale for reduced fertility as contributor to welfare ends.

Over the past decade, as family planning programs have emerged as the major action deliberately undertaken to reduce fertility rates in developing countries, a number of criticisms have been made of their efficacy for that purpose. Since family planning is a key element in the current effort to slow population growth in such countries, the criticisms need to be noted:

- that whatever family planning can contribute to fertility decline is insufficient to the need
- that observed declines in the presence of family planning efforts would have occurred anyway, in a trivially longer time
- that family planning can perhaps accelerate an

existing decline, slightly, but cannot initiate one in a traditional society
- that family planning can "work" only in relatively advantaged societies, where it is less needed
- that family planning can "work" only among the relatively better-off sectors of a developing population, who would soon come to it anyway, but not among the uneducated rural masses that make up such countries
- that family planning programs can perhaps "skim the cream" of available motivation in such societies but cannot generate motivation and hence have no staying power
- that expressions of interest in family planning found in fertility surveys are not valid indicators of subsequent behavior
- that current norms as to family size leave little room for family planning interventions toward fertility decline
- that family planning interest, such as it is, is found too late in the reproductive career to make much difference from a demographic standpoint
- that for the various reasons above a new contraceptive technology will not make much difference either
- that only a massive social and economic transformation and the attendant structural changes can bring about the necessary decline, in the absence of state impositions.

These are serious criticisms, seriously made.[3] We do not organize this report to address them one by one, but they do underlie and inform the subsequent description and analysis of the record.

The demand side of the equation is usually reflected by fundamental social and economic characteristics of a society. The sharp differences in birth rates between developed and developing countries—below 25 or even 20 in the former, 40 and above in the latter—reveal a strong association between fertility and what is referred to as "modernization," that is, better health, widespread education, higher material standards of living, nonagricultural employment, emancipation of women (into roles alternative to childbearing), lessening of familial and kinship ties relative to secular institutions. Moreover, the fertility decline of the West was initially achieved without family planning programs—indeed, generally in the face of institutional and governmental opposition—and without modern means of fertility control. Accordingly, is it reasonable on historical or comparative grounds to expect much effect from manipulating the supply side of the matter?

Unfortunately, the historical record is too ambiguous to provide firm guidance on the question. To begin with, the early nineteenth century West and the late twentieth century Third World are sufficiently dissimilar to limit easy generalizability from the one to the other.[4] At the least, today's empirical record would seem to take precedence over the historical and cross-cultural inference. Beyond that, however, the closer one looks the less definitive the historical record is on this point. The pre-conditions for substantial and sustained fertility reduction—what are coming to be called the thresholds—are not at all firmly established in the sense that one can say that specified levels of certain social characteristics, or combinations thereof, lead to a fertility decline of a specified magnitude.

There is no question that from a long perspective, broad developmental changes and fertility declines go together, but that is not conclusive in assessing trends and policies in the current perspective of a few decades. Teitelbaum has recently summarized the evidence as follows:

> When the available data on the 19th-century decline in European fertility are analyzed on a systematic basis, some major propositions of transition theory are empirically supported, but only those at a high level of generality. From a broad macrohistorical view it is correct to say that in the two centuries from the mid-1700's onward there were widespread and substantial declines in marital fertility which were associated with major social and economic transformations in European societies. However, the more specific and explanatory propositions derived from transition theory cannot explain all of the salient features of the European experience. In particular, the theory fails to explain fundamental phenomena such as variations in pre-transition levels of fertility and in the timing of onset and the pace of the fertility decline which eventually became universal.[5]

Teitelbaum's summary is based mainly on the findings of the European Fertility Study of more than 700 areas of Europe, which finds instances of fertility declines where they should not have occurred according to the theory and instances of sustained fertility where it should have fallen. For example, the modern fertility decline in Bulgaria began when infant mortality was high and most of the population were illiterate peasants. Fertility decline in parts of France began before the spread of industrialization and urbanization and prior to or simultaneous with the declines in mortality, whereas the declines in Germany and England began only decades later when most relevant development indicators were much higher.[6] "Hungary provides a remarkable proof of the possible adoption of increasing degrees of voluntary control of marital fertility in the absence of any fundamental modernization of the underlying socioeconomic structure."[7]

There is also increasing evidence of fertility patterns implying voluntary control of fertility in parts of Europe long before the modern fertility decline.[8] On the other hand, for example, in some of the Soviet Socialist Republics birth rates are currently high (and may even have increased since 1926), although development and mortality decline have been considerable.[9]

As the European Fertility Study of the transition in several hundred local areas of Europe has shown, many areas that are culturally similar (for example, in language or on an ethnic basis) have also moved together with respect to fertility, either more or less rapidly than other areas in the same countries, without reference to the socioeconomic developmental indices central to transition theory. This suggests that barriers to diffusion *across* cultural lines and channels for diffusion *within* cultural groupings were operating so as to affect the adoption of birth control, one way or the other. Such cultural factors may reflect structural elements not captured by the conventional development indicators, but they may also indicate communication barriers and channels that may need to be overcome or utilized by family planning programs. In any case, as Teitelbaum points out: "Unlike much of 19th century Europe, most modern developing countries have the administrative and technological infrastructure (for example, central planning and administration, widespread publications in multiple languages, improved transportation, telecommunications, radio and T.V., and postal systems) to enable them to better permeate such barriers."[10]

In short, there is some indication that something more than mechanistic effects from developmental variables are at work. In his most recent overview of the comparative experience in Europe, Ansley Coale, Director of the European Fertility Study, concludes that:

> our re-examination of the demographic transition gives no clear indication whether or not birth control programs in countries at an early stage of modernization can be successful . . . There is no convincing basis for asserting that a program . . . would inevitably be a failure in a rural poorly educated population.[11]

In sum, the position is widely held that family planning programs cannot "succeed" in the absence of considerable social change of a modernizing character and are unnecessary in its presence. But the historical and comparative record, insofar as applicable, seems to leave room for debate on the matter and certainly for policy judgment. Accordingly, we here take the empirical position of seeking to determine under what conditions family planning programs of various characteristics and strengths have achieved what results.

Which returns us to our central concern: what is the record?[12]

Program and Performance

As of 1973, 32 of 117 developing countries had official policies to reduce population growth rates, typically implemented through family planning programs (Table 11.1). The 32 countries – 19 in Asia, 7 in Africa, 6 in Latin America – are only 28 percent of all developing countries but they contain 75 percent of the total developing world population. Another 31 countries (26 percent of all developing countries and 16 percent of the total developing world population) provided official support to family planning activities for expressed reasons other than demographic. Thus, for whatever reasons, family planning programs have been established by countries with the large majority of the population of the developing world in a relatively short time, as a novel ingredient in the developmental mix. Whatever their demographic impact, they have had sufficient attractiveness to win acceptance from societies and governments of varied characters as the policy of choice with regard to fertility reduction. Two points about this array: (1) Virtually all of the larger countries of the developing world are included: only two countries with populations over 25 million are missing—Ethiopia and Burma; (2) The policies are quite recent in adoption, with median dates of 1967 for the first column[13] and 1969 for the second; and since implementation does not follow immediately on adoption, many of these programs are still quite young. In addition, in the past decade or so, there have been a number of experimental and demonstration programs, roughly 40 of them of some consequence.

Our appraisal of the performance of such programs begins with two measures:

1. new acceptors in 1973 as a percentage (a) of all married women of reproductive age (MWRA, usually age 15–44) or (b) of the residual target population, that is, MWRA minus those already practicing fertility control at the time, from whatever source (and unless otherwise noted, acceptance refers to new acceptors throughout); and

2. program users as a percentage of all MWRA; program users are those who, at a given time, are using a method of fertility control provided by the family planning program, that is, acceptors modified by continuation rates over time. Acceptor data are typically provided by the service statistics collected by the program; MWRA data are estimated from census figures; the residual target is estimated from MWRA derived from demographic sources, prevalence information provided by sample surveys, and continuation rates derived from clinical and field studies.[14]

We say that the appraisal begins with these two measures because beyond them are further measures that are still more difficult to secure, on technical grounds—not only the effect on "averted births" or on fertility measures (in one sense[15] the objective) but also the thorny twin issues of the substitution effect (to what extent would the observed fertility behavior have occurred anyway, in the absence of the program?) and the indirect effect (to what extent did the program stimulate fertility control that was then provided from nonprogram sources?).

What national family planning programs have done in recent years, operating under real-life conditions, is illustrated in the following tabulation

TABLE 11.1. Developing countries, by family planning policy and population size, as of 1973

Population (millions)	Policy to reduce growth rate	Support to family planning, nondemographic reasons
100 and above	China India Indonesia	Brazil
50–100	Bangladesh Pakistan Mexico	Nigeria
25–50	Philippines Thailand Turkey Egypt South Korea Iran	
15–25	Colombia Morocco Taiwan	South Africa Zaire North Vietnam South Vietnam Afghanistan Sudan Algeria
10–15	Sri Lanka Kenya Nepal West Malaysia	Tanzania Venezuela Uganda Iraq Chile
Under 10	Ghana Tunisia Dominican Republic Hong Kong Laos Singapore Jamaica Trinidad & Tobago Mauritius Botswana Fiji Barbados Gilbert & Ellice	Cuba Khmer Ecuador Rhodesia Guatemala Mali Bolivia Haiti El Salvador Honduras Dahomey Paraguay Nicaragua Costa Rica Panama Liberia The Gambia

Source: Dorothy Nortman, "Population and family planning programs: A factbook," *Reports on Population/Family Planning*, no. 2 (6th edition, December 1974), Table 8, pp. 26–35.

limited to these first two measures, and thus representing a first cut at appraisal:

1973 Acceptors as percentage of: Residual target (MWRA minus users)	All MWRA	Country	Program users as percentage of MWRA	All users as percentage of MWRA
15.7	8.9	Taiwan	21	55
14.9	6.9	Hong Kong	27	55
13.4	9.5	South Korea	24.5	30.5
9.5	7.1	Thailand	17.7	24.8
7.9	5.7	Colombia	14	31
3.7	3.0	Egypt	16.8	20.5
3.2	2.7	Mexico	1.0	13.1
1.6	1.5	Morocco	2.4	6.2

Source: Dorothy Nortman, "Population and family planning programs: A factbook," *Reports on Population/Family Planning*, no. 2 (6th edition, December 1974), Tables 16 and 22, plus necessary calculations.

Perhaps the most striking element in that illustrative tabulation is its range—from about 15 percent of the residual target or 10 percent of all MWRA down to 1-2 percent; from about 25 percent program users down to a percent or two; from countries in which the program directly accounts for most contraceptive practice to countries in which it accounts for well under half. Thus, under current conditions of political will, social readiness, administrative capacity, professional interest, fertility control technology, and available resources—under such realistic conditions, that is about what such programs can do, or at any rate have done. These are the limits of performance for this period: from 1-2 percent of the target up to 10-15 percent per year, from a small cumulative percentage of practitioners of family planning up to 20-25 percent within the program. And once a program has "reached its level," there is a certain stability to such performance—contrary to some early expectations that it would quickly "skim the cream" of motivation and then decline. Here, for example, are data on program acceptance from the residual target, in percentages, for a few representative programs:

	1969	1970	1971	1972	1973
In two stronger programs					
Taiwan	9.0	14.0	18.0	16.0	16.0
South Korea	17.0	18.0	15.0	13.0	13.4
In two weaker programs					
India	2.0	u	2.7	3.0	2.6
Egypt	3.5	4.8	5.1	5.6	3.7
In three growing programs					
Thailand	2.7	4.5	8.3	9.7	9.5
Philippines	–	–	7.0	10.0	11.0
Indonesia (Bali)	1.0	3.7	7.1	11.0	12.9

Source: Indonesia (Bali) from *SFP*, April 1975; % of MWRA, fiscal years; others adapted: Dorothy Nortman, "Population and family planning: A factbook," *Reports on Population/Family Planning*, no. 2 (6th edition, December 1974). u = Unavailable.

Programs seek to bring together acceptors and methods. We review them in some detail before turning to overall performance.

. . . By Acceptors

Although the characteristics of acceptors vary from country to country, acceptors tend to be older and to have more children than the average married women of reproductive age (MWRA) (see Tables 11.2 and 11.3). For example, the median acceptor in most countries has three or more living children and is aged 27–30 years. In a country with high fertility and little birth control, it is not surprising that interest in family planning begins to arise when the couples are under demographic pressure, that is, when they have all or even more than the children they want, often in the middle or late childbearing years. This was also the general pattern when birth control was initiated during the early period of the demographic transition in Western Europe.

Are acceptors, then, too old and with so many children that their birth control practice can have little effect on their own or their country's fertility? The answer is generally "No," but the argument is not all one-sided. Certainly, some late-beginning acceptors might have had no more children, even without birth control. This is particularly a problem in the case of incentive programs, since some couples who are sterile or too old to have a demographic motive may accept contraception just to receive the incentive. For example, a significant minority of the program sterilizations in India may have represented such a response by couples unlikely to have more children.

However, the argument that the program reaches only older women (e.g., over 30) and of higher parity (e.g., over three) and that therefore program acceptances are of doubtful demographic importance appears not to be well founded, as the following observations indicate:

1. In most developing countries a large proportion of births occur to women over age 30 and are of fourth and higher parities. Preventing a substantial number of those births can have and has had a substantial effect on overall fertility. For example, between 1961 and 1970, 79 percent of the decline in total fertility in Taiwan was the result of lower birth rates for women over 30. Among 17 developing countries with total fertility rates of 5,000 or more (i.e., roughly equivalent to 5 children per woman), the total fertility accounted for by age-specific birth rates of women aged 30 or older ranged from 34 percent to 45 percent with an average of 40 percent, according to a recent UN publication. In an earlier UN study with data for 37 high-fertility countries, the total fertility attributable to birth rates of women at ages 30 and over averaged 41 percent.[16] A large part of the difference in the birth rates for the developing and the developed countries is a result of more higher-parity births in the developing countries, usually but not always to older women. For example, it has been calculated that if all births beyond the fourth (30 percent of the total) were averted in India, the birth rate would immediately drop about 10 points, from under 40 to under 30.[17] Women with higher-parity births (especially if they are still relatively young) are likely to be more fecund than the average, and thus capable of producing many more children. Adoption of birth control can prevent additional higher-order births.

2. Even if the median age of acceptance is 30 or the mean parity is four, this still means that a substantial minority of acceptors are in prime reproductive ages (e.g., 25–30) and with fewer than four children.[18] The median of the tabulated medians is just about 27 years. Moreover, in some populations, younger and lower-parity women

TABLE 11.2. Wife's median age among acceptors, by contraceptive method

Country and year	All methods	Orals	IUDs	Sterilization
Colombia 1973	26.2	25.4	26.5	
Dominican Republic 1972		24.1	25.9	
Ghana 1973		28.8	30.7	
Hong Kong 1972	26.5	25.5	29.5	
India 1970			32.8	34.5
Indonesia 1973	28.7	28.3	29.4	
Jamaica 1973	24.1			
Kenya 1970		28.0	29.3	
South Korea 1972			32.8	34.2
West Malaysia 1972	27.4	26.7	30.0	33.5
Mauritius 1969	26.8			
Mexico 1973		27.8	27.8	
Philippines 1973	29.5	28.9	29.0	
Singapore 1973	25.3	24.4		
Sri Lanka 1973	28.6			
Taiwan 1972		28.8	29.6	
Thailand 1971		29.5	29.2	
Tunisia 1972			30.9	
Turkey 1971			29.2	

Source: Nortman (1974), Table 20.

TABLE 11.3. Median number of living children among acceptors, by contraceptive method

Country and year	All methods	Orals	IUDs	Sterilization
Colombia 1973	2.9	2.7	2.9	
Dominican Republic 1972		2.7	3.5	
Ghana 1973		3.9	4.4	
Hong Kong 1972			2.9	
India 1970			3.4	M 4.0 F 4.4
Indonesia 1973	3.2	3.0	3.5	
Jamaica 1973	3.0			
Kenya 1970		4.1	4.8	
South Korea 1972			3.6	3.7
West Malaysia 1972	3.1	2.9	4.1	5.6
Mauritius 1969	3.2			
Mexico 1973		3.7	3.7	
Philippines 1973	3.3	3.2	3.5	
Sri Lanka 1973	3.3			
Taiwan 1972		3.0	3.2	
Thailand 1971		3.4	3.6	
Tunisia 1972			4.3	
Turkey 1971			3.4	

Source: Nortman (1974), Table 21.

TABLE 11.4. Percentage currently using contraception by education for married women aged 20–39 years

Country and year	Wife's education: No formal	Primary	Junior high	Senior high and over	All wives	Number of cases
Ankara[a] 1966	22	43	53	65	37	552
Calcutta 1970	21	44	47	65	40	947
India 1970	8	19	*	36	12	10,246
Korea 1971	20	24	24	26	24	1,620
West Malaysia 1966–67	4	11	23	39	9	4,242
West Malaysia 1970	12	19	29	36	18	13,449
Mexico City 1971	5	21	45	47	24	486
Philippines 1968	10	15	21	32	17	25,604[b]
Taiwan 1967	26	33	45	51	32	4,300
Taiwan[c] 1970	39	43	60	63	44	2,491
Thailand (urban) 1970	30	43	50	47	42	1,080
Thailand (rural) 1969	6	14	–	–	13	642

Note: See Appendix 1, item 6 of the source publication for definitions. Sterilization included as contraception.
– = Fewer than 20 cases in the category.
* = No such category.
[a] Defined as "ever used contraception."
[b] Frequency weighted: urban respondents multiplied by 4 and rural respondents multiplied by 12.
[c] Taiwan 1970 data refer to ages 22–39.
Source: Ronald Freedman and Lolagene C. Coombs, *Cross-Cultural Comparisons: Data on Two Factors in Fertility Behavior* (New York: The Population Council, 1974), p. 61.

have had average or higher than average acceptance rates. In Bali, for example, in 1973–74 acceptance rates were highest at age 25–29, and 55 percent of all acceptors were women under 30. Between 1971 and 1973 the Balinese acceptors with fewer than four children increased from 43 percent to 57 percent.[19]

3. In countries with trend data, there has been a significant shift downward over time in the age and parity of acceptors.[20]

Nevertheless, it is undoubtedly true that fertility reductions would be greater in most circumstances if most of the acceptances came at young ages and low parities. In developing countries, where mortality is still moderately high, replacement fertility will be more than two children for a time. For example, with a female life expectancy of 50 years a total fertility rate of 2,840 is required to produce a net reproduction rate of 1.0.[21] However, in order to attain permanent zero-growth fertility levels with low mortality, it is obviously necessary for the average couple to have about two births, and this leaves little latitude for many higher-order births if most couples want at least one child (as they do). But in developing countries with average completed parities near six, a reduction to three or four by eliminating higher-order births is clearly a move in the right direction. With the possible exception of some parts of China, we have no examples of a sudden shift from six to two children. A move from six to two is likely to pass gradually through four, so programs that can help reduce the average parity to four make a substantial contribution to reduced fertility.

Do the family planning programs reach only or predominantly the more "modern" couples, for example, the better educated, wealthier, and more urban? Although systematic data are lacking for many countries, most of the evidence available for most countries indicates that the more modern couples have rates of contraceptive practice significantly above average—for example, the better-educated (see Table 11.4). In general, the less contraception is practiced within a society, the more it tends to be limited to urban and better-educated groups, to an elite. In some countries, however, while the more modern couples are likely to find and use fertility control first, through their own resources, a family planning program appears to bring contraception to the less modern and more disadvantaged who may wish to limit fertility but apparently need the organized program effort to bring them information services and to legitimize the idea.

Thus, in Taiwan and Korea, while it is true that the practice of contraception is positively related to being "modern," the acceptance rates in the program do not differ consistently by such criteria and in some cases the rate of acceptance is greater for the more traditional strata. (That is now the case in Bali as well.) For example, in 1968, when Taiwan's family planning program was in full swing and the Philippines' had not begun, the educational level of women of childbearing age in the Philippines was substantially greater than that in Taiwan, but the practice of contraception was greater in Taiwan at every educational level and age; at that time, women with no education in Taiwan had a higher rate of contraceptive practice than the upper educational stratum in the Philippines. Similarly, while urban Thailand had a higher educational level than Taiwan in 1970, rates of contraceptive practice were lower at most educational levels. Moreover, the Taiwan program narrowed the educational gap over the years: in 1965 the proportion who had ever practiced contraception ranged from 19 percent with no education to 60 percent with senior high school or more, whereas in 1973 the equivalent figures were 71 percent and 79 percent.[22] The recent decline in fertility in Taiwan is mainly attributable to a decline in marital fertility for women at each educational level, rather than to a significant improvement in educational levels. In such places as Taiwan, Korea, Bali and East Java, a large majority of the acceptors are rural, poorly educated, and poor, because these are still the largest groups in the population, so even if acceptance rates in these groups are lower than those in the more advanced strata, the predominant proportion of acceptors will come from the disadvantaged sectors.

Nor is it at all clear that a fundamental modernization of the family must precede the widespread adoption of birth control to avert high-parity births. In Taiwan, large-scale adoption of contraception has occurred while traditional familial values and practices persist. For example, the proportion ever using contraception among women aged 35–39 is very little different whether the women hold traditional or "modern" familial attitudes: whether the parents chose the husband (69 percent) or the wife did (75 percent), or whether the wife expects to live with her married sons all her life (67 percent) or never (78 percent). A majority of the Taiwanese couples still live in extended households with the husband's parents and/or married brothers if those relatives are alive; they place a high value on male heirs; and so on—but they still practice fertility control.

In many countries a significant number of couples say they want no more children but are not using birth control[23] (see Table 11.5). Such responses are regarded by some as indicators of a large potential demand for family planning services, by others as an invalid response to superficial surveys. The truth probably varies with circumstances, which will only become better known as a result of follow-up studies in contrasting situations, but a number of observations can be made:

1. This is not a universal response. The fact that there are relatively few such respondents in some African countries where mortality and desired family size are both very high may confer greater credibility on responses in, for example, Asia. The response does not appear to be a simple reflex of respondents giving the interviewers what they think the interviewers expect of them.

2. There are denominator problems that tend to magnify the apparent discrepancy. At any time, when *X* percent say they want no more children but are not practicing, that *X* contains a proportion of sterile or presumed sterile (about 5 percent), of currently pregnant (perhaps 15 percent), of women in postpartum amenorrhea or with husband absent (probably over 10 percent)—all of whom are not at need. The discrepancy is clearly there, though not so great as normally inferred. In India, for example,[24] about 40 percent of MWRA say they want no more children but are not practicing; of them one-fifth, or 8 percent, are subfecund, perhaps an equivalent proportion is currently pregnant and a substantial part of the remainder, or 18 percent, do not know a single method of fertility control—leaving only, say 6–10 percent "in contradiction."

3. Women who say they want no more children but are not using contraception are not necessarily giving an invalid response. The response to a single question about an attitude (e.g., how many children do you want? or, do you want more children?) is, in probability terms, a modal sample response

TABLE 11.5. Percentage of all wives who want no more children and are not currently using contraception, by wife's age

Area and year	Wife's age				All ages	Number of cases
	20–24	25–29	30–34	35–39		
Ankara[a] 1966	26	36	28	37	32	552
Calcutta 1970	13	20	30	42	26	947
Delhi 1968–69	9	14	18	24	16	5,242
India 1970	20	35	50	58	41	10,246
Rural East Java 1972	5	19	27	43	24	1,418
Jakarta 1968	17	30	57	54	38	811
Korea 1971	7	18	35	48	30	1,622
West Malaysia 1966–67	11	18	28	44	25	4,242
Mexico City 1971	12	31	44	50	35	486
Philippines 1968	18	34	46	60	42	28,964[b]
Taiwan 1967	7	19	33	37	25	4,300
Taiwan[c] 1970	6	17	26	30	22	2,491
Thailand (urban) 1970	14	17	19	31	21	1,080
Thailand (rural) 1969	28	39	52	66	50	642
Belgium 1966	6	3	6	12	8	2,567
Great Britain 1967–68	3	3	4	9	5	1,088
Hungary 1966	5	10	15	24	14	5,309
United States 1965	11	12	13	16	13	3,593

Notes: See Appendix 1, item 3 of the source publication for definitions. Sterilization included as contraception except in Belgium and Great Britain.

The numerator is the number of women who *both* want no more children *and* are not using contraception; the denominator is all married women in the age range. This should not be confused with the proportion who are users among those who want no more children.

[a] Defined as "percent wanting no more children *and* never used contraception."

[b] Frequency weighted: urban respondents multiplied by 4 and rural respondents multiplied by 12.

[c] Taiwan 1970 data refer to ages 22–39.

Source: Freedman and Coombs (1974), pp. 56–57.

from an underlying preference ordering (e.g., among women who say they want three children some strongly prefer four or five to two if they cannot have three, others the reverse). Such measures as the Coombs preference scales have demonstrated that respondents with similar first preferences (e.g., two, three, four) vary significantly with respect to their position on an underlying preference-order scale, not only between countries but also by social strata within countries. How people react behaviorally will be affected by variation in their underlying attitudes. (One version of the Coombs preference scale has been shown to predict fertility and contraceptive behavior in the United States. Another version is significantly related to contraceptive behavior in a Taiwan study. In both Taiwan and the United States these effects are after adjustment for the effect of first preference statement about desired number of children and other variables. The scales have also been tested in Korea, Malaysia, the Philippines, and Hungary.)[25]

4. This is not the only attitude at work. Some women do not act because of the pressure of other attitudes (e.g., in Taiwan data those who have fewer than two sons expect to have more children than they want more often than those with more sons). And among the salient counter attitudes are those about contraception itself, as immoral or illegitimate.

5. People do not act instantaneously to make behavior and attitude correspond. Taiwan in 1965 had a large percentage who wanted no more children but were not using contraception. It could have been said that such a discrepancy indicated that the attitude was "invalid." But the fact is that

while attitudes toward wanting no more children changed little, the percentage among them who neglected contraception decreased steadily. Similarly for the recent decline in fertility and massive adoption of effective fertility control by low status groups in the United States: many said they were having unwanted children in the early 1960s and with a big national program and abortion, they acted. It took time for people to learn about and accept the new contraceptive behavior. If this was so under favorable climate and program, it would take longer where supply and environment were less favorable.

6. Sometimes a general charge is made that attitude statements about desired number of children are invalid, whether West or East. The validity of such attitude statements as predictive of behavior to reduce fertility has been demonstrated for Taiwan, admittedly a favorable situation. The overwhelming majority of Taiwanese wives who said they wanted no more children in 1967 had none in the following three-year period, while the great majority of those who said they wanted more children had at least one.[26] Moreover, in 1965, 48 percent of the Taiwanese wives over 30 said they wanted no more children but were not using contraception,[27] and it may then have been said that the discrepancy between attitude and behavior was so great as to render the attitudinal measurements meaningless. Yet by 1973, just eight years later, the proportion had decreased to 20 percent, and that despite an increase in the proportions wanting no more children, because there was an even larger compensating increase in contraceptive practice among those who wanted no more. Similarly, in India "the proportion of women using contraception among those who wanted no more children is nearly five times greater than the corresponding proportion among those wanting more children" (19.9 percent versus 4.5 percent).[28]

7. Another possible explanation is that the discrepant cases have a poor supply situation at acceptable psychological and economic costs: lack of information or lack of supplies through reasonably convenient and legitimate channels. For some, this will prevent or delay acceptance.

8. Finally, there are undoubtedly situations in which the numerical response is invalid, either in a whole survey because it is badly done, or because the population wants unlimited numbers of children, or because individuals give invalid answers for any one of the reasons that may produce *some* invalid answers to any question on any survey.

The issues of the discrepancy and its reduction by improvement in information and service, then, are empirical and must be resolved by: (a) narrowing the gap by removing the "ineligible"; (b) using additional questions or such devices as the Coombs scale to help classify the cases into those more or less ready to be acceptors, by indicating the intensity of their initial responses and whether they lean toward smaller or larger families; (c) testing by optimal program services; and (d) inquiring among the residual discrepant group to establish, as far as possible, whether the initial response was invalid or whether there are countervailing attitudes or other barriers.

Finally, the fact that the average number of children of acceptors is almost always above three and usually close to four raises the question of whether a change in norms and values about desired number of children must precede any large-scale adoption of contraception. It is generally assumed that the sequence of change goes like this: developmental change in education, women's status, economic level, and so on, will lead to a change in familial institutions; this will, in turn, lead to a change in desired family size; and then, as by-product, some form of birth control will be adopted. While this may indeed be the sequence in some places, in others a different pattern, namely, a fairly large-scale adoption of contraception prior to significant change in family size preferences, has been observed, although following development and mortality decline. If mortality falls to low and stable levels, then the result is a much larger number of surviving children, in many cases more than the traditionally preferred or needed number, and that results in growing pressure on institutions and facilities traditionally organized on the assumption of much lower survival rates.

In Taiwan, for example, between 1965 and 1970, preferred numbers of children changed very little but the percentage ever practicing contraception increased from 28 percent to 56 percent among women aged 22–39 and from 38 percent to 72 percent among women over age 30 (who were mainly responsible for the rapid fertility decline during this period). It appears also to be true in rural Thailand that in a recent period contraceptive practice increased and fertility decreased without change in the desired number of children.[29] As we know in other fields, behavior can affect norms as well as the other way round: as the knowledge and use of contraception spreads, norms about family size may be affected; knowing what is possible by way of fertility control may lead some couples to consider seriously the idea that they should have fewer rather than more children.

These examples are cited not as models of an inevitable or universal sequence, but as illustrations of the idea that there are alternative pathways to demographic change. Adoption of contraception may come earlier rather than later in the process, making fertility reduction possible through the reduction of higher-parity births. Once contraception is adopted, the transition to still lower fertility as the desired number of children declines will presumably be easier. In societies where many couples have learned that they can limit the number of their children to four, others should more easily be able to make the decision to limit the number to two, since they will have learned that reproduction need not be left to fate. In such a case as Bali, where the proportion practicing contraception increased very rapidly from 16 percent to 32 percent in just two years, it is unlikely that there was a change in desired family size of equal proportion just at that time. Unfortunately, there are few cases in which we have time series of the kind needed to monitor parallel trends in developmental change, contraceptive practice, preferred family size, and fertility.

. . . By Methods

The uptake of family planning and its performance in affecting fertility can be seen as influenced by three factors: the social setting that generates motivation (through helping to set group or class norms to which individuals respond by various cost-reward calculations of a highly subjective character[30]); the public program or private or commercial system that provides information and service; and the methods of fertility control thus provided. We briefly turn now to this last matter, to the technology of fertility control, since in many quarters it is strongly argued that "there is no technological solution to the population problem" and at the same time a substantial proportion of external funding in the population field is devoted to the search for an improved technology.

As noted above, there are five methods of fertility control included in fertility-reducing efforts around the world: IUD, orals, condom, sterilization, and abortion.[31] Their "general availability" in developing countries in 1973 is summarized thus:[32]

All 5 methods	2 countries (China, South Korea)
4 methods (excluding legal abortion)	3 countries (Singapore, Taiwan, Thailand)
3 methods (excluding legal abortion and sterilization	9 countries (Barbados, Colombia, Egypt, Hong Kong, Jamaica, Philippines, Sri Lanka, Trinidad & Tobago, Venezuela)
2 methods	8 countries (Dominican Republic, El Salvador, Tunisia, Indonesia, India, Nepal, Pakistan, West Malaysia)
1 method (oral contraceptive)	5 countries (Guatemala, Iran, Mauritius, Mexico, Morocco)
0 methods	5 countries (Bangladesh, Ghana, Kenya, Laos, Turkey)

Thus, on average only slightly over two methods are "generally available" in this set of countries, and the certain methods (abortion, sterilization) are the last to be included as compared with the "probabilistic" methods. Among the efforts in the developing sector, as illustration, the condom is a major method in India (the Nirodh program) and via subsidized commercial schemes (in Kenya and Sri Lanka); the pill in the programs in West Malaysia, Egypt, and Thailand; the IUD in Taiwan and South Korea; sterilization in India; and legal abortion in China.

As the developed world is currently demonstrating, this combined technology is sufficient to support replacement-level fertility; indeed, much less will do with sufficiently high motivation, as shown in the 1930s in Western countries. Eventually, across the entire world the technology of fertility control must realize an efficiency, now experienced in developed societies when couples are trying to prevent births, of about 1 in a thousand—that is, 3,000 to 3,500 sex acts in a reproductive period of 30 to 35 years resulting in, say, only three or four known pregnancies and only two or three planned live births.

For purposes of family planning programs, the technology of fertility control could be improved in three ways: by improving acceptability or continuity or effectiveness. Improving the effectiveness of current methods—already quite effective if used properly—would not make a major contribution; the relatively few additional points of effectiveness that might be gained would not be programmatically powerful, especially when compared to the potential effect of the other two qualities. Continuity of use can be critical; for example, as we shall see an annual acceptance rate of 5 percent of nonusers with 30 percent discontinuing each year (e.g., the IUD) would stabilize at about 15 percent current use and four points off the birth rate, whereas the same 5 percent acceptance with only 5 percent discontinuing (e.g., sterilization, with "discontinuation" referring to older users aging out of the period of fecundity) would take ten points off the birth rate in about a decade—and it would take only four years to take ten points off the birth rate with twice the acceptors. Or consider the IUD in Taiwan or South Korea: if every woman who had an IUD inserted there had retained it, except those wanting another child (i.e., if there were no removals or expulsions), then about 35–40 percent of both societies would now be practicing effective contraception from that source alone. At the same time, the continuity of a particular method is not so important as the continuity of the practice, as those who discontinue switch to other methods of birth control to keep their fertility at low levels. This has been the case in Taiwan and South Korea for a large majority of those originally accepting the IUD. It is continuity of practice that is critically important—which means that the single-act-plus-continuity method of sterilization is particularly important in such countries as India and Bangladesh, where logistical and motivational problems for switching methods are severe, even if each sterilization achieves only 1–1.5 averted births.

Moreover, any method that extends acceptability through its intrinsic attractiveness is obviously a valuable adjunct, and particularly when it is able to generate its own programmatic activity or delivery system expansion, as with the IUD in Taiwan in the early 1960s. The impact of a new technology upon program uptake is illustrated by a few country programs where a method new to that society was introduced (Figure 11.1).[33] In Taiwan each new method seemed to add another layer of use to the existing practice, presumably by attracting a new clientele; in South Korea, the pill was partly introduced through newly established Mothers' Clubs; in Thailand the large increase in pill use at the end of the 1960s resulted from the administrative decision to allow pill distribution by nurse/midwife field workers without doctor's prescription; in Hong Kong, with relatively easy logistics, there was a deliberate programmatic decision to substitute the pill for the IUD as the method of choice more readily administered, especially to younger women for spacing purposes; and in India the condom added another layer of use to that achieved by the other two methods.

As for abortion, that is certainly a major method of fertility management around the world though it is not yet an active programmatic method except perhaps for China. India has recently legalized induced abortion under liberal conditions though it is not prepared to make it programmatically available throughout the country; and greater use of the method may develop in Bangladesh and South Korea. Its importance in developed as well as developing countries is shown in a recent computer simulation concluding that:

> . . . it is unlikely that any population has ever attained a low level of fertility (TFR = 2.2 or less) without the use of induced abortion, legal or illegal. A TAR (total abortion rate) of about 1.0 is a plausible minimum estimate for countries with moderately effective contraception and a TAR of 0.2 for countries with highly effective contraception . . . Barring a major breakthrough in contraceptive technology or major modifications in human sexual behavior, levels of fertility required for population stabilization cannot be easily obtained without induced abortion.[34]

Thus it would appear that an improvement in the technology of fertility control, in the form of an attractive new substance, device, or mode of administration (e.g., vaccination) might make a nontrivial difference, particularly if it had high continuity and did not require medical intervention—for example, a reversible immunization without side effects that could be administered by subordinate personnel. In the end, however, any supplied method needs a delivery system, not

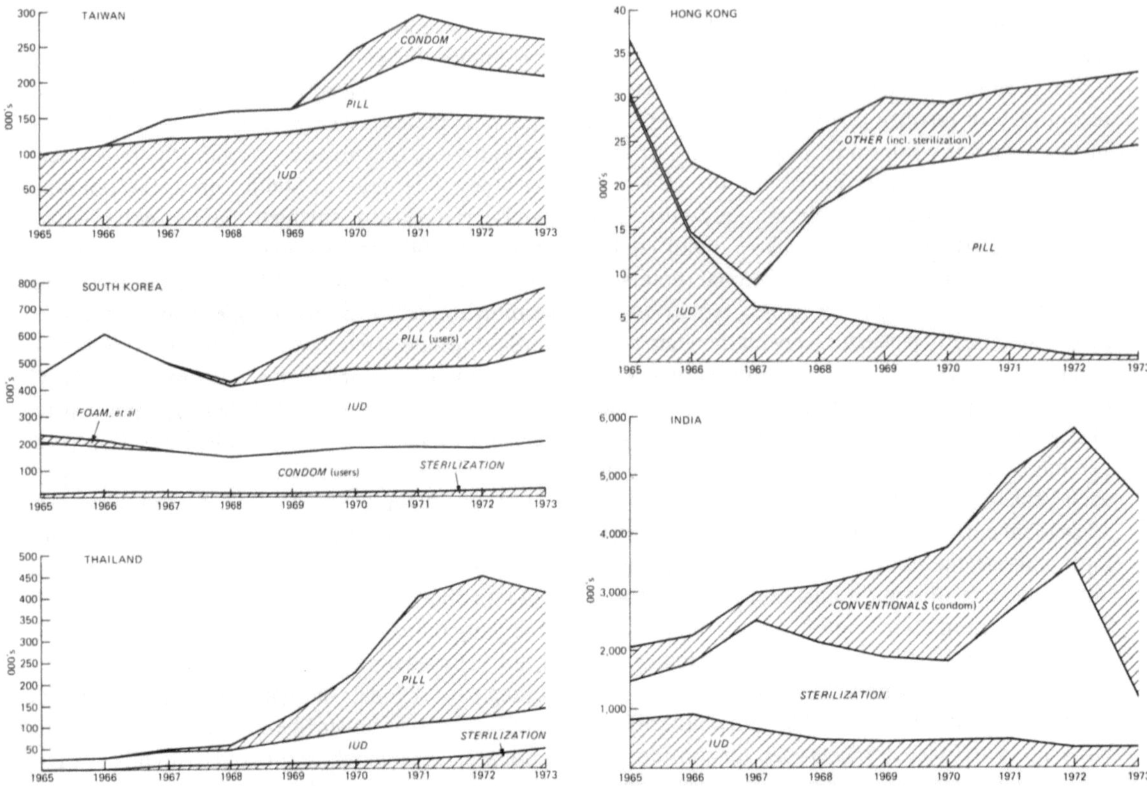

FIGURE 11.1. Acceptance by "new" method in several countries.

necessarily governmental. Indeed, it is worth stressing an elementary point: that if and as socioeconomic development or some aspect thereof does increase motivation for fertility control, some form of delivery system is needed for the more modern means—whether commercial sector or private sector or both. The public sector version is called a family planning program; the stronger the total system, the better.

The argument that improved contraception could facilitate a fertility decline is based on the assumption that motivation to limit family size is usually not a simple dichotomy of "yes" or "no"—want more children or want no more. It is true that without any motivation to limit family size or with very strong motivation, the nature of contraceptive technology is likely to be irrelevant. In the former case no methods will be used, and in the latter case even a method like coitus interruptus may be sufficient. It is likely that motivation has been at one of these extremes at certain periods in some societies but it is unlikely that this simple dichotomy is a universal phenomenon.

Motivation to have more or fewer children, like most other motives in individuals or collectivities, reflects an underlying preference order or distribution. Whether the motivation results in implementing action depends on how it is balanced against competing motives. Distributions of motives and competitions between motives, both within and among individuals, are likely to be particularly relevant during a period of social change when new values are being adopted by some and not by others and when those who are beginning to hold the new values are under cross-pressure from competing values slower to change. Currently it is clear that there are competing pressures between the desire to have fewer children and the desire (motive) to have two sons (e.g., in Taiwan and South Korea).[35] Such related motives were complementary for a long time under high mortality; they may not change at equal rates in the short

TABLE 11.6. First preference for number of children, by Coombs Number Scale: Value positions for Malaysia and Taiwan

First preference for number of children and country	Percent distribution of IN scale values[a] (higher number indicates bias toward relatively large number of children) IN values 1 Small family bias	2	3	4	5	6	7 Large family bias	Total percent	Number of cases
2 Children									
Malaysia	0	8	10	39	20	6	16	100	79
Taiwan	0	19	21	55	6	0	0	100	1,020
3 Children									
Malaysia	0	1	6	22	48	15	9	100	82
Taiwan	0	4	7	30	42	17	0	100	1,453
4 Children									
Malaysia	0	0	0	9	53	26	12	100	215
Taiwan	0	1	2	20	41	34	2	100	1,136

[a] IN denotes the I-scales for preference for number of children.
Source: Data from a forthcoming study under the auspices of a subcommittee of the Committee on Comparative Fertility of the International Union for the Scientific Study of Population.
Data on Malaysia collected in Selangor state by the Malaysian Department of Statistics. Data for Taiwan collected by the Taiwan Institute for Family Planning.
For references for the Coombs scales, see footnote 25.

run during a period of social change, and it is the short run (e.g., a decade) that is at issue here.

The point we are making can be illustrated concretely with data for two countries on the conventional first-preference statements about desired family size compared with the Coombs preference scales reflecting the underlying order in which the first preferences are imbedded (see Table 11.6). As these data illustrate, in each country the first preference statements arise out of an array of possible alternatives, and the underlying preference structure revealed by their ordering can be quite different for the same first-preference statements. In Malaysia those who say they want three children have an underlying preference structure that indicates a bias toward larger numbers of children than is the case in Taiwan. Those who say they want three or four children are more likely to be using contraception in Taiwan than in Malaysia, and fertility rates are lower and are falling more rapidly in Taiwan than in Malaysia (and the family planning program is stronger).

The point of this excursion into questions of motivation and measurement is that in the current situation in countries like Taiwan, Malaysia, and probably many other (but not all) developing countries, people who say they want three or four or *X* children are indicating their first preferences among a range of more or less acceptable numbers. The strength of the motivation to limit family size to the preferred first number depends on the nature of the underlying distribution. Whether behavior will be implemented depends also on the nature and strength of competing motivations. It is plausible that in this situation one element that will encourage people to have fewer rather than more children, within the acceptable range, is a contraceptive with as many as possible of the desirable features listed in the accompanying box. More broadly, the whole supply system (including the family planning program, commercial outlets, the medical network, etc.) can make a difference given the distributional character of the motives.

In short, contraceptive technology and family planning programs are elements in a larger complex of competing motives and means in a situation of social change. There is no empirical basis for the simplistic assumption that the motivation

Contraceptive Criteria

Intrinsic quality

1. *Medical safety:* required, above a very high level (but not necessarily 100 percent).
2. *Effectiveness:* not necessarily 100 percent, but the higher the better, and under field, not laboratory, conditions; effectiveness of the contraceptive system as well as the single method.
3. *Continuity:* the longer the better. Continuing effectiveness, at will, but with effective *reversibility* as well.

Social acceptability (under conditions of field use)

4. *Personal* (motivational): for example, simplicity and ease of use, independence from sex act, free of "nuisance" side effects, one-time administration for long-lasting effect, protection of privacy, male and/or female, appropriateness to life cycle.
5. *Cultural:* for example, tie to local customs, concern over private parts, resistance to superstition, concern with menstruation.
6. *Religious:* for example, Catholics and rhythm (or licit variant), Muslims and menstruation, several religions and abortion.
7. *Sexual:* for example, non- or positive effect on libido and pleasure.
8. *Medical:* for example, preference for mode of administration, non- or positive effect on normal physiological functions.
9. *Organizational and logistic:* for example, non-reliance on supply lines, non-need for (male) doctors, positive diffusibility through word-of-mouth, self-administration, ease of access.
10. *Economic:* for example, costs to individuals and/or society.
11. *Political:* for example, welcome to outside products, symbolic issues.
12. *Philosophical:* for example, free decision.

itself and the probability of implementing such complex motivation fall into simple dichotomies during periods of rapid social change that now characterize more and more of the developing world.

. . . By Setting and Effort

As we have seen, there is considerable variability in the overall performance of family planning programs; we turn now to the conditions that underlie such variability. How is the differential performance to be explained? More particularly, as reflective of the basic controversy, how much is attributable to differences in social setting as against differences in programmatic effort?

It is generally acknowledged that social setting —as reflected in "modern" levels of infant/child mortality, popular education, standard of living, status of women, urbanization, family structure—matters to fertility in a fundamental way. In the broadest cut, for example, that is shown by the sharp differences in such factors between countries with crude birth rates under 25 and over 40.[36] At first glance, this would seem to suggest that only social modernization could effect such fertility reduction, at least at the indicated levels. However, the means of fertility control are also much more available to the population at large in the one than the other set of countries, and there is a transitional period to account for as well. So a key question remains: are observed fertility control and fertility declines due entirely (or virtually entirely) to social modernization and not at all to direct intervention upon fertility, as in family planning programs? As a first approach to the answer, let us look at the record of national programs to see how program acceptance rates vary in countries simultaneously classified by social setting and by programmatic effort (Table 11.7)—and with the caution that in the present state of the art, and probably the visible future as well, the precise quantification of different influences upon fertility behavior is technically not possible.

The most striking finding in this tabulation is the joint effect of setting and availability upon acceptance—from about 15 percent in the doubly favored upper left to 2 percent in the doubly deprived lower right, and with a regular progression in both directions in between. Both factors appear to be important: if anything, program effort somewhat more. Note also that all the strong programs are in high settings and that there is only one high country with a weak program—a country without a fertility-reduction policy and with other constraints as well. (Another special case is Fiji, where the numerator contains only IUDs and sterilization since only those methods are provided in public facilities; the government program also heavily subsidizes orals and condoms in the private sector, and if they were included the Fiji figure

TABLE 11.7. 1973 Acceptors as percentage of estimated nonusers, by social setting and program effort

Program effort	Social setting: High		Middle		Low		Mean Range
Strong	Singapore	24.6					
	Costa Rica	18.2					
	Taiwan	15.7					
	Hong Kong	14.9					14.8
	South Korea	13.4					7.0–24.6
	Jamaica	10.0					
	Fiji	7.0					
	Mean	14.8					
Moderate	Trinidad and Tobago	10.0	Philippines	11.2	Iran	10.8	
	Chile	7.0	Thailand	9.5	Indonesia	6.3	
			Mauritius	8.8	India	2.6	
			Sri Lanka	8.0			
			Colombia	7.9			7.1
			Tunisia	5.2			2.6–11.2
			West Malaysia	4.0			
			Dominican Republic	4.0			
			El Salvador	4.0			
	Mean	8.5	Mean	7.0	Mean	6.6	
Weak	Venezuela	6.5	Honduras	6.1	Egypt	3.7	
			Ecuador	3.5	The Gambia	2.2	
			Mexico	3.2	Kenya	2.0	
			Guatemala	1.7	Ghana	2.0	
			Turkey	0.9	Bangladesh	1.8	2.5
					Morocco	1.6	0.3–6.5
					Nepal	1.5	
					Pakistan	1.0	
					Nigeria	0.3	
	Mean	6.5	Mean	3.1	Mean	1.8	
	Mean	12.7		5.6		3.0	6.7
	Range	6.5–24.6		0.9–11.2		0.3–10.8	0.3–24.6

would be substantially higher, and hence more fitting to the category.)

For comparative purposes, an unpublished tabulation like Table 11.7, but limited to the available countries from column 1 of Table 11.1 only (family planning for fertility reduction), shows only trivial differences in the average values: .7 average difference within the cells, .65 in the margins. And if all the countries in each cell are weighted by population size, here is the outcome:

Program effort	Social setting: High	Middle	Low	Total
Strong	14.5			14.5
Moderate	7.3	8.7	3.6	4.5
Weak	6.5	2.5	1.1	1.6
Total	12.4	6.1	2.9	4.0

Furthermore, the social setting seems to have an effect on the infrastructure itself—on how much of a family planning program the country's administrative capacity can support—and in this way has an indirect effect on fertilty by affecting the strength of the programmatic intervention.[37] But this relation is only moderate; there is a considerable range of program variation within similar social setting levels. (The correlation between social settings and program effectiveness is .33 using tau and .44 using lambda). The fact is that, except at the extremes, we find considerable variation in program strength within levels of social setting, so the ability to mount an effective program is not simply a reflection of developmental levels; among other things, political interest and will are closely involved.

It should not be surprising that the social setting works through the program to affect program acceptances—after all, these data represent acceptors in the program. But there is nothing inevitable about the relationship: program effort could be expended with relatively little effect, and there are some examples of that. The data in the tables are consistent with the simple idea that input affects output, yet in this field that is a relationship often denied.

The preceding discussion of Table 11.7 is based on an inspection of the relationships shown by the cross-tabulations. In an attempt to quantify the relationships, we subjected the data of Table 11.7 to a regression analysis. To do this, we went back to the original quantitative data from which the trichotomous classifications of Table 11.7 were derived. The correlations of these indicators with acceptance rates (when squared) can be interpreted as indicating the percents of the variation in the acceptance rates that are associated with social setting and with program effort. The results of this analysis are as follows:

Percent of variations in 1973 acceptance rate associated with:	
(1) Social setting considered alone (the multiple correlation with the three indicators—infant mortality, school enrollment, and per capita gross domestic product)	51.3
(2) Program effort alone	62.1
(3) Social setting and program effort together (multiple correlation with the three social setting indicators and the program effort scores)	70.0
(4) Net effect[a] of the social setting (3) - (2)	7.9
(5) Net effect[a] of the program effort (3) - (1)	18.7
(6) Joint effect (3) - (5+4)	43.4

[a] The net effect is the difference between the squared total multiple correlation and the squared zero-order correlation of the other variable.

Both social setting and program effort have strong positive correlations with acceptance rate, and the correlation for program effort is somewhat greater. By these calculations program effort accounts for about one-fourth the total influence of the two variables, even without attributing to it any of the joint effects of the two variables.

Such a regression analysis was also done using separate dummy variables to represent the trichotomous categories of social setting and program strength in Table 11.7 (i.e., not going back to the initial individual scores). That resulted in the same total correlation, but with a greater net effect for program effort and a somewhat lesser net effect for social setting.

Whichever analysis is considered, none of these numerical values should be taken too literally in view of the small number of cases and the necessary crudeness of some measurements. However, we used the best data available to us, we have constructed the measures independently of each other, and we have included all countries with family planning programs for which we could obtain data or make reasonable estimates (and similar results, with a somewhat different list of countries, were reached in a regression analysis in a World Bank Staff Report, *Population Policies and Economic Development*, 1974, Appendix B).

The quantitative analysis is consistent with the conclusions reached by inspecting the cross-tabulations in Table 11.7: program effort has a significant relation to acceptance rates that is independent of the social setting. Unfortunately, given the limitations of the data base and the fact that we have made a cross-sectional rather than a longitudinal analysis, we cannot assert unequivocally that we have demonstrated that this measured association is the effect of program effort. At the least, however, we can say that the results are consistent with such a conclusion, and that it is reasonable to pursue the question with better data.

For 27 of the countries in Table 11.7 we were able to find data on current contraceptive use,[38] whether the contraceptor was ever an acceptor in the family planning program or not. While subject to other limitations enumerated for the data in Table 11.7, these data are much less subject to the "substitution effect." That is, the results of the Table 11.7 analysis can be criticized on the grounds that program acceptors are simply substituting the method they adopted in the program for a method they would otherwise have obtained in the private sector. Table 11.8 minimizes this possible problem so far as contraception is concerned, since it deals with contraception wherever it is obtained.[39]

TABLE 11.8. Contraceptive users as percent of married women of reproductive age, circa 1973, by social setting and program effort

Program effort	Social setting: High		Middle		Low		Mean / Range
Strong	Singapore	62					
	Taiwan	56					
	Hong Kong	55					50.8
	South Korea	30					30–62
	Mean	50.8					
Moderate	Chile	18	Colombia	31	India	14	
			Thailand	22	Iran	14	
			Mauritius	21	Indonesia	5	
			Philippines	12			
			Sri Lanka	12			14.3
			Tunisia	10			4–31
			West Malaysia	9			
			Dominican Republic	4			
	Mean	18.0	Mean	15.1	Mean	11.0	
Weak			Mexico	13	Egypt	17	
			Guatemala	6	Pakistan	13	
			Ecuador	3	Morocco	5	
			Turkey	3	Bangladesh	4	6.5
					Ghana	3	2–17
					Kenya	2	
					Nepal	2	
			Mean	6.3	Mean	6.6	
Mean		44.2		12.2		7.9	16.5
Range		18–62		3–31		2–17	2–62

The results in Table 11.8 (and in the regression analysis based on it), considering all contraceptive use, are roughly similar to those in Table 11.7. There is a considerable joint effect, but social setting and program effort have independent effects. As before, program effort accounts for about one-fifth of the total variation in contraceptive usage, even without attributing to it any of the joint effects of the two variables:

Percent of variation in 1973 rate of contraceptive use associated with:	
(1) Social setting considered alone (the multiple correlation with the three indicators—infant mortality, school enrollment, and per capita gross domestic product)	55.5
(2) Program effort alone	60.5
(3) Social setting and program effort together (multiple correlation with the three social setting indicators and the program effort scores)	73.9
(4) Net effect[a] of the social setting (3) – (2)	13.4
(5) Net effect[a] of the program effort (3) – (1)	18.4
(6) Joint effect (3) – (5+4)	42.1

[a]See footnote *a*, p. 140.

With the reservations previously detailed for the acceptor analysis, both the rough quantitative analysis and the inspection of Table 11.8 are consistent with the earlier conclusion that program effort has a significant relation this time to total contraceptive use, that is independent of the social setting.

The findings in Tables 11.7 and 11.8 are indeed remarkable. We would place greater reliance on them if we had the data as time-series articulated with properly lagged time-series on changes in social setting and program strength. Unfortunately, such data are not yet available cross-culturally. Tables 11.7 and 11.8, nevertheless, are consistent with the idea that program effort makes a difference not only to program acceptances but to the general practice of contraception.

. . . By Effect on Birth Rates

Now that we have reviewed acceptors, methods, and acceptances, we come closer to the core of the matter: what effects do family planning programs have on reducing birth rates? That is an essential question so far as population policy is concerned. Again we are handicapped in reaching a firm answer, partly because of lack of data but also because of technical difficulties in disentangling the impact of this one factor from a complex of simultaneous events; or in determining how much of a program's apparent effect on fertility reduction is merely a substitution for what would have happened anyway by other means, given favorable development trends; or in measuring the indirect effects of program activity upon the practice of fertility control; or indeed in satisfactorily conceptualizing the very notion of cause in such situations (for example, if *X* percent of fertility reduction can be tied to program-supplied fertility control, how much of the *X* was "caused" by the program as against the facilitating social factors?). Thus the picture is somewhat blurred, but nevertheless, as a contribution to both technical and substantive progress on the matter, we present our tentative conclusions based on the available evidence.

An approach to the problem is to consider how birth rates vary in relation to variations in social setting and in program effort, as before for acceptance. There is no doubt of the correlation between setting or effort on the one hand and birth rate on the other (see Table 11.9).[40] In each direction the differences are quite consistent. Together, favorable setting and effort are associated with a birth rate in the mid-20s in the upper left and their opposites with a birth rate of twice that in the lower right. This is obviously a rather crude set of data, apart from the fact that the categories are necessarily broad; a number of birth rates are estimates of questionable validity; and questions can be raised in some instances about the temporal order of the program inputs and the birth rates. However, the classifications and the birth rates were obtained independently and represent all the countries for which data were available. The table does suggest that, within development settings, better availability of fertility control measures is associated with lower birth rates—and it is well to remember that the developed countries differ from the developing not only in socioeconomic measures related to fertility but in such availability as well. At the least, this justifies a systematic effort over time to get adequate data for all major programs with which to approach the important questions we have here addressed with inadequate data.

The data in Table 11.9 were subjected to the same kind of regression analysis previously carried out for acceptance rates. The results of that analysis are as follows:

Percentage of variation in 1972 birth rates associated with:	
(1) Social setting considered alone (the multiple correlation with the three indicators—infant mortality, school enrollment, and per capita gross domestic product)	61.3
(2) Program effort alone	71.4
(3) Social setting and program effort together (multiple correlation with the three social setting indicators and the program effort scores)	76.6
(4) Net effect[a] of the social setting (3) - (2)	5.2
(5) Net effect[a] of the program effort (3) - (1)	15.3
(6) Joint effect (3) - (5+4)	56.1

[a] See footnote *a*, p. 140.

According to this analysis, both social setting and program strength have a strong (negative) correlation with the level of the birth rate, and the correlation of program strength is greater. The net independent effect of the program strength is also greater, being associated with 15 percent of the variation in birth rates without considering the joint effects of the two variables.

When we did the regression analysis again using separate (dummy) variables to represent each of

TABLE 11.9. Estimated crude birth rates, circa 1972, by social setting and program effort

Program effort	Social setting: High		Middle		Low		Mean Range
	Costa Rica	32.0					
	Jamaica	31.5					
	Fiji	29.0					
	South Korea	28.0					
Strong	Taiwan	23.8					25.8
	Singapore	22.2					20–32
	Barbados	20.4					
	Hong Kong	19.8					
	Mean	25.8					
	Chile	26–28	Dominican		Iran	48	
	Trinidad and		Republic	45–50	Indonesia	40–45	
	Tobago	25.1	Philippines	42–45	India	37–39	
			El Salvador	41.0			
Moderate			Colombia	38–42			36.8
			Tunisia	38.0			25–50
			Thailand	37.0			
			West Malaysia	33.0			
			Sri Lanka	29.5			
			Mauritius	24.9			
	Mean	26.1	Mean	37.2	Mean	42.8	
	Venezuela	40–45	Honduras	49.0	Nigeria	53–57	
			Ecuador	45–48	The Gambia	50–52	
			Guatemala	43–48	Afghanistan	50	
			Paraguay	45	Dahomey	50	
			Mexico	43–45	Kenya	50	
			Turkey	37.0	Liberia	50	
					Morocco	50	
					Sudan	50	
Weak					Algeria	48–50	47.0
					Tanzania	48	34–57
					Ghana	47–50	
					Bangladesh	45–50	
					Haiti	45–50	
					Pakistan	45–50	
					Nepal	45	
					Zaire	45	
					Egypt	34–36	
	Mean	42.5	Mean	44.5	Mean	48.2	
Mean	27.4		40.1		47.4		40.2
Range	20–45		25–50		34–57		20–57

the trichotomous categories of Table 11.9, the total correlation of the birth rate with both program strength and social setting decreased slightly (R^2 fell from .76 to .74). However, the net effects of the two predictors were about equal—about 8 percent each without allocating their joint effect.[41]

We began this report with the assumption that the social setting would be the major influence and the big question was whether the programs had a significant independent influence. In this perspective, accounting for 8–15 percent of the variance is not inconsequential, especially since the independent effect of the social setting is no greater. Again, we must emphasize that with the limitations of the data base and the cross-sectional character of the analysis, causal inferences are unjustified. The

TABLE 11.10. Percentage declines in the crude birth rates, 1960–73, by social setting and program effort

Program effort	Social setting: High		Middle		Low		Mean Range
Strong	Hong Kong	45					36.2
	Singapore	43					20–45
	Taiwan	39					
	South Korea	37					
	Barbados	33					
	Jamaica	20					
	Mean	36.2					
Moderate	Trinidad and Tobago	34	Mauritius	35	India	10	15.2
			West Malaysia	20	Iran	0	0–35
			Sri Lanka	19			
			Colombia	17			
			El Salvador	15			
			Tunisia	13			
			Thailand	11			
			Philippines	8			
			Dominican Republic	0			
	Mean	34.0	Mean	15.3	Mean	5.0	
Weak	Venezuela	17	Turkey	23	Egypt	19	6.9
			Guatemala	17	Bangladesh	0	0–23
			Mexico	0	Ghana	0	
					Kenya	0	
					Morocco	0	
					Nepal	0	
					Pakistan	0	
	Mean	17.0	Mean	13.3	Mean	2.7	
Mean		33.5		14.8		3.2	16.4
Range		17–45		0–35		0–19	0–45

results are consistent, however, with the hypothesis that program strength has an influence, so that it is also worthwhile to pursue this problem further with better data.

The most pertinent question we can ask is whether program strength is associated with a decline in birth rates independently of the effect of social setting. We must emphasize that, however close they come to the heart of the matter, the data in Table 11.10 on birth rate declines involve much more questionable estimates than the data on birth rates. In certain instances, the decline shown may be smaller than the probable error in estimating the birth rate level itself. Furthermore, errors are more serious for birth rate declines than for birth rates, since the difference between a 5 and a 10 percent decline in the birth rate represents a much larger relative variation than the corresponding differences in the birth rates. But since these are the best data at our disposal, since changes (declines) in birth rates are "closer" to the program's impact than the rates themselves, insofar as the temporal connection is concerned, and since the components are not estimated in a way that would produce biased relationships predictable in advance, it seems worthwhile to undertake the exercise if only to indicate what we would like to do with better data. On the basis of inspection of the cross-tabulation (Table 11.10), within levels of program effort, the birth rate declines are greater in higher social settings; within social setting, the declines are greater with more program effort.

The results of a regression analysis like those above yielded the following results:

Percentage of variation in birth rate declines associated with:	
(1) Social setting considered alone (the multiple correlation with the three indicators – infant mortality, school enrollment, and per capita gross domestic product)	51.3
(2) Program effort alone	60.7
(3) Social setting and program effort (multiple correlation with the three social setting indicators and the program effort scores)	68.1
(4) Net effect[a] of the social setting (3) - (2)	7.4
(5) Net effect[a] of the program effort (3) - (1)	16.8
(6) Joint effect (3) - (5+4)	43.9

[a] See footnote *a*, p. 140.

Given the small number of countries for which data are available and the questions about the data, the size of the quantitative measures should not be taken too literally. However, the results are consistent with the reading of the cross-tabulation: each variable is correlated with the birth rate decline within categories of the other variable. We do not attribute any weight to the fact that the net program effect is greater than the net social setting effect, since the comparisons were reversed when we used separate (dummy) variables to represent each of the trichotomous categories of Table 11.10.

In the case of Table 11.10, the question of temporal priority is especially serious, since the fertility declines are available for the period 1960–73 and in most cases the program effort was not significant until the later part of that period. We can say that countries with the largest fertility declines generally had the stronger programs, usually contemporaneously with a major part of the period of decline. But there are elaborate indirect mechanisms at work here, and we need much better data on the timing and amount of program input and output and better fertility data, year by year, to sort out the full lines of influence.

We indicated earlier that there is no consensus on just which aspects of development set off changes in reproductive behavior, but that it is becoming increasingly clear that not all aspects of development are equally relevant and that they do not necessarily follow a parallel course. In this perspective, it is of interest that in three of the four sets of the regressions based on Tables 11.7 to 11.10, the net regression coefficients are largest for education and smallest for gross domestic product. In the fourth case (contraceptive use–Table 11.8), the largest net coefficient is for infant mortality, and gross domestic product ranks second. So, in all four regressions the net effect for gross domestic product (our economic measure) is smaller than that for either infant mortality or school enrollment or both.

The birth rate is so intertwined in a complex of social and demographic variables changing at different rates for different groups within the society that unimpeachable empirical measures on selective impacts or reasons for change are difficult to come by, on technical grounds, and hence relatively rare. That is so for historical trends and for shifts in developed countries as well as for the present situation in developing countries. If the fertility effect of family planning programs were always of overwhelming magnitude it would shine through; if it were always zero the question would not survive. In the middle-ground cases, while problems of data and measurement remain, we find plausible evidence that family planning programs make a difference that matters.

Beyond that, however, we can estimate the broad parameters of the necessary relationship between fertility control on the one hand and birth rates on the other through a combination of empirical observation and model construction. Empirically, we know that the practice of fertility control is closely associated with the level of the crude birth rate within the following range: 5–10 percent of current practice within a society is associated with a crude birth rate of 40–50, as in Morocco or Nepal or Guatemala; and 60–70 percent of practice is associated with a crude birth rate under 20, as in the United States and Europe.[42] On that scale, a 30 percent level of practice is approximately associated with a crude birth rate of 30: roughly, 2 points of additional use mean 1 point off the birth rate. We take that condition – "the 30/30 rule" – as our criterion for the following exercise.

Although any such criterion is arbitrary, we find this one attractive for two reasons. First, for the "typical" developing country with a birth rate around 40, achieving a rate of 30 in a reasonable period of time—say, eight to ten years—would be a distinctive achievement under any form of intervention, development or family planning, or under the impact of "natural processes," for that matter. Seldom have declines of that magnitude been observed in large societies. Second, any country achieving the 30/30 condition, like Fiji or South Korea currently, is in all likelihood well established on the road to demographic transition,[43] and the normal processes of modernization and diffusion are likely to carry the society farther down that road.

In any case, that is the criterion used here for illustrative purposes. Given a representative age/marital distribution for developing societies, given the "standard" mix of acceptors primarily by age (average: 30.4) and parity (average: 4.1), and given the "standard mix of fertility control methods and their continuation rates" (70 percent at one year), what is required?[44] If we enter these assumptions into the designated model, what do the indicated performances yield in fertility effect?

Percentage new acceptors of nonusers annually	Fertility effect
15	About 10 points off CBR of 40–42 in 8 years, and stabilization there, with about 30% current use
10	About 6–7 points off, and stabilization, with about 25% current use
5	About 4 points off, and stabilization, with about 15% current use
2	Too small to measure

Thus, to get a crude birth rate of 30 from a start of around 40 or slightly above, in say a decade of program build-up and operation, would require sustained annual performance at the level of 15 percent of current nonusers, or about 10–12 percent of all MWRA with the current mix of methods. That performance is now obtained, with considerable effort, only by the best programs in the most advantaged settings like Taiwan and South Korea. Thus, that level of performance tends to establish the upper limit against which family planning programs can be evaluated. Given the indicated assumptions in the model, performance at the 10 percent level of nonusers would get the birth rate down only to the mid-30s, with no decline thereafter, and the 5 percent level would reduce it still less. The performance in Table 11.7 weighted by population size (as on p. 139) and based on today's mix of acceptors and methods will yield a decline in the crude birth rate of only about 3 points before stabilizing. Moving below a crude birth rate of 30 requires even higher uptake of contraception, from whatever stimulus and whatever source, or higher continuation rates, or more abortion, or some combination thereof.

Alternative Means of Fertility Intervention

This has been a review of the record of family planning programs as the major policy instrument used by governments in achieving fertility reduction in developing countries. But it is not the only conceivable such instrument, and indeed a number of other proposals have been put forward as more effective and/or more efficient. Reviewing them is not our intent here, nor would that be altogether possible at this juncture on data and other grounds, but it may be useful to set down the alternative paths, by way of inventory for comparative purposes.

If a country seeks to reduce fertility, there are approximately 20 means that can in principle be used—that is, reasonably specific actions that have been responsibly proposed or are currently being tried:

Family Planning		
1.	Family planning program	Provision of information, supplies, and services for voluntary fertility control via modern contraception and various delivery systems; many examples operating today

1a. Family planning program plus sterilization	. . . and adding sterilization, male and/or female, on an equivalent basis, as in India
1b. Family planning program plus abortion	. . . and adding induced abortion, on an equivalent basis, as in China
1c. Family planning program plus stepped-up informational and educational campaign	. . . and adding energetic propaganda for smaller families, as in South Korea, Singapore, China
1d. Family planning program plus incentives	. . . and adjusting incentives/disincentives, in money or in kind, in antinatalist direction, as in Singapore, Taiwan, India tea estates, and vasectomy camps
1e. Family planning program integrated into maternal and child health	. . . organized as integral part of MCH, e.g., as in current efforts in Indonesia, the Philippines, Turkey
1f. Family planning program integrated into general health	. . . organized as integral part of total health infrastructure, as in Narangwal
1g. Family planning program integrated into community development	. . . organized as part of rural improvement and community development, as in Gandhigram
Development	
2. General development	Reliance on social change, modernization, development, social-structural transformation, "new international economic order" to reduce fertility rates "automatically" in the process
2a. Threshold:[45] infant and child mortality	. . . with special reference to reducing infant and child mortality, as a necessary precondition to fertility reduction, e.g., Heer[46]
2b. Threshold: popular education	. . . with special reference to extending popular education, particularly for girls, as a necessary precondition, e.g., Rich[47]
2c. Threshold: income redistribution	. . . with special reference to poverty reduction, particularly at the bottom of the income pyramid, as a necessary precondition, e.g., Kocher,[48] Cassen[49]
2d. Threshold: women's status	. . . with special reference to emancipation of women from traditional (i.e., childbearing and rearing) status, and opening of other opportunities and particularly moneyed employment, e.g., sewing factories in Egypt[50]
Legal Channels	
3a. Age at marriage	Increase in minimum age of marriage for women, to at least 20 and preferably beyond, as in China, Tunisia
3b. Social security system	Development of obligation by the state for provision of welfare to the aged, in order to reduce need for children (sons) for that purpose
3c. State requirement	Governmental imposition of a limit to childbearing, as in proposals by Davis or Boulding[51]
Other	
4a. Youth corps: male	Development of a work program away from home, for young men, in order to delay marriage and "modernize" attitudes
4b. Youth corps: female	. . . Same for young women
5. Population education	Incorporation of population materials into primary and secondary school curricula, for long-term effect, as in the Philippines
6. Community organization and/or "pressure"	Provision to local community of means, autonomy, and incentives for collective development so that members have common stake in low fertility; systematic efforts to develop community consensus and peer pressure in antinatalist direction, as reportedly in China, McNicoll[52]

All such means must be appraised against the same criteria as family planning programs: acceptability to governments and societies, administrative feasibility in implementation,[53] and effectiveness within a reasonable time period: for example, the target of 10 points off the birth rate in 10 years. In the end, any evaluation of the record of family planning programs must thus be a comparative one: if they are not altogether useless or positively harmful, how competitive are they with other realistic means when judged against such criteria?

Conclusion and Commentary

The major findings in this review were signalled in the underlined statements. Here is a compressed and paraphrased reprise:

- For several reasons, the historical record of fertility decline in the West is not a firm guide as to the potential efficacy of programs organized to provide modern fertility control to the populations of developing countries.
- Family planning programs have been undertaken by a number of developing countries as the prime instrument of their policy of fertility reduction.
- Under realistic current conditions, such programs have reached between 1–2 percent and 10–15 percent of the target per year, and achieved prevalence of up to 20–25 percent.
- Acceptors tend to be older and of higher parity but that does not dispose of their demographic impact or their potential effect upon the birth rate. The programs reach the lower educated, the rural residents, and the poor, all of whom would normally come to modern fertility control in a tardy fashion; the discrepancies between expressed interest and actual behavior are complex and empirical; and substantial fertility control can go on at present in a typical developing country without any shift in norms of family size.
- The efficacy of the technology of fertility control, for program purposes, depends not only on the acceptability of the method, particularly as generator of program activity, but upon continuity; improvements in these respects could make a nontrivial difference.
- The complexities of motivation, methods, and program do not resolve into simple dichotomies in periods of social change like the present, so there appears to be some room for innovative intervention.
- Country performance is associated with both social setting and program effort, in about a 7-to-1 ratio from the doubly favored to the doubly deprived areas. The social setting also affects the quality of the programmatic infrastructure; still, the program effort has a clear, substantial, and independent effect upon performance.
- Program effort appears to be associated along with social setting in both level and decline of birth rates, but for technical reasons definitive answers are not available, particularly with regard to the substitution effect—which is probably present to some (unknown) degree but unlikely to be of sufficient magnitude to account for the entire impact of moderately good programs.
- To take 10 points off a birth rate around 40 in a decade requires sustained program performance at about the current level of the best programs; performance at about a third of that level will take off only about 4 points in that time.
- Some programs currently pursued in favorable or moderate settings have apparently been able to expedite an existing fertility decline; others have had no appreciable impact and/or were not broadly or energetically implemented. And the same can be said in summary of the several demonstration projects in the field.
- Two special cases are deserving of the most careful international attention: China, which may provide a test of fertility reduction in a country with little urbanization and relatively low living standards but with a combination of low mortality, intensive political commitment to fertility control permeating the local community and the structure of small groups, together with equity in what is available and other institutional changes, for example in status of women; and Indonesia, which may provide a test of the potential for program effect under poor developmental levels and extreme population pressure but in the presence of strong political and organizational commitment.
- In the end, the proper appraisal is the comparative one: what alternative use of equivalent resources, under realistic conditions, would have achieved more impact toward fertility reduction?
- Realistic alternatives to family planning programs, as specific paths to fertility reduction, need further exploration by the same criteria of acceptability, feasibility, and effectiveness. They are not now available, except in broad terms of "development."

That is a brief summary of the foregoing material. We have tried to limit ourselves, in this report, to such findings and their empirical base. But on a public matter of this complex character, policy is rarely determined solely on the basis of scientific evidence, however it may be read; if for no other reason, the evidence is rarely complete or definitive enough for that. Beyond such evidence is empirical experience, and beyond that informed judgment. In the end, policy-making comes down to their judicious combination. In that context, we highlight a few residual considerations of importance to any final judgment about the record of family planning programs—a kind of personal commentary and assessment.

We began this report with a brief discussion of the evidence on the demographic transition in the West, and we have occasionally referred to ways in which developing countries differ from Western countries when the latter were at a similar stage of development. At this point, a review of such differences may be useful.

As compared to the situation of the developed countries prior to their fertility declines, the developing countries differ in a number of ways that affect their demographic trends[54]:

1. Fertility levels were initially much higher.
2. The mortality decline has been much more rapid.
3. As a result, the rates and amounts of population growth have been unprecedented.
4. High fertility has meant a much younger population with a greater built-in momentum for population growth.
5. There is much less opportunity for emigration to siphon off population growth.
6. The results of those trends are: (a) to make educational progress more difficult because of the much larger numbers and higher rate of growth of population of children; and (b) to make employment less available for women because the rapid growth of the total labor force places great pressure on job opportunities, given first to men.

At the same time, there are some points of difference from the Western experience that may facilitate earlier and more rapid fertility decline:

7. The small family norm that exists in many countries now was not available earlier in the West as a model and basis for cultural diffusion.
8. There is greater potential for fertility decline by increase in age at marriage.
9. The elite and, to an increasing extent, the masses in developing countries are aware of living standards and life styles (including smaller families and birth control) in societies elsewhere that transcend local and familial bounds. While perhaps ambivalent about just what they want, there is increasing evidence of strong aspirations for something better as the existence of other possibilities becomes known.
10. Governments have more competence to permeate subnational ethnic/linguistic barriers.
11. The means of contraception are more numerous and more effective.
12. Governments are increasingly committed to lowered fertility (whereas earlier most social institutions, including the political, were pronatalist in character), and as one result:
13. Family planning programs exist.

Factors 7–13 presumably should facilitate fertility decline, given some (unspecified) minimum of development in certain respects. Factors 1–6 are important because they make for greater pressures on traditional institutions. The unusually rapid mortality decline and the resulting rapid growth of population in many developing countries (especially at the younger ages) must be exerting pressures on traditional economic and social institutions, especially in situations of high density on the land. This may be why there is a very rapid uptake of family planning in Indonesia, in response to a strong family planning program and despite rather poor progress on other development fronts. It may also be relevant that in some places (e.g., Sri Lanka and Kerala) fertility has fallen with substantial gains in mortality and in education, but without much economic progress. The special role of education is in linking those educated to a wider world that transcends local and familial institutions. This should be particularly effective when it occurs in a population increasingly aware that the risks of losing their children through death are greatly reduced. Education is no substitute for development on other fronts, but it may stimulate interest in those other changes—including the demographic.

In attempting to go beyond the mechanistic versions of transition theory, a number of scholars have stressed the possibility that what sets off a fertility decline is a change that threatens a traditional cherished value (e.g., land for one's sons)[55] or a change that opens up new opportunities[56] (e.g., the opportunity for upward mobility in a changing economy). It is worth noting that in the regression analyses reported above, education and mortality had a considerable association with acceptance rates and birth rates, but a measure of economic product per capita was less important.

We suggest the possibility that the combination of low mortality and more education may create a triggering situation—the education making the population aware of the potentiality of change, and of future prospects (as against present requirements) and the lower mortality making it possible for them to consider having fewer children without changing basic familial institutions very much (because the number of *surviving* children need not change). Knowing that change is possible (through education) is no substitute for the desired change, but it may very well lead to actions and ideas (note the student unrest) to attain that change.

Mortality decline did not always precede fertility decline in the West, but the amount and rate of mortality decline in the current developing countries is so much greater than at any previous time in history that it might well have a special "shock" effect. Mortality decline has in fact preceded all the fertility declines among developing countries in the postwar period. It is probably not enough in itself (although we cannot be sure of that under all circumstances), since so many developing countries have had the mortality decline without much sign yet of fertility decline. Mortality decline plus some elements of development may be enough in some circumstances, and education may be one of those additional elements. It would appear that this combination might be a particularly suitable environment for an energetic family planning program to be effective. Let us make it clear again that we are convinced that the wider the range of development progress, the more likely the decline in fertility, with or without a program. What we are suggesting is that, short of that and during the time required for the broader range of movement, countries with something less—for example, mortality decline and educational progress—may be in a position to make progress with a well-organized family planning program.

What can be done may also be affected by the nature of the culture in ways that we do not fully understand. As we pointed out earlier, cultural enclaves in Europe appeared to follow quite different patterns in the demographic transition. Some observers have speculated that the Chinese-Korean-Japanese cultural area may be particularly favorable to fertility decline. Whether Buddhism provides a more favorable setting than Hinduism is an important and interesting question. (And beyond culture into climate, is it accidental that most of the world's high fertility is found in tropical areas?) The point is that to stress structural factors without reference to cultural factors may be incorrect in view of the available evidence.

Throughout this paper, we have tried not to speak of the "success" or "failure" of family planning programs, since those judgments can be made only against explicit or implicit criteria. Whether current programs have "succeeded" or "failed" depends on the scale against which they are measured, and such scales are readily available in widely diverse verdicts on the record:

> Family planning programs are a "success": They have done a lot in some countries, have not really been implemented in countries where not much has happened, are impressive when viewed comparatively against other social interventions seeking to change mass behavior, and anyway have no realistically competitive alternatives in public policy.
>
> Family planning programs are a "failure": They do reasonably well only where the social setting has modernized to the point where people would control fertility anyway in a trivially longer time (if that), they cannot have any substantial effect in the large poor countries where fertility reduction is most needed, the expressions of interest (such as they are) are not genuine in anticipating change in behavior, and they divert attention and support from what is really required.

In our belief, such views taken by themselves are mistaken, often mischief-making. There is something to be said for each; family planning programs are neither sufficient nor worthless. The record is mixed.

It is hard to see how it could be otherwise on a matter of this complexity. Family planning programs can do some things, cannot do everything. If hastening a trend or effecting a notable increase in fertility control in an unlikely population within a short time will do, then several have succeeded; if achieving replacement-level fertility in "not too long" or cutting a high birth rate in half in a decade is required, then programs have failed. The *fully* versus *only* judgment remains to be made, against explicit standards. Protagonists in the debate agree quite broadly about several of the facts of the matter but disagree essentially about what the standard is—expectations, "requirements" for "solving the population problem," the criteria for "success" and "failure."

Consider, for example, the intermediate target, for developing countries with birth rates of 40+, of aiming for the 30/30 position—a prevalence of 30 percent practice of modern fertility control resulting in a crude birth rate of approximately 30, which would in turn generate its own momentum in the desired direction. By the historical record, lowering such a birth rate by 10 points in 10 years would be a notable achievement indeed. It would appear that present programs, or some better versions thereof, can, or could, achieve nontrivial results in unlikely social settings, but are not likely to achieve the 30/30 state from a standing start around a crude birth rate of 40 within a decade: an uptake of 6–8 percent of the target population per year would be good performance in an unfavorable social setting, and that would go only about half the way. By the 10-points-in-10-years criterion, current efforts in the most needy countries will not suffice.

But even short of that, so far as the empirical record is concerned, the fact remains that a number of the "failed" family planning programs may have failed for lack of implementation—for lack of political will or administrative capacity rather than programmatic response. In many countries, perhaps most, the administrative capacity to reach the target appropriately and continuously may be absent; what would happen if it existed is not known.

For a country seeking reduction in fertility as a means to a better life ahead, what are the alternatives? If family planning is not "enough," what other policy channels are open? General development ("Take Care of the People and the Population Will Take Care of Itself") or specific thresholds like women's status or popular education or income redistribution are being strongly advanced at present, in the post-Bucharest spirit. There can be little doubt that such fundamental social changes would also affect fertility downward, but they too take time and effort, not to mention (far larger) funds; and they are, after all, the ends for which fertility control is a means, not the other way round. It is precisely the drag that population growth places on such development that is the problem: the question is, can fertility be lowered significantly as a prior aid in the process? As Teitelbaum says,

> [reliance on development] fails to provide adequate answers to two questions of fundamental scientific and policy significance:
>
> 1) Sufficiency: Will the moderate levels of development to which many developing countries can realistically aspire in the medium-term future be sufficient to establish the preconditions for 'natural' fertility decline?
>
> 2) Timeliness: If such declines do occur, will they occur soon enough and at a pace rapid enough to compensate for the sharply increased pace of mortality decline and higher initial fertility levels of these countries as compared with transitional Europe?[57]

Incidentally, it seems necessary to stress, post-Bucharest, that family planning programs are not to be considered as substitutes for development and that the latter is to be sought for its own sake. As it is gradually achieved, it will surely affect prospects for fertility decline in a favorable direction—just as the fertility decline being sought through family planning programs will affect the prospects for development. Moreover, as is now becoming more clear, fertility reduction can occur under varied developmental conditions and there are transitional opportunities: not everything changes at just the same rate. And beyond the joint effect of development and family planning appears to be only some version of community commitment or "pressure," as reportedly in the Chinese case.

That circumstance signals the first of two needs for further exploration in this field—the need for greater concern with the non-family planning alternatives for public policy, *in programmatic terms*. They have not sufficiently emerged, and need to be sought in a systematic and imaginative manner. They will not easily be found—it is not clear that many such alternatives are realistically there, given political and other considerations—but the stakes are high.

The second need is for fuller knowledge about the record itself. At several points in this report we have had to say, in effect: don't know. In this respect, neither the data bank nor the technical apparatus is sufficient to the task. The fact that they are also deficient with regard to the historical fertility decline in the West only underlines the point. There are several specifics:

- Better outreach measures for individual programs—that is, measures that will tell, by various standards, how much actual coverage the program has achieved in various sectors of the society.
- More sophisticated work on the validity or "meaning" of favorable attitudes as predictive of fertility-related behavior.
- More work on the central issue of fertility effectiveness, beyond initial acceptances.
- Better annual data on the family planning inputs, the acceptances, developmental indicators, and the detailed components of fertility and nuptiality (preferably separately for the persons who use no birth control and for those who use it inside and outside the program).
- More work on the substitution effect.
- More penetrating analysis of the issues contained in Tables 11.7 to 11.10—that is, the relationships among social setting, program effort, and fertility.
- More work on cost effectiveness as related to fertility outcome.
- More work on the timing problem, that is, if the programs have "expedited" an ongoing fertility decline, by how much?
- More work on the fundamental conceptual problems of assigning "cause" in such an intricately interwoven network of events.

The fact that these are difficult matters, previously resistant to technical solution, only makes the effort more urgent.

Finally, at the core is time. What is the timetable? There is a shorter term and a longer term.

In the short term of a decade or so, the problem of a family planning program can be seen as not to change people's norms on such a key issue of their lives, very difficult if not virtually impossible in the absence of any substantial change in life conditions, but rather to provide information on how people can achieve their own norms and provide services to make that prospect real. In our judgment, in the past decade or less the field has learned that fertility *can* decline without substantial, certainly without commensurate, decline in family size norms. The sequence is of considerable policy importance. The received view is that development leads to changes in family structure and the functions of children, which in turn lead to changes in desired family size and that in turn, finally, leads to the adoption of fertility control. But we are now learning that development and mortality decline lead to the survival of more children than the numbers traditionally experienced as valuable, as a result of which fertility control may then be adopted to avoid the additional unwanted children, not because of any significant change in the norm of desired numbers. By this rationale, fertility control may well be adopted sooner rather than later in the entire process, as part of a feedback loop well before a society is fully modernized. After all, even in high-fertility countries, fertility is already 40–60 percent below the highest known levels, not to mention biological capability, so some degree of control is already there.

The longer view provides a fitting close. Family planning programs have themselves served, with their health and humanitarian elements, to energize the issue of rapid population growth, and to do so in a relatively short time on a relatively stigmatized subject. But in the long run they contribute to more than just fertility reduction or demographic measures. They are redistributional in the larger sense, since they disproportionately serve the poor and the deprived through their contribution to maternal and child health, to women's status, to income equalization. So they too are part of the desired social revolution, a "threshold" for development and not merely fertility reduction. In any case, on such an issue, "some of our colleagues are impatient when change from year to year cannot plainly be discerned in the statistics. Historians consider change to have been rapid when there was a perceptible difference in the behavior of successive generations."[58]

Footnotes

[1] A number of such reviews have already been done, including some by ourselves: e.g., Ronald Freedman and John Y. Takeshita, *Family Planning in Taiwan: An*

Experiment in Social Change (Princeton University Press, 1969); and Bernard Berelson, "An evaluation of the effects of population control programmes," in *Population and Its Problems*, The Wolfson College Lectures 1973, H. B. Parry, ed. (Oxford: Clarendon Press, 1974), pp. 133–168. See also the forthcoming volume edited by C. Chandrasekharan and A. Hermalin, *Measuring the Effect of Family Planning Programs on Fertility* (Ordina Editions, 1975).

[2]"Supplied or programmed" to differentiate these means from *coitus interruptus*, or withdrawal, which is still widely used in some parts of the world; and from rhythm, or periodic abstinence, which is only rarely a program method (e.g., Mauritius and the Philippines, for Catholic clientele). There is a sense in which all five of the major means are modern: the oral and the IUD are of quite recent development, indeed it is an open question whether family planning programs would have been developed to their present state without them; abortion technique was recently modified by the "suction" technique; and both sterilization and condom have recently had marginal improvements.

[3]By way of illustration, these are among the critical commentaries: *Action Pack* (distributed by the World Population Year Secretariat of the UNFPA, 1974); Samir Amin, "Development strategies and population policies: Underpopulated Africa," in *Population-Education-Development in Africa South of the Sahara* (meeting of experts, Dakar, UNESCO Regional Office for Education in Africa, November-December 1971); Ahmed Bahri et al., "A new approach to population research in Africa: Ideologies, facts and policies," (Paper issued at the African Population Conference, Accra, December 1971); Judith Blake, "Demographic science and the redirection of population policy," in *Public Health and Population Change: Current Research Issues*, Mindel C. Sheps and Jeanne C. Ridley, eds. (University of Pittsburgh Press, 1965), pp. 41–69; Michael Carder and Robert Park, "Bombast in Bucharest: Report on the World Population Conference," *Science for the People* (January 1975): 17–19; Rick Casey, ed., "A frustrated consensus," (Report on the consultation on population policy, cosponsored by the Canadian Inter-Church Project on Population and the Center of Concern, Montreal, October 1973); Kingsley Davis, "Population policy: Will current programs succeed?," *Science* 158 (10 November 1967): 730–739; Garrett Hardin, "The tragedy of the Commons," *Science* 162 (13 December 1968): 1243–1248; Philip Hauser, "Family planning and population programs: A book review article," *Demography* 4 (1967): 397–414; Philip Hauser, "Population: More than family planning," *Journal of Medical Education* 44, no. 11, part 2 (November 1969): 20–29; W. T. Li, "Temporal and spatial analyses of fertility decline in Taiwan," *Population Studies* 27, no. 1 (March 1973): 97–104; Pierre Pradervand, "The Malthusian man," *New Internationalist*, no. 15 (May 1974): 20–24, and Letter of Correction to Editor (9 September 1974); William Rich, "Smaller families through social and economic progress," (Monograph no. 7, Overseas Development Council, January 1973); N. B. Ryder, "Realistic pathways to fertility reduction in developing countries," (Paper presented at the annual meeting of the Population Association of America, April 1974); Paul Singer, "Population growth: The role of the developing world," (Paper presented at the World Population Conference, in IUSSP Lecture Series on Population, Bucharest, 1974).

[4]For an excellent summary of the major points of difference between the historical and modern situations as related to fertility decline see Michael Teitelbaum, "Relevance of demographic transition theory for developing countries," *Science* 188 (2 May 1975): 420–425.

[5]Teitelbaum, p. 424.

[6]From a more general discussion in Etienne van de Walle and John Knodel, "Demographic transition and fertility decline: The European case," (*Proceedings* of the International Union for the Scientific Study of Population, Sydney, 1967), pp. 47–55.

[7]Paul Demeny, "Early fertility decline in Austria-Hungary: A lesson in demographic transition," *Daedalus* 97 (1968): 519.

[8]E. A. Wrigley shows such conditions for Colyton, England, in late medieval times: "Family limitation in pre-industrial England," *Economic History Review*, 2nd series, 19, no. 1 (April 1966): 82–109. Ronald D. Lee has recently carried out a sophisticated econometric analysis from which similar conclusions can be drawn for parts of Europe: "Natural fertility, population cycles and the spectral analysis of births and marriages," *Journal of the American Statistical Association* 70, no. 350 (June 1975): 295–304. See also Gösta Carlsson, "The decline of fertility: Innovation or adjustment process," *Population Studies* 20, no. 2 (November 1966): 149–174.

[9]Personal communication from Ansley Coale cited in Teitelbaum, footnote 4.

[10]Teitelbaum, p. 424.

[11]Ansley Coale, "The demographic transition," (*Proceedings* of the IUSSP International Population Conference, Liège, 1973), p. 69.

[12]This is as good a place as any to signal the limitations of the available data to support a complete appraisal of the record. Indeed, that state of affairs, due to gaps in the scientific methodology and lack of trained personnel, is at bottom responsible for continuing controversies as to the facts. In this respect, the population field is not unique.

> Unfortunately, the increase in data availability has not been accompanied by an adequate improvement in statistical quality. In many cases the growing interest in the subject has simply led to the proliferation of crude estimates for various countries, based on data sources which may be the best available but are

simply not good enough. (Three major sources of error in this field: the inadequacy of the concepts, the difficulty of measurement in practice, and the inaccuracy of sample estimates.) Because of these problems, available estimates in most underdeveloped countries are, at best, approximations of the underlying distribution. Estimates for different countries, and even for the same country at different points of time, are typically based on noncomparable data sources, making intercountry and intertemporal comparisons very hazardous.

These limitations present a familiar dilemma in empirical analysis. The data are very weak, but they are also the only data we have. An extreme response to the problem is to reject any use of most of the available data for analytical purposes. The approach adopted . . . is less puristic. We assume that until better data become available, cautious use of existing data—with all its limitations—provides some perspective on the nature of the problem.

These paragraphs deal with income distribution. They could apply as well to population. (Quotation from Montek S. Ahluwalia, "Income inequality: Some dimensions of the problem," in Hollis Chenery et al., *Redistribution with Growth*, published for the World Bank and the Institute of Development Studies, University of Sussex (Oxford University Press, 1974), pp. 4–6.

[13]This median date may be advanced one year by two technical re-datings—Hong Kong moved in 1973 from the second column to the first and Bangladesh re-adopted in 1971 the policy that earlier applied to the area as East Pakistan. If both are put back to their earlier datings, the median becomes 1966.

[14]Continuation rates vary by method of fertility control, by motivation of the users (e.g., stoppers over spacers), and often by place or social setting. As rough order of magnitude, the current ranges of continuation per year in developing societies are estimated as follows: sterilization 95–100 percent, orals 30–70 percent, and IUD 55–85 percent. Data are not available for condom use, and the concept does not apply to abortion. In field programs, continuation rates tend to be lower in settings in which competing methods (including induced abortion) are readily available and in settings where energetic efforts are undertaken at mass recruitment, thus cutting relatively lower into the motivational scale. Note that program use" usually refers to continuation by people not by method; that is, users can continue by switching (i.e., discontinuing) particular methods. The continuation rates usually cited refer to the first "segment" of use (e.g., the continuation rate for a first IUD insertion) rather than to the birth control practice of the couple once they have adopted a method in the program. For example, in some countries (e.g., Taiwan and Korea) there is evidence that once couples have entered a program (e.g., by a first IUD insertion), they continue to control their fertility at low levels even after terminating the use of the first IUD by adopting other methods, abortion, or a reinsertion of the IUD. How much such "extended use" exists in a particular country is an empirical question. The point is that the often-cited first segment continuation rates are a conservative estimate of the possible program effect. This is another illustration of the complexity and difficulty of securing unimpeachable data on these matters.

[15]We say "in one sense" to signal that although family planning programs can be evaluated against their effect on the birth rate, as their immediate objective, their ultimate or "real" objective is of course to improve welfare prospects by means of fertility reduction. In the post-Bucharest period, it seems necessary to make this elementary point in order to make clear that such programs are not justified solely on grounds of fertility reduction.

[16]*The Determinants and Consequences of Population Trends*, vol. 1 (United Nations, 1973), table IV.7; *Population Bulletin*, no. 7, "With Special Reference to Conditions and Trends of Fertility in the World," United Nations, 1965, table 7.6.

[17]Calculations by Anrudh Jain, (Personal communications, May 1975).

[18]For example, in the Philippines in 1972, while the median age at acceptance was 29.9 and the average number of living children was 3.8 at acceptance, 25 percent were under age 25 and another 26 percent were aged 25–29; and 31 percent had fewer than three children and 31 percent had just three.

[19]I. B. Astawa, S. Waloeyo, and J. E. Laing, "Family planning in Bali," *Studies in Family Planning* 6, no. 4 (April 1975): 86–101.

[20]Of ten developing countries with data for at least three time periods, in nine the median age of acceptors declined; and in all nine cases with parity data, the parity declined. Data from Dorothy Nortman, "Population and family planning programs: A factbook," *Reports on Population/Family Planning*, no. 2 (6th edition, December 1974), tables 20–21.

[21]This estimate, taken from the Model-West female tables in A. J. Coale and P. Demeny, *Regional Model Life Tables and Stable Populations*, (Princeton University Press, 1966), is interpolated to obtain NRR of 1.0 with mean generation length of 27.

[22]R. Freedman, L. C. Coombs, M. C. Chang, and T. H. Sun, "Trends in fertility, family size preferences, and practice of family planning: Taiwan, 1965-1973," *Studies in Family Planning* 5, no. 9 (September 1974): table 30.

[23]A statement by the respondent that she wants no more children probably has more reliability and validity than an answer to a question about her preferred number of children. In the table, all respondents who said that such matters were "up to God, up to fate," or that they could not answer the question were classified as wanting more children, so the figures cited are conservative estimates of the proportion who want no more children.

[24]D. V. N. Sarma and Anrudh K. Jain, "Preference about sex of children and use of contraception among women

wanting no more children in India," *Demography India*, no. 1 (1974): 104.

[25] L. C. Coombs, "The measurement of family size preferences and subsequent fertility," *Demography* 11 (November 1974): 587–611; C. H. Coombs, L. C. Coombs, and G. H. McClelland, "Preference scales for number and sex of children," *Population Studies* 29, no. 2 (July 1975): 273–279. The theoretical and feasibility tests of the scales in the United States, Hungary, South Korea, Philippines, Taiwan, and Malaysia were conducted under the auspices of a subcommittee on comparative fertility studies of the International Union for the Scientific Study of Population and analyzed by L. C. Coombs and C. H. Coombs. All indicated a variability of scale positions for specific first preferences. The results will be reported for the subcommittee in a forthcoming publication by L. C. Coombs.

[26] R. Freedman, A. Hermalin, and M. C. Chang, "Do statements about desired family size predict fertility? The case of Taiwan, 1967–70," *Demography* 12 (August 1975): 407–416.

[27] Freedman, et al. (1975), Table 30.

[28] Sarma and Jain (1974), p. 97.

[29] John Knodel and Pichit Pitaktepsombati, "Fertility and family planning in Thailand: Results from two rounds of a national study," *Studies in Family Planning* 6, no. 11 (November 1975): 402–413.

[30] For example, see T. W. Schultz, ed., *Economics of the Family: Marriage, Children, and Human Capital* (University of Chicago Press, 1974).

[31] This listing omits withdrawal, which is still widely practiced in some societies though not promoted by organized programs; and rhythm, which is also practiced but, as noted, only rarely included as a program method, as in Catholic efforts in Mauritius and the Philippines. It also omits an injectable (Depo-Provera) with limited use and some medical questions.

[32] Adapted from W. Parker Mauldin, "Assessment of national family planning programs in developing countries," *Studies in Family Planning* 6, no. 2 (February 1975): 33, table 2.

[33] Data from Nortman "Factbook," various editions.

[34] Christopher Tietze and John Bongaarts, "Fertility rates and abortion rates: Simulations of family limitation," *Studies in Family Planning* 6, no. 5 (May 1975): 119. The TAR is counterpart to the TFR, i.e., the total number of abortions summed from lifetime experience at age-specific rates under consideration.

[35] Freedman et al. (1975), and Freedman and Coombs, eds. (1974).

[36] For example, see Berelson in Parry, ed. (1974), tables 1.9.2(a), (b), (c).

[37] For an analysis thereof see K. S. Srikantan, "Comparison of 20 program countries: Family planning programs, associated socio/economic infrastructural factors and fertility," (New York: Population Council, April 1975, manuscript).

[38] Data reported in W. B. Watson and R. J. Lapham, eds., "Family planning programs: World review 1974," *Studies in Family Planning* 6, no. 8 (August 1975): table 3. Figures there for 1972 and 1974 abridged for this tabulation.

[39] It is, of course, possible to argue that the program substitutes for almost all private sector contraception. But this is implausible, since it appears probable that if private sector services were readily available a significant portion of the users would be using them for reasons of convenience, privacy, etc. In fact, we know that in a number of the countries there is considerable private sector use. Possible substitution for abortion is not taken into account in either table.

[40] Table 11.9 includes more countries than Table 11.7 because plausible estimates of birth rates are more available than data on acceptance rates. For quite a few of the countries, especially those with high birth rates, these are crude estimates. However, even if the birth rates for the countries err by 5 points or so, it will have little effect on the results of the regressions since we have no reason to believe that the errors are systematically related to the social setting or program effort. Most of the large errors are probably concentrated in the lower right cell of the table where the true figures are as likely to be above as below those cited, but are in any case likely to be high.

[41] K. S. Srikantan (1975) has done a much more complex analysis of a larger body of data on a cross-sectional basis that relates a large number of social and demographic indicators to program output (acceptors) and to birth rates for 20 countries. His conclusions are broadly similar: socio-demographic development indicators are powerfully related both to program outputs and to birth rates, but he finds that a significant part of the socioeconomic influence operates through the program output and that the program output has, in addition, a separate independent association with the birth rates. Again, in the work of Dr. Srikantan, questions of temporal order can be raised about some of the data. Further questions can be raised about the application of a large number of different sets of data to just 20 countries (the universe of countries with suitable data). Both our crude tabulations and his more sophisticated analysis indicate that, apart from the dominant influence of development, there appears to be independent association of program input with birth rates.

[42] See "World Population: Status Report 1974," *Reports on Population/Family Planning*, no. 15 (January 1974): 34.

[43] For a revealing analysis of the timing of fertility decline—the later begun, the faster achieved—see

Dudley Kirk, "A new demographic transition?" in *Rapid Population Growth* (Washington, D.C.: National Academy of Sciences, 1971), pp. 123–47, and specifically the table on p. 132.

[44]For a full description of the model from which these figures are derived, see Dorothy Nortman and John Bongaarts, "Contraceptive practice required to meet a prescribed crude birth rate target: A proposed macro-model (TABRAP) and hypothetical illustrations," *Demography*, 12, (August 1975): 471–89. That model contains a range of assumptions as to initial age-sex-marital distribution, marital rates, mortality levels and trends, age-specific birth rates with and without various mixes of contraception and various continuation and effectiveness rates. From that complex array, we selected the indicated regimen, realistic for a "typical" developing society, to illustrate the rough order of magnitude of what is involved.

[45]By "threshold" is meant the attainment of a designated pre-condition for fertility decline. It is perhaps fair to say that there is no scientific consensus on what the thresholds are, at what values, or even whether there are any of general applicability across a range of diverse countries.

[46]David Heer and Dean O. Smith, "Mortality level, desired family size and population increase," *Demography* 5 (1968): 104–121.

[47]Rich (1973).

[48]James E. Kocher, *Rural Development, Income Distribution, and Fertility Decline*, (New York: The Population Council, Occasional Paper, 1973).

[49]Robert H. Cassen, "Economic-demographic interrelationships in developing countries," in *Population and Its Problems*, Parry, ed., pp. 216–238.

[50]Aziz Bindary, "Egypt studies a new plan of action," *Studies in Family Planning* 3, no. 8 (August 1972): 193–194.

[51]Kingsley Davis, "Zero Population growth: The goal and the means," in *The No-Growth Society*, Mancur Olson and Hans H. Landsberg, eds. (Norton 1973), pp. 15–30; and Kenneth E. Boulding, "The shadow of the stationary state," *The No-Growth Society*, pp. 89–102.

[52]Geoffrey McNicoll, "Community-level population policy: An exploration," *Population and Development Review* 1, no. 1 (September 1975).

[53]Including costs, a complex issue that we do not deal with here in any detail. Some elementary data, to indicate order of magnitude:

Official population assistance of all official development assistance	2–2.5%
Annual per capita budget of family planning programs (23 countries)	$0.15
Family planning in total national budget (17 countries)	11%
Family planning in health budget (17 countries)	2.7%

Source: First figure derived from Statistical Annex of DAC Chairman's Report, OECD, 1974. Other three derived from Nortman *Factbook*, Tables 9–12.

For fuller information on costs, see *Status Report*, pp. 40–41. For economic analysis of the matter, see Gavin Jones, *Population Growth and Educational Planning in Developing Nations* (Irvington, 1975), especially pp. 220–227; and Warren C. Robinson, *Population and Development Planning*, (New York: The Population Council, 1975), passim. Also note this evaluation of whether the expenditures on the Indian family planning program have been worthwhile despite its limited success:

> The question is, had there been no family planning programme, and the population grown by 1 m. a year more, would that Rs. 435m invested in other things have generated Rs.7 per head for the larger population? The answer is, No. If the Rs.435m were invested every year in the rest of the economy instead of the family planning programme, the capital stock would be about Rs.3,000m bigger after six years, which on very generous assumptions would yield an extra Rs.1500m of income in 1972/3, or about Rs.2.5 per head. Every assumption we have made favours non-family planning investment, including the low estimate of number of births prevented at high cost, and the thoroughly optimistic figures for the income yielded by alternative investment. Yet per capita income is higher by preventing a million births annually than by investing generally in development—though not all that much higher. Various authorities have estimated the value of a prevented birth in India—the highest estimate was Rs.7,800, the lowest Rs.690. All we have tried to do is to show that funds expended on family planning would not have made a bigger impact on income per head if spent elsewhere. [from Cassen, forthcoming.]

[54]See Teitelbaum; and also R. Freedman, "The transition from high to low fertility: Challenge to demographers," *Population Index* 31, no. 4 (October 1965): 417–429.

[55]See, e.g., Demeny (1968) in footnote 7.

[56]Kingsley Davis, "The theory of change and response in modern demographic history," *Population Index* 29, no. 4 (October 1963): 345–366.

[57]Teitelbaum, p. 424.

[58]John C. Caldwell, "The containment of world population growth," *Studies in Family Planning* 6, no. 12 (December 1975):431.

Part VII—Ethical Considerations

12
Government Efforts to Influence Fertility: The Ethical Issues

Written with Jonathan Lieberson

In the past twenty years or so "the population problem" has been added to the world's agenda not simply as the subject of scientific study and public discussion but also impinging on policy intervention. In the international arena, the United Nations has held meetings, including the first intergovernmental World Population Conference at Bucharest in 1974, passed resolutions, sponsored programmatic efforts, and established a special organization to concentrate on the issue (the United Nations Fund for Population Activities). National governments, both developed and developing, have set up various commissions on the subject and beyond that have adopted policies and organized programs to influence demographic trends. Private foundations, universities, and voluntary organizations have devoted substantial resources to research, training, technical assistance, service, and information distribution. In short, there has been, one might say, a minor revolution in the field—spotty in space and time, trendy in its ups and downs, filled with visions, revisions, and fashions, controversial as to both ends and means, but still maintaining a dynamic vitality of its own.[1]

At the heart of this development, certainly the sole stimulus at the outset and the major one today, is the definition of "the population problem" as the unduly rapid rates of population growth in the developing world, resulting from the sharp decline in mortality after World War II and the continuation of high fertility (the "demographic gap"). Rapid growth is not considered the villain "in and of itself" but only insofar as it retards national efforts toward development, modernization, a better standard of living for the world's poor, human welfare—in sum, insofar as the quality of human life is being burdened or threatened by the quantity.

Population growth can be reduced in only three ways: raise mortality, promote migration, lower fertility. The first is unacceptable and the second infeasible.[2] Thus, lowered fertility has become a proximate goal of development policy in many countries (that today include the vast majority of the population of the developing world); and despite a recent broadening and softening of that goal for various political and other reasons, the goal itself remains. Meanwhile, as ironic counterpart to the growing theme, some developed countries concerned about their "too low" birth rates have taken policy steps to try to raise fertility among their populations or particular subgroups thereof. To our best knowledge, all married couples in the world today have the "human right" (as expressed in international resolutions and documents, e.g., Teheran and Bucharest) to have the number of children they want, subject only to some appropriate language about parental responsibility, and, moreover, have the legal right as well. But fertility behavior is subject to various cultural "controls" and to an increasing number of government interventions as well, both pro- and antinatalist.

If a government decides to intervene to influence fertility behavior for demographic reasons, either antinatalist or pro-, what can it do? What policies

---

Reprinted with permission from *Population and Development Review* 1979; 5(4):581–613, The Population Council, New York, NY.

are available? There are numerous ways to describe the array of possibilities, but by class of actions (as against the wide variety of specific implementations in particular settings) there are not many. For present purposes they can be listed thus:[3]

1. *Manipulate public and private access* to modern methods of fertility control, including not only oral contraceptives, IUDs, and condoms but also sterilization and abortion.
2. *Change the perceived socioeconomic determinants* of fertility behavior: popular education and literacy, infant/child mortality and life expectancy, industrialization and urbanization, income and income equity, status of women, housing, among others.
3. *Make propaganda* and/or limit opposing views.
4. *Manipulate incentives and disincentives* in the desired directions, through child assistance stipends, maternity leaves and costs, tax benefits, direct monetary subsidies to individual families for "correct" fertility behavior (e.g., fees for vasectomies), community incentives or disincentives for "correct" fertility behavior (e.g., roads or schools).
5. *Exert sociopolitical pressure or impose direct sanctions*, from minimum age at marriage to limits on family size.

This paper seeks to explore the ethical implications of such interventions: What are the current government efforts to affect fertility that raise ethical questions, how are they to be appraised from the standpoint of ethical acceptability, and what is the general rationale informing that appraisal? In short, we are concerned only with the *ethical issues* involved in *what the state should and should not do on demographic grounds* (understanding that such actions are not ends in themselves but are a means toward larger concerns of human welfare).

In order to stay close to the reality of the matter, we limit the examples for discussion to actual policies being undertaken (with a side glance at proposals being made). We deal exclusively with the ethicality of the policies, not with their effectiveness. As it happens, all of the policies under discussion are indeed effective in nontrivial degree, so this is not simply an abstract philosophical exercise but rather an attempt to join philosophy and public affairs in the realm of real-world decisions with important human consequences, individual and collective.

We base our discussion here on three premises: (1) that current fertility trends are considered undesirable in many places, certainly not optimal, and particularly the "too high" rate in developing countries; (2) that governmental intervention to change trends is as legitimate in this connection as it is in other spheres affecting human welfare;[4] and (3) that completely benign measures (e.g., provision of fertility information or services, enhanced development efforts) may be insufficient in some settings to achieve the demographic and welfare goals considered appropriate or even necessary.[5]

We hasten to add that we know that none of these premises is universally accepted by knowledgeable and respected specialists: some believe that fertility trends are not much of a problem, some believe that government ought to stay out of this arena altogether, some believe that benign measures properly taken will be sufficient to the task. Without arguing the matter or even asserting our own views, we consider it enough here simply to observe that all three premises are now accepted in significant degree in the real world and that remedial actions of importance are now being taken. So whether the premises are correct or not, whether they are only perceptions or facts, they are having real consequences for people and, hence, call for review on that ground alone.

The question then becomes, for example: If family planning programs on the one hand and general or selective development on the other are for different reasons not enough to achieve the "necessary" fertility reduction in the time available, what then? To that point, some knowledgeable observers believe that whatever success in reducing fertility has recently been achieved in the three largest developing countries (China, India, and Indonesia), all at low levels of socioeconomic development, is attributable significantly to incentives and pressures; and further, that similar records, such as they are, cannot be expected in countries of similar socioeconomic setting without similar "hard" measures. So "what then" is not merely an academic question, but, to some, a living issue for the next years—an observation offered analytically, not normatively. Indeed, the recent Report of the Select Committee on Population of the US House of Representatives contains a section on "Ethical Issues" that raises more questions than it settles in seeking to delineate "compulsion" in this field. As the Committee asks: "Is the right of parents to determine the number of children an absolute one? Is it always unethical for a government to use compulsion to restrict population size?"[6] In short, however the solution of "the population problem" may be defined, what if it cannot be achieved without some form of incentive or pressure or sanction? Where do the ethical rights lie then?

Note that we make a clear distinction between government policy to affect fertility and cultural conditions that affect fertility. The cultural milieu consists of several accepted practices, often of a pronatalist character, deriving from the long history of arrangements supporting human survival, that have a strong but often unremarked influence on fertility behavior: religious proscriptions, kinship requirements, early marriage as protection against premarital sexuality, the role of women, breastfeeding practices, divorce and remarriage traditions, marital needs to demonstrate fecundity or virility, son preference, sex roles, even fashion. Such traditional practices are typically taken for granted by the participants, are considered of the nature of life, and are usually not experienced as influences on fertility much less as unethical interventions; so pervasive are they that it is not easy to conceive what "absolute freedom" from the cultural setting would mean with regard to fertility. One demographer has argued that societies need not invent or impose antinatalist incentives if they would only eliminate the existing pronatalist ones:

> What kinds of reproductive policies can be pursued in an effort to reduce long-term population growth? The most important step toward developing such new policies is to recognize and understand the existing ones, for we already have influential and coercive policies regarding reproductive behavior. . . [in the] complex social organization and system of incentives that encourage mating, pregnancy, and the care, support, and rearing of children. These institutional mechanisms are the pronatalist "policies" evolved unconsciously over millennia to give societies a fertility sufficient to offset high mortality. The formation and implementation of antinatalist motives must be based, therefore, on an analysis and modification of the existing pro-natalist policies. Many of these new [anti-natalist] policies will entail a *lifting* of pressures *to* reproduce, rather than an *imposition* of pressures *not* to do so.[7]

But can a cultural practice be called a "policy" in the same sense as a government intervention? How indeed can it be changed in a reasonable time except through such intervention?—as the author's own remedial examples seem to acknowledge. In all likelihood, current fertility trends are determined more by cultural practice than by government policy, whether pronatalist or anti-. But here again we limit ourselves to state policy, often developed in direct opposition to established cultural practices.[8]

At all times we seek to anchor the ethical discussion in real-world problems and policies, as we move toward informed conclusions. We say "move toward" because we are under no illusion that such questions can be definitively answered, especially across the wide range of cultural and political situations and attendant ethical positions that characterize today's world. Indeed, it is in the nature of the case that such issues are never "settled"—whatever that might mean—but only ventilated, sorted out, and framed for further discourse. Where we think we see a clear position, we state it; where we remain puzzled by the counterarguments, we acknowledge that. We hope this spirit of "thinking through" shows: an attempt at enlightenment. We trust that issues are somewhat clearer at the end of this exercise than at its beginning—as indeed they are to us personally as a result of this inquiry.

The Policy Situation

We begin by putting the ethical question to the above list of policy options. Only one option, promotion of socioeconomic determinants, does not raise questions in this connection, if for no other reason, because such policies are not normally pursued on demographic grounds (though they can have demographic effects). Efforts at development or "modernization" may on occasion raise their own similar ethical issues as, for example, when the liberation of women or certain forms of secularism are pushed against people's desires or pushed too fast and hard to be assimilated by the traditional culture (Iran—the current tragic illustration). Similar ethical issues can be raised with regard to governmental interventions for development or "modernization" in their impact upon traditional cultures, but they are outside our purview here. To our best knowledge, the following array contains the types of government programs now or recently in effect that have raised questions of ethical propriety in the field.

Limited Access to Fertility Control

This includes limitation on demographic grounds of legal access to certain methods of fertility control that are generally considered medically acceptable: for example, induced abortion in many countries (e.g., Catholic), sterilization in many countries (e.g., Muslim and Latin), the oral contraceptive in Japan (in order, some think, to protect the profitable medical monopoly on induced abortion). A 1973 review[9] listed only two developing countries out of 33 surveyed that had "general availability" of the five modern methods (oral contraceptive, IUD, conventionals [condoms], sterilization, abortion); and as of mid-1975 another study[10] found abortion fully legal (though with various conditions) in only 11 of 93 countries. Sudden withdrawal of legalized abortion in Romania at a time when it was the major instrument of fertility control, and discouragement of other modern methods, on demographic grounds, had a dramatic demographic effect.[11] Withdrawal of federal government funding of legal abortion for the poor in the United States has had demonstrable results with class and ethnic differentials.[12]

Official Promotion of Propaganda

This occurs often with nonencouragement or limitation of opposing viewpoints; it includes propaganda exhorting that changed family norms for reasons of the individual and collective benefit, in countries with official policies to change fertility, typically in the absence of equivalent support for opposition views but also without restriction of such views, except in a few more authoritarian regimes. This has been a strong element in a few countries (China, Indonesia, South Korea, India and Israel earlier) but not in most. Where information and education shade off into persuasion, and persuasion into pressure, is a sticky question, but usually distinguishable.

Incentives and Disincentives

Whether immediate or remote, direct or indirect, individual or community, incentives and disincentives have a long pronatalist history in the developed world and in recent years have been introduced in the developing world as well, as a possible "third way" to expedite fertility decline beyond family planning programs ("not enough") and general development ("too slow"). Among typical incentive efforts are these:[13]

1. Direct monetary stipends, pronatalist: Child assistance subsidies and maternity costs and leaves, for a combination of demographic, family welfare, and redistributional motives, in such Western European countries as France and Sweden, have long been in practice, but with unproved demographic effect.[14] Family allowances and maternity and birth payments sharply graduated by birth order from about 5 percent of average annual wage for the first child to about 40 percent for the third, and then up further in some countries but down in others, in such Eastern European countries as Bulgaria, Czechoslovakia, Hungary, and East Germany, have been of relatively short duration and of unknown demographic effect.[15]

2. Direct monetary stipends, antinatalist: Direct monetary payments for vasectomy have been most widespread in India, both in the regular program and in special vasectomy camps, with other incentives in kind plus occasionally a large payoff lottery. Such direct and immediate payments are limited to sterilization because of the administrative difficulty, probably the impossibility, of monitoring the continuation of such methods as the pill or the IUD. The payments in India ranged from about Rs. 100 in cash and kind in the camps to one-sixth that amount under the normal family planning program.[16]

3. Deferred monetary incentives, pronatalist: East Germany provides low-income couples with interest-free loans at marriage for home furnishings with 20 percent cancelled with the first birth, 30 percent with the second, and the remaining 50 percent with the third, if within eight years.[17] Similar low-interest loans for housing and furnishings are offered in Czechoslovakia and Hungary, substantially forgiven with births.[18]

4. Deferred monetary incentives, antinatalist: In the Taiwan educational bond scheme, couples with two or fewer children received annual deposits to their name in a blocked savings account available only toward the costs of higher education for their children; if a third child was born to the couple the account was reduced to 50 percent, if a fourth child, to zero.[19] In the India tea estate program, a joint savings account was set up in the name of the company and the woman, into which the company paid about Rs. 5 each month the woman was not pregnant. The account, which with accumulated interest would amount to nearly a year's earnings at normal retirement after 30 years' participation, is available to the woman at the end of her childbearing years but part is forfeited with the fourth child and the total with the fifth.[20]

5. Indirect incentive for late marriage: In China disincentives for early marriage are reported through the use of wage level, housing allocation, and university admission.[21]

6. Mixed program of incentives and disincentives: Paid maternity leave for first two children but not for third and subsequent; preference in choice of primary school limited to first three children in a family but extended to the fourth and higher if a parent is sterilized; removal of large family priorities for highly valued public housing; permission to sublet rooms to families with three or fewer children; construction of few large flats; increased delivery charges in public hospitals for higher birth orders by factors of 2 to 5 from first child to fifth and subsequent, and charges for antenatal clinic visits for mothers of two or more children; special monetary consideration following upon sterilization; increased tax relief only for first three children and less for the third—all in Singapore.[22] (Similar treatment of maternity leaves and child allowances for government employees occurs in a few other countries.)

Pressures and Sanctions

In the very nature of the case, it is not always possible to secure an authoritative, complete public account of precisely what such interventions are meant to be or how they actually operate in certain situations and over large territories. What follows is an effort to suggest what went on or goes on by way of fertility intervention under this heading.[23]

With regard to grant of marriage license: As part of a "model city" project in the Philippines, a municipal ordinance required proof of family planning counseling before issuance of a (compulsory) marriage license. A legal opinion from a university law center considered the proposal unethical and unconstitutional, but through subsequent efforts of government departments "more than 200 municipalities have passed ordinances requiring family planning counseling as a precondition for the issuance of marriage licenses."[24]

With regard to later age at marriage, which contributes on the average to lower fertility, China apparently manages to enforce a later age than the legal minimum (18 for females and 22 for males) by promoting and realizing minima of 24 and 26 (with some differences in rural and urban areas) through "propaganda, heavily backed by pressure of public opinion."[25] Virtually all countries have laws regulating minimum age at marriage, and a recent compendium finds that at least 54 countries have changed such laws in the past generation.[26]

With regard to fertility control and family size, the three main current instances of operational interventions that can be classified under this heading—on occasion, pressure shading into sanction—come from the three largest developing countries, China, Indonesia, and India.

In China, use of birth quotas is reportedly widespread.[27] Provincial authorities allocate local population growth targets based on national population growth plans. At the local level, the allowable births are allocated on a priority basis. Married couples without children have first priority, followed by those with one child over age two, followed by those with one younger child, and so on. Local officials maintain detailed records of all couples' contraceptive practice. Permission to plan a birth is conferred on a couple on the basis of group decision at public meetings. Strong peer pressure is placed on those who become pregnant out of turn to have an induced abortion.

In Indonesia, too, there appears to be a well-organized political-bureaucratic transmission of targets from top to bottom (especially in Bali and East Java) that results in peer pressure at the village level.[28] Family planning is a community affair in the 3,500 *Banjar*, or hamlets. A map of all houses in the banjar is prominently displayed in the meeting hall, identifying the method of contraception used in each household. Contraceptive practice is discussed at each monthly meeting of household heads, and nonusers are asked to justify their behavior. In some banjars, the banjar leader daily sounds a drum to remind women to take their oral contraceptives.

A comprehensive description of precisely what occurred as pressure or even "coercion" exerted on fertility behavior during India's Emergency, culminating in 1976, does not to our knowledge exist.[29] What can be said with assurance is that there was an intensive drive, at least in some areas of India, with high targets set by the central government increased in some states; that district commissioners were required to achieve given sterilization targets by whatever means they could find; and that the means often included exercise of their power over permits, licenses, school entry, appointments, and employment, as well as further dispersal of the target to teachers and other local-level governmental employees who used their own means, sometimes including paid agents and, apparently infrequently, physical force. The total campaign added up to a substantial exercise of pressure to secure candidates for sterilization.

Based on this array, a few preliminary observations can be made, of an empirical not (yet) normative character.

To date, most government intervention with regard to fertility behavior, not detailed here, has been benign. That is, it has been informational, developmental (with respect to presumed determinants, good in their own right, though not instituted on demographic grounds), and programmatic (with regard to family planning services) to the end of increasing fertility options for individual couples rather than limiting them—particularly under conditions where that increase in available options is expected to decrease fertility itself.

No legal sanctions limiting family size on demographic grounds or governmentally inspired "heavy" coercion have been used to control fertility behavior in developing countries, except sporadically and temporarily in India under the Emergency and infrequently elsewhere with regard to marriage age or requirements.[30] Such sanctions are used to limit access to methods of fertility regulation on other than medical or moral or religious grounds and specifically on demographic grounds, but as part of an effort to raise fertility not lower it (e.g., Romania). Indirect efforts to lower fertility through legal sanctions are infrequently used, and even there, as in the notable Singapore case, the impact is considered to derive more from the official declaration of an appropriate public norm than from a sanction to be scrupulously enforced.[31]

Nonetheless, certain problematic issues from the standard of ethical permissibility or propriety remain. The ethical issues, whatever they are and however they are to be applied, arise from only three categories of government intervention actually being applied at the present time:

- Limitations imposed on access to modern methods of fertility control, on demographic (not medical) grounds
- Incentives and disincentives of various kinds, offered but not compelled (and restricted to the ultimate actors, i.e., not including fees to doctors or field workers)
- Peer pressure organized and guided by the political apparatus.

As we have noted, much more has been proposed, but only these are now somewhere in effect.[32]

Ethical Issues Raised by Particular Policies

Now that we have presented the various types of policies that have raised ethical questions in the population field, we turn to the question of what is "right" and "wrong." We remind the reader that just as our previous discussion has been confined to policies already in effect, so our discussion of ethical acceptability is similarly limited, though the ramifications to other proposals will be obvious.

In what follows, our discussion reverses the customary order in ethical literature. Instead of first presenting a grand design—the "basis" or "foundations" of ethics—and then deriving particular consequences for the issues in question in the population field, we shall first offer our views concerning the propriety of the particular policies we have surveyed one by one, setting forth and anticipating certain problems with our approach as we go along. Then, in the following section, partly by way of justification and partly by way of further articulation of our view, we shall sketch out what kinds of answers in general we would give to the grand questions of procedure and substance. Nothing we shall say entails that answers to problems arising in "population ethics" can be divorced from larger ethical questions; indeed, one merit of our approach is that it keeps the discussion close to the decisions at hand and allows us to elucidate certain general features of justification in ethics.

First, the problematic policies and our assessment of the issues they raise.

Limitations on Access to Methods of Fertility Control

Limitations on access are not ethically permissible as a means of pursuing demographic goals in our view: they impinge upon the autonomy of the individual couple and restrict the couple's options and effective choice and freedom to decide, and they can be circumvented by the rich more easily than the poor.

There is one qualification and one distinction to be drawn here. The qualification is that we do not claim that there are absolutely no conditions under which a government might not justifiably impose limits on access: there may be medical grounds that justify the banning of a birth control pill or Depo Provera. (If this be derogatorily called "paternalism," some regard it as justified paternalism.[33]) The central issue here is whether limits on access are justified or implemented *for demographic reasons* and whether the decision to enforce them is generated in such a way as to allow for public participation and discussion. In the absence of these proper conditions (as in the Romania case), limitations on access seem to infringe unnecessarily upon the autonomy and liberty of individuals to decide for themselves, with the best available knowledge and technology, whether they wish to bear children.

But we must add a distinction here as well. We do not claim that government has an obligation to provide free and equal access to all means of fertility control. That is a different point from our claim that government has an obligation not to limit access on demographic grounds. Note in this respect that traditional family planning programs are, in both design and effect, discriminatory in favor of the poor—in bringing them an opportunity (service) disproportionately available in their societies to the better-off. This form of discrimination is of course generally approved, both as to intent and effect. Note also that in most developing countries, the "garden variety" of family planning programs (i.e., without pressures) was instituted in a nonopen society without public participation in the policy decision; in this case, however, the ease of declining to participate in the program itself gives the individual couple autonomy of decision.

Incentives

We regard positive incentives (rewarding for "correct" fertility behavior) as ethically permissible provided certain circumstances are fulfilled as noted below; and we regard the use of negative incentives (withholding or penalizing for "incorrect" fertility behavior) as acceptable under the same circumstances, provided safeguards for the protection of innocent third parties who might be adversely affected are guaranteed.

A variety of objections may be thought to arise against incentive programs, whether such programs are positive, negative, or mixed, direct or remote, individual or community directed. In the main, the objections fall into two categories: (1) incentives infringe upon freedom of choice by (unduly) influencing the options of parental decision makers, and (2) incentives can be unjust.

With regard to the first, let us note that by definition incentives are rewards or penalties, tangible or intangible, given to a couple or group in order to induce some specific fertility behavior. As such, they are expressly designed to alter parental choice; their use would otherwise be unnecessary.

In our view, positive incentives serve to enlarge options, not diminish them, and hence can serve both freedom and (interclass) justice. The individual is presented with a choice he did not have in the absence of the incentive; since he can decline the incentive, he has lost nothing from his previous state but has gained an option—the incentive rather than his normal fertility behavior.[34] If the incentives, positive or negative, are simply offers to an individual or group that can be taken up or turned down according to desires and preferences, and if the individual or group possesses adequate knowledge concerning the options and the consequences of choosing one or another without loss of the prior alternative—if these conditions are met, if (in other words) an *effective* choice exists, then in our view no specifically ethical problem is present. Whether these conditions are met in the particular case is a question of empirical fact, not of ethical principle.

As for the assertion that incentives impugn human dignity by monetizing children, the most telling response is that that has long been common practice and by the parents themselves: for the children's presumed economic value as workers and social security in poor countries, for their costs as against alternative benefits and expenditures in other countries. Balancing children against affluence is a familiar choice, and both couples and societies typically choose the latter when the choice presents itself.

The discriminatory, or unjust, quality of incentives is more complicated and more difficult (though it would not seem to be an issue in a situation in which the individual was effectively free to decline the incentive). First let us distinguish between discriminatory intent and discriminatory effect: a policy aimed at parity, not class, need have no intent to discriminate by class, yet have such an effect since the poor will be more attracted to an incentive of given size than the rich.[35] By definition, the poor are less well-off than the rich, so that it follows that given incentives will vary in attractiveness to the two groups. This is not a powerful objection to incentive programs as such. Indeed, what is usually overlooked in this charge is that the effect of the incentive itself is precisely as a device to redistribute wealth from richer to poorer. Small? Yes, but then the ethical impact must be commensurately small.

To turn now to special problems concerned with negative incentive programs, the chief one is the possible effect on third party innocents born in disregard of the disincentives. Since negative incentives penalize those who engage in fertility behavior beyond a specified limit, the possibility of disadvantages unfairly thrust upon innocents is particularly acute. The potential disadvantages fall into two groups: first, the effects of entry into a society implementing disincentives—socioeconomic status, housing, schooling, and general welfare affected adversely; and second, psychological or internal effects in the form of intra-family reactions to innocents on the ground that they cost the family something—subsequent regret, unfair preferment, and other attitudes causing low self-esteem and reduced self-worth. Such effects may not be large in disincentive programs that can be realistically envisaged (i.e., feasible), but they exist nevertheless and should be safeguarded against. There are clear cases that must be corrected—for example, if the Nth+1 child were deprived of public education—but the multiple ramifications of the problem of innocents are so subtle and difficult to place under standardized control that they constitute a *prima facie* reason in favor of employing positive incentives in preference to disincentives. In short, the innocent party must not be unduly harmed by the working out of policy—and the Singapore experience has shown that is achievable in design and in practice.

In sum, our view is that positive incentives are usually permissible—provided that means of resolving a population problem are not sufficiently effective in their absence and that those who are affected by the incentives possess sufficient knowledge of and understand the consequences of accepting them. The potentially discriminatory effects of such programs should be reduced as far as possible through adapting and readapting program design to varying situations. Positive incentives are, all things considered, to be preferred to negative ones (and mixed programs) on the ground that the potential harm to innocents entailed by the use of negative incentives may be a present danger.

Finally, there is the problem, essentially administrative in our view but apparently ethical to others, that incentive programs lend themselves to corruption and abuse. That is probably so. But let us distinguish between a policy and a particular application of a policy. The latter may be disastrous, a gross abuse of the former. Once again, it is obvious that incentive programs may be abused or corrupted (as reportedly in India),[36] but so can any policy involving monetary transfers—indeed, any policy at all. But not all policies are inevitably abused to the point of ethical inadmissibility. Instead, they are usually supplemented by qualifying conditions as to the circumstances of their application, and abuse, far from being part of the policy, is not even inevitable given decent administration. Similarly, the incentive can be misused through deceit: some people who accept incentives do not intend to or cannot have further children anyway. But in such cases the ethical onus seems to us to fall on the dissemblers for accepting the incentive, not on the state for offering it.

It is not surprising that such programs cannot be rigidly safeguarded from corruption or abuse in all possible circumstances. But this, we think, means not that they should never be used but that intelligence and diligence must be introduced in implementing them in each particular case. The same can be said of virtually any public policy.

Politically Organized Peer Pressure

In our view, a mixed picture emerges of the ethical acceptability of such efforts. Politically organized peer pressure seems to us permissible only under certain conditions, to be enumerated shortly.

A few preliminary points must first be made. First, it is not precisely clear how to delimit such efforts from milder policies: government information, guidance, and education shade off, sometimes imperceptibly, into "soft" then "hard" persuasion and that into peer pressure, either because larger and larger groups in the society accept the views being disseminated or earlier "failures" lead governments toward stronger and stronger measures. Ordinarily, we do not raise special difficulties when government takes the role of informant or educator or regulator—but where does that allowance end? Is it possible to set limits on this role so that government may engage in information-giving but not in generating peer pressure that is "politically organized"? So there is a difficulty at the outset in discriminating the effects of government involvement in public concerns.

Another point that is pertinent here concerns culture. We are each born into a culture that approves or condemns certain behavior. As we have noted, cultural practices are not "policies," but they are often the residue or deposit of deliberate actions undertaken by prior dominant powers. If we are to be consistent we must note that much that passes for "culturally determined" beliefs and attitudes is politically determined. Consider attitudes toward nuptiality, mortality, and other vital areas of life: many of them are the effects of prior government enactments that have crystallized cultural practices into law, which in turn reinforce or solidify the practice itself.

In order to clarify these complex issues, let us confine ourselves to a program of politically organized peer pressure deliberately designed to promote demographic goals, whether pro- or antinatalist, whether going against the grain of cultural practices or not. The issue is to provide ethical appraisal of such a program regardless of whether it is appealing to the cultural heritage, whether it is likely to be effective, and whether it makes use of existing practices. Is there any perfectly general judgment that can be made or laid down for such an appraisal? We think not, but we do suggest that there are at least three conditions that ought to be satisfied before any such program is put into effect.[37]

First, no such program ought to be considered until every reasonable effort has been made to exhaust the possibilities of using "softer" measures, such as purely voluntary family planning supply programs, efforts to affect relevant socioeconomic factors, provision of positive incentives, or negative incentives harmless to innocents. The reason for this course is to maximally reduce the possibility of harmful effects and to invoke policies with potentially harmful effects only if the problem under consideration is of both sufficient gravity and sufficient recalcitrance. In each such case, we would require both that softer measures be tried out or contemplated before resorting to measures that are harsher, and that an official determination of serious consequences from fertility trends without further intervention be made and balanced against the consequences of using "harsher" measures. The justification of this "stepladder" approach will become clearer as we proceed, although it seems to us intuitively secure on its face.

The second condition is also a matter of procedure. We would require that members of the community to be affected be involved, whether directly or through their representatives, in an open and fair discussion as to whether to institute the program in the first place. Of course there are snags here: the form, duration, and consequences of such programs are often a matter for expert judgment. But the fundamental point we wish to make is that affected citizens should, at the very least, be able to "talk back," to be heard up the line, regarding such issues as quotas, means, time, urgency, degree, and so on—and especially in nonopen societies.

The third condition follows upon the second. Not only should community members be reasonably involved in the formulation of this policy; they should also be reasonably and adequately protected from penalty for subsequent individual dissent. Although of the greatest importance, this requirement is difficult to satisfy: a person who dissents from community consensus arrived at through village councils or meetings is liable to exposure to subtle forms of harassment, harm, humiliation, loss of status, and other pressures that are difficult to detect, not to mention the overt withholding of ration cards and the like (another form of injury to innocents). The consenting members of the community are apt to regard the dissident as malingering, unpatriotic, or selfish. We believe, however, that on ethical grounds politically organized programs of peer pressure should not be instituted where freedom or safeguard is absent for dissidents. Furthermore, it seems to us that the most effective means of ensuring the right to dissent is through consulting community members in each case in order to ascertain the most appropriate method of protection. In Indonesia, for example, identification of contraceptive users and nonusers on a public bulletin board does not seem to us excessively harmful, whereas marching dissidents up and down the village street in humiliation for nonconformance does; but the villagers themselves may very well see the matter differently. (This whole issue raises the profound question of "whose ethics" are to be observed, to which we later turn.)

Given the official nature of such political organization of peer pressure, particularly in nondemocratic or nonopen societies, there is obviously considerable room for abuse. All the more reason to insist on these conditions as safeguards. With them, however, the practice can be seen as an attempt, under difficult circumstances, to move societies ahead guided by major reliance upon the development of community consensus—on fertility in this case, as on agriculture, schools, roads, or water supply in other cases. If it can be done with due (ethical) regard for the community's members—in both the policy's origination and in its outcome—it seems to us ethically admissible.[38] These three conditions do not eliminate the possibility of deleterious effects stemming from the use of such peer pressure to reduce fertility; hence, we stress again, such programs ought not be employed unless an extraordinarily serious problem is present, and schemes should be devised that carry the least possible moral risk with them.

We have now cited our views on the three types of government policies employed today in the realm of fertility performance that entail possibly objectionable intervention from the ethical viewpoint. Limitations on access we have seen as generally impermissible, positive incentives as generally permissible except under unusual circumstances, negative incentives as generally permissible if harm is not visited upon innocents, and peer pressure programs as permissible only under the specified conditions. In each case, we have observed, the seriousness of the problem at hand must be considered in accordance with our "stepladder" or hierarchical conception: employ less severe measures where possible and only ascend to harsher measures if the problem at hand, as a matter of (established) fact, is clearly grave enough to warrant it.

The Ethical Framework Used to Assess Policies

So far, we have presented our position on the ethical acceptability of the three types of interventionist policies now in effect. In order to clarify and strengthen this position, we must note that it is tied to, and not meant to be isolated from, a conception of a moral society. This should be apparent from our discussion of the conditions under which the various interventions are in our view ethically admissible. Still we need to provide a sketch of the background we have in mind that underlies and informs our specific judgments. The following is the ethical framework within which we have worked.

Decision Not System

We consider that there is no overriding "correct" ethical system or universally "approved" ranking of human rights that is ready and waiting for application to specific events;[39] but that ethical issues arise out of a perception of specific conflict, disagreement, disparity: between ethical values (e.g., where freedom and equity may be in conflict) or between ethical values and other goals (e.g., personal freedom vis-à-vis perceived public welfare, as in the case of reproductive voluntarism vis-à-vis population growth as burden on development or population decline as burden on productivity and power).

Our view is not a "system" but an eclectic combination of insights of a common-sense kind gathered from central schools of ethics. It does not accord with Natural Rights theory, or Contract theory (at least in its modern versions), or Utilitarianism, but tries instead to collect the central claims of these diverse views in a serviceable manner. It seems to us to be an intuitive view as it stands—no doubt in need of amendment, improvement, and further articulation, but sound at the core.

It is customary in the moral literature to provide a "justification" for one's views. Have we given a "justification" for our views? The issue is a tangled one. Suffice to quickly make the following points here: it is not clear exactly what is desired by way of "justification," and the familiar views on the subject seem to us to rest upon a mistaken view of ethics.

To the first point, the term "justify" is radically unclear. Ordinary justification of a moral view consists in describing it further to another person who shares a set of fundamental views, perhaps unarticulated; there is no need for more. Then there is a sense of justifying a view to another person who does not share the same set of fundamental views and must be persuaded of their validity. Finally, although there are a variety of other senses of the term, there is extraordinary justification, which a long tradition in moral philosophy has endorsed: it consists in satisfying certain logical or deductive standards and deducing from a base of absolutely certain or self-certifying moral premises the views in question, thereby forestalling any possible problems that might arise in time. Our position is that there is generally no *need* to justify our views in any way other than "ordinary justification," unless parties to the discussion demand otherwise—a rare situation. This first point is one that rejects what is known as "foundationalism" in ethical theory.[40]

But we also have a second claim to make: it seems to us that ethical theory is properly concerned with action and therefore with choice.[41] Construing ethics as a conflict-resolving discipline, we not only see no need, in the absence of substantive and genuine problems at hand, for justifying (in any sense) what is unproblematic, we also suspect there is little need for the kind of theory that it has been the traditional aim of ethics to provide, namely a system of "pure" ethics, which is then to be "applied" to cases at hand. If ethics is to be seen as we have seen it, there is no incompatibility with providing systematic views—where they are needed, where problems are "big" enough to require "big" justifications—but their role is no longer to specify eternal truths of morality or supreme laws but simply to aid in reflection upon how to act. Thus, the distinction between "pure" and "applied" ethics ceases to play any role. In this sense, ethics is just a branch of decision-making. In our view, ethical inquiry is always a question of "What is to be done?" and whatever "system" comes into the picture depends upon the problem to be resolved. Otherwise, we need not scratch where it does not itch. As the last paragraph of a noted book on the subject claims: "Morality is made to minister to the good lives of individuals and not to interfere with them any more than is necessary. Morality is made for man, not man for morality."[42]

Twin Criteria

We consider that the proper ethical appraisal rests upon two foundations: (1) procedural, that is, how is the policy formulated and implemented, with regard to the citizen's degree of participation in the process thus affecting him, from the macro level (the "open" as against the "closed" society) to the micro level (deliberations and determinations within the village or community); and (2) substantive, that is, what "ethical values" are taken into account, for example, freedom, justice, enhancing options for both individuals and collective.[43]

There are two central questions concerning the ethical status of any government intervention. The first is: What sort of governance is in question? How are decisions affecting its citizenry reached and implemented? This is what we call the "procedural" question; it concerns how government operates, whether it takes into account the preferences of those governed, and how it reaches decisions and puts them into effect. In brief, is it an "open" society—with free speech, free dissent, free organization, and so on—or not? The second question is: Granted some procedure for arriving at decisions, what sorts of considerations have entered into the decision in question? This is a "substantive" question; it concerns the issue of whether the decision is right, acceptable, "good," based on "correct ethical values." In any discussion of government policy, these two questions figure prominently, but they are logically independent. They frame the discussion of our prior appraisals.

In our view the ethical society would realize acceptable or proper answers to these two questions. Such a society would be one based on something like voluntary or consensual agreements—no doubt an idea very hard to render clear, but serviceable in any case. The purpose and end of such a society would be to ensure personal liberties and, through the deliberate construction and maintenance of desirable standards, to create institutions to promote goals for the society as a whole that could not be realized if its individuals acted in isolation.

This idea is familiar enough, but precisely because of its clichéd familiarity it is frequently empty of any determinate meaning; the specific problems that arise in bringing such a society about in actual circumstance are left unexamined. In particular, the key issues of reconciling private and public goals and desires, of overcoming tensions between pursuing private liberties and fostering certain public aims such as justice and welfare, are clouded by appeal to sterile generalities.

Although we do not pretend to offer detailed accounts of specific social problems or issues, we wish to pinpoint one important aspect of the society we are describing. As we see it, conflicts of the sort just described are ineliminable in a so-called open society. On the other hand, what is distinctive about such a society, at least ideally, is its adherence to a method or procedure for resolving conflicts. The liberal ideal of a democratic society consists primarily in the guarantee that such a procedure—vague and risky as it is—is ensured, and that it acts as a mediating and controlling influence in settling disputes between the plural emphases, influences, and desires existing in the society. Once this point is grasped, the radical tensions usually attributed to democratic government are modified, softened, rendered less angular.

And because the procedural and substantive questions we have raised earlier are so thoroughly interlaced in our conception, the diverse ways in which democratic processes absorb public interest and lead to constructive change are brought into play, again at least in theory. With the exception of paradoxical cases (such as voting out democracy per se), the presence of a public method for resolving conflict through open and fair discussion without appeal to injurious force renders possible the weeding out of unsatisfactory results and fosters increased attention upon informed and intelligent decision-making with the best available knowledge and a broad sensitivity to moral considerations.

A particularly prominent effect of the presence of the procedure or method we have described concerns the twin notions of "freedom" and "coercion." Summarized in these "fighting words" are a host of issues and problems that cannot be fully discussed here, but a few words might be said about both. The familiar choice presented in the policy literature—that voluntarism is good and "coercion" bad—is clearly simplistic. We are all of us "coerced" daily by both culture and law, in countless accepted ways, so one should be aware of, so to speak, the small c and capital C versions, and the continuum between. The term itself is neutral: the issue turns on what end is served by a coercive policy and the participatory conditions under which it is implemented.

In any government decision, there are specific values that must be considered—"freedom" or "liberty" is among them, as is "welfare." But traditional discussions, fixated on a false conception of ethics, have erected out of these values rigid distinctions and absolute priorities that can only hinder responsible decision-making. Once fixed and absolutely prior indexes or criteria are set up, it is no wonder that difficulties arise as to their reconciliation. In the case of "freedom," much political theory has shifted between two major senses of the term—"freedom from" interference, "freedom to" some good. As we see the matter, freedom is a highly valued consideration in ethical thinking but enjoys no rigidly defined status, in either of these two senses. In particular, freedom (in both senses) functions as an ideal, adjusted to circumstances as they arise, not as a rule set for all space and time. There is, in our view, no "right" of a "natural" sort to freedom from all interference or to any particular set of goods, such as education, health care, and so on.[44] What must be stressed, rather, is the search for freedom in determinate situations; there is no way in which we can set down a rule that anticipates the character of all such situations so that we can claim that liberty must always be recognized in this or that form or degree. That this is so links up with our earlier discussion of "real" or "effective" choice, a species of "positive" freedom or "freedom to" certain goods.[45] Although we can say with confidence that both freedom from government interference and freedom to determine family size are values that must be considered in any policy affecting population rates, it is impossible to lay down once-for-all standards. "Real" freedom is an ideal, one of enlarging options and choices open to the individual, consistent with the liberties of others in the society.[46]

Essentially the same point should be made about the values taken into account in decision-making that concerns public or social goals. Once we free ourselves from old-fashioned conceptions of welfare as a crude Utilitarian summation of individual pains and pleasures or some transcendent expression of Public Will (as in the "Organic" theory of the state), we can view welfare as a goal to be determined by public discussion and the competitive claims of individual preferences. Depending on the circumstances, the aims or goals will differ. The so-called clash between private and public pursuits is not a theoretical necessity, only a persistent fact. Ideally, the twin aims of securing personal liberties and promoting public goals would be mutually reinforcing; they would both be construed as instruments for improving a whole composed of the demands of both citizens and "government." The picture that would emerge would be one of mutual benefit between these two aims: the promotion of justice, welfare, and other goods would create and augment private options and liberties to enjoy further goods; personal liberties would be protected and strengthened in the process of participating in decision-making, a process grounded in the force of persuasion and constructive criticism.

Of course, such a process is, as we have noted, bound to encounter serious conflicts in practice—which brings us to the contrary notion of "coercion." Should persuasion and argument fail to be effective—an occurrence that would hopefully be rare in a society habituated to those tools of dispute-settling—coercive means might be necessary. Now "coercion," like its relative, "freedom," is seriously vague. Like "freedom," its meaning varies from place to place—although there is a core meaning that appears to be invariant: just as "freedom" conveys "being left alone," so "coercion" conveys "being forced to do something." Furthermore, there are several key senses of the term any society must take into account.

For our purposes, we distinguish just two, broad and narrow. The broad sense identifies coercion with any compulsion or constraint, socially determined or not. It is clear that this sense is entirely useless in political theory, for according to it, arguments, contracts, traditions, beliefs, cultural practices, "fate" are all "coercive." The narrow sense excludes all forms of coercion in the broad sense except those that are deliberately instituted or invoked by human beings in relation to others, and further narrows the term to the use of force (direct, implied, threatened) initiated to alter behavior by diminishing the accessibility or desirability of the behavior by some means—whether by threats, pressures, sanctions, violence, or otherwise. Even this description is quite vague[47] but it will do for our purposes. It covers a spectrum of possible activities, from stern warnings and subtle pressures to direct violence. The important point to notice is that it is, thus far, ethically neutral.[48] No condemnation of coercion per se can be made in this sense unless a specification of the end or reason for invoking it is given. This raises the difficult problem of the justification of coercion. When a violent mob is restrained or a potential murderer is threatened with severe punishment should he kill, the use of coercion is rarely questioned; there are undoubtedly many cases of justified coercion.

Settlement Through Informed Judgment

We consider that there is no automatic or absolute or fool-proof way to "settle" the kinds of issues we have been discussing, save through continuing judgmental review and renewing consensus on a specific problem in a specific culture, with consideration to right procedures and values; and the facts of the matter are closely involved in ethical judgments.

The general view we have taken is that government does play a moral role in promoting the welfare of its citizens, and therefore can intervene in this area—the degree of intervention determined by the demands of the problem situation, and by the best available knowledge on the subject as well as on the consequences of doing nothing. Both the liberties and the autonomy of the individual member of society as well as the good of the society as a whole have been stressed in our account.

As we view the matter, the balance between the competing claims of these considerations, if any, should be struck according to the character of the problem situation; there is no absolutely general rule we can invent that would settle a ranking once and for all. We regard both autonomy and welfare as values, but there are no perfectly general ways of ranking or balancing them, so that the individual "rights" are not absolute "trumps." Nor is there any science by which to weigh N units of personal freedom against M units of the public good; that is where our twin criteria come in to facilitate a correct judgment.

On the side of the individual, our view would stress his autonomy but point as well to the knowledge of the consequences of population growth as it affects both his own future autonomy and that of future members of his society. The individual does not live in a self-sufficient area bounded by "natural rights" but in a network of relations, not only with living others but also, in an attenuated sense, with future members of his society. While the future people may not have present "rights" or easily identifiable claims to specific moral consideration, there is no doubt that they must be taken into account in governmental decision-making—a point we meet daily in discussions of conservation, nuclear energy, and arms treaties.[49]

On the other hand, we have also emphasized that a government that routinely overrides individual claims to moral attention is ethically unacceptable. Only in extraordinary circumstances—to be specified in context—is severely coercive governmental intervention in the lives of its citizens acceptable; the specific decision whether to intervene must be made by consideration of the costs and benefits of a specific policy. The "stepladder" approach provides the framework or skeleton, and only that, for such decision-making; the determinate "costs," "benefits," and other data must be filled in each time anew, with intelligence: is there a "population problem" that warrants governmental intervention? in what degree? are the facts reasonably established for policy judgment, and reasonably communicated and understood for the judgment of the citizenry? does the magnitude of the proposed solution somehow match the magnitude of the problem itself?[50]

Earlier we invoked a hierarchical or "stepladder" approach to interventionist policies in the population field. The ethical ideal controlling that approach was this: granting the primacy of the democratic procedure of institutional criticism, "voluntary" means should be employed whenever possible to settle disputes; only if such means cannot be employed or have been exhausted in the presence of a serious problem threatening the maintenance of the society should nonvoluntary means be employed. Now "nonvoluntary" is not synonymous with "coercive" in the sense we are using; what matters, however, is that the degree of coercive policy brought into play should be proportional to the degree of seriousness of the present problem and should be introduced only after less coercive means have been exhausted. Thus, overt violence or other potentially injurious coercion is not to be used before noninjurious coercion has been exhausted. This "stepladder" seems to us congruent with the ethical ideals for government we set down earlier.

The most extreme deviation from our ideal would be the situation in which an area or population is so conflict-ridden that as the saying goes, "ethics does not apply." It is all very well, it is said, to plead for rational persuasion and, if necessary, reconstruction of institutions so that universal participation in a democratic life is possible, but this is patently impossible or impracticable in most current circumstances where most needed. In old-fashioned language, the "circumstances of justice" do not apply.[51] As the argument goes, there are always emergency cases calling for action; we cannot either afford the leisure or require a justification for intervening, and ordinary constraints on action must be suspended. In response to this view, as applied to population, we do not know of any actual circumstance today in which this argument applies; but, more important, we do not feel that much trust should be placed in it. Even if "coercive" measures were necessary in some cases, it would not be the case that "ethics does not apply," but rather that a "disaster ethic" would have to be invented or articulated, as for example now exists in time of war but is put aside in time of peace. That such an ethic exists is apparent in any case: there are measures we would most likely "never" take in dealing with even a crisis situation, for example, randomizing medical care so as to raise mortality rates. Nor do we consider it likely that "population" will be perceived as sufficiently threatening in the next years to justify such actions: the disease will be downgraded before that cure is prescribed.

Ethical Consistencies

We consider that just as the problem must be initially defined in its local site, so should the ethical appraisal be initially made with a view to local values, traditions, customs. Beyond that, however, a wider view may be—indeed should be—introduced in order to test ethicality against broader procedural and substantive considerations. And while we consider it salutary to seek logical consistency in ethical positions on similar issues—here, those related to population—we recognize that historical and social considerations make that virtually impossible at a given time and tend to lead to "least common denominator" ethics if pushed too far.

The first issue is a sticky one: *whose* ethics are to apply? We write out of a Western, individualistic mode; most of the world's population lives with different political and philosophical traditions. There is no question of our "imposing" our values on others; neither is a moratorium imposed on our own observation, comment, and criticism.

It seems to us intuitively correct—especially in light of what we have spoken of earlier as the primacy of procedural aspects of government decision-making—that our attitude should be as follows. Just as before, when we introduced a "stepladder" of permissible interventions as compared with the gravity of the problem at hand, so here another "stepladder" may be introduced, this time with regard to our attitude toward other societies. First, assuming the problem is not catastrophic, we should attempt to justify to the members of the other society ethically acceptable means of arriving at government decisions and feel free to recommend specific means of resolving population problems, particularly when asked. Second, if the problem is grave and direct access to the members of the society is not possible, we should at the very least provide our best information and policies to the dominant powers of that society. This second step seems to us to be in accord with our earlier views: it is grounded in the idea that autonomy and self-determination should be respected and provided with institutional frameworks for expression.

Finally, largely unremarked in this connection—though striking when recognized—are the several ways in which governments now intervene, indeed exercise control through sanctions and force, in *all* the other major areas of demographic behavior without normally raising questions of politico-ethical propriety:

with regard to nuptiality: legal requirements of monogamy, legal establishment of age at marriage, and certain other conditions for marriage, e.g., health status of the partners;

with regard to mortality: various requirements and standards with regard to health practices—required (coerced?) vaccination, spraying, and other public health measures;

with regard to migration: limits on international emigration and especially on immigration; forced emigration and even expulsion of legal residents, typically those of the "wrong" ethnic character; limits on internal migration, e.g., pass laws or internal passports, induced or enforced resettlements, incentives/disincentives to regulate internal migratory streams usually in order to reduce rural-to-urban migration

—not to mention a whole array of related matters like prohibition of child labor, compulsory education, and so on. Note that the forms of government intervention used for these demographic events are identical with those used or proposed for fertility, that is, propaganda, incentives, pressures, legal sanctions. Further, while some of the policies involved with migratory sanctions have been criticized on ethical grounds,[52] those dealing with nuptiality and mortality do not generally raise such questions in their constraints on individual behavior for the common good.[53]

Still the legal form and the ethical content would *in abstracto* seem to be identical: for the good of the society as a whole, what differs in requiring that the citizen be limited to one spouse at a time or to three children? We see no fundamental ethical or philosophical difference between sanctions on monogamy or vaccination on the one hand, and sanctions on fertility on the other—only sociological and historical differences. The former are more familiar and (presumably) more proven out to serve the public good (or at least are so perceived), but in principle they are no less congruent with or invasive of ethical values in abstraction. To put it another way, the procedural and substantive criteria have been met in the earlier cases but not (yet?) with regard to fertility. Nor would we wish to be understood as necessarily supporting an ethics-by-precedent, for that would flow toward a least-common-denominator ethics by its internal dynamics.

In summary, the ethical framework permeating our appraisal of present practice includes these themes: (1) no single ethical system applied to specific cases; (2) no ethical precedents automatically applied to fertility from other aspects of population; (3) no absolute or formulated way to decide such issues; (4) ethics as a branch of decision-making, arising out of conflict; (5) the double criteria of procedure and substance; (6) the centrality of the facts (knowledge); (7) the utility of the "stepladder approach," within and between nations; and (8) appeal to, and cognizance of, *their* ethics but not without outside comment and appraisal.

Coda

What *should* governments do to "control" population growth through fertility? In the best of all possible worlds it would be enough for them to do three things: maximize the flow of full information about the consequences of fertility behavior, both individual and collective; maximize the capacity of people to regulate their fertility by medically approved means, in accordance with individual conscience; and minimize undue pressures on fertility behavior either way. Those conditions are met today for a small fraction of the world's population—and that fraction, incidentally, has very low fertility. If these conditions were met, then let the demographic chips fall where they may—the trade-offs between child-bearing and other ends in life would then have found their free and rational level.[54]

The trouble is, this is not the best of all possible worlds, so we must settle for less-than-optimal solutions in order not to get worse. This essay has been our effort to pick a way through the maze of ethical issues enmeshing "the population problem" and chart a decent and humane path.

There is no need here to summarize the position or the argument, except perhaps in signpost form, as simple reminder. First we identified three current policies used by governments to intervene on fertility that have raised ethical questions—limitations on access to modern means of fertility control; incentives and disincentives; and peer pressure organized by the political apparatus. Then we appraised the policies and gave our ethical judgments. Finally, we presented the broad rationale within which those judgments were made.

The trouble is, again, that in a field like this, solutions do not come prepackaged. Tradition, culture, decree, law, bureaucratic practice—all these (and more) function actively in the concrete situation and make a complex mix indeed, where the shading runs from information to propaganda to heavy persuasion to incentives to pressure to compulsion to sanction to force.[55] Nor is it very helpful to frame the issue as exclusively one of private interest versus the public good, and then come down on one or the other side, or even easier, find that they are really the same in the end.[56] They are not the same, and adjusting them poses severe difficulties; indeed, the Nobel prize was awarded for the demonstration that an unambiguous collective decision determined by individual preferences and certain intuitive conditions is impossible.[57]

The problem arises precisely because public and private goals are, or are perceived to be, in disharmony; private decisions about fertility do not add up to the net, let alone the optimal, benefit of the collectivity. How to balance them out, in a politico-ethical as well as an efficient manner, is the task. That is why we stress the procedural aspects of the task, along with the increase of personal options. The open society is a great, and risky, social invention; but most of the world we speak of is closed. Ethical issues are easier in an open society, where citizens can fight back against government policy, as India has shown. Hence we stress, as with peer pressure, the community's right to participate and dissent under nondemocratic conditions at the national level.[58]

Finally, nothing is final: no once and for all, no definitive answers. Nor is finality forthcoming on the factual side either: how serious is a given level of fertility or growth?—even that elementary question is answered variously by seemingly qualified scholars. Nor, despite mankind's search to date, have the ethical answers seemed to hold. The most we claim, and the least we expect, is that this essay has made the discourse a little more sophisticated, more pointed, and more enlightening.

Notes

1. For a general overview, see "World Population: Status Report 1974," *Reports on Population/Family Planning*, no. 15 (January 1974). And for a summary of present status, see Bernard Berelson, W. Parker Mauldin, and Sheldon Segal, "Background paper on population," prepared for the World Population Conference at Bellagio, 1979.

2. Though perhaps this last should be qualified in view of the forced out-migrations in Africa and Southeast Asia, and the illegal migrations into the United States from Latin America; but how much is their motivation demographic?

3. For a much fuller listing that compresses into these categories, see Bernard Berelson, "Paths to fertility reduction: The policy cube," *Family Planning Perspectives* 9, no. 5 (September/October 1977):213–219.

4. For the argument to this effect, see for example Simone Veil, "Human rights, ideologies, and population policies," *Population and Development Review* 4, no. 2 (June 1978):314–316 on "Is a state justified in adopting a population policy?"; and the *Report of the Symposium on Population and Human Rights*, Amsterdam, January 1974, in preparation for the UN World Population Conference, especially paragraphs 17, 18, 39, 40, 41, 42. On the other hand, an increasingly strong position is being put forward in the ethical and political-philosophy literature these days in support of the limited function of the state as "traffic policeman" or "night-watchman," notably by Robert Nozick in *Anarchy, State, Utopia* (New York: Basic Books, 1974).

5. In a recent query among members of the American professional population association, 34 percent believed that "coercive birth control programs should be initiated in at least some countries immediately," and 19 percent were undecided; 56 percent believed that "if world population continues to grow at its present rate, coercive birth control will have to be initiated within the next fifty years," and 18 percent were undecided; and 42 percent believed that "the United States should press a country with a high birth rate to establish a family planning type of program before socioeconomic aid is provided." See *P.A.A. Affairs* (Fall 1978):2.

6. *World Population: Myths and Realities*, Report prepared by the Select Committee on Population, October 1978, pp. 7, 42–45.

7. Judith Blake, "Population policy for Americans: Is the government being misled?" *Science* 164(2 May 1969):528.

8. The matter does raise interesting ethical questions about whether what is tolerated or approved by cultural practice (like peer pressure, perhaps its most powerful means of influence) is impermissible if deliberately emphasized in government interventions. Can culture itself be unethical? The historical and comparative answer is obviously Yes.

9. W. Parker Mauldin, "Assessment of national family planning programs in developing countries," *Studies in Family Planning* 6, no. 3 (February 1975):33.

10. Christopher Tietze and Marjorie Cooper Murstein, "Induced abortion: 1975 factbook," *Reports on Population/Family Planning*, no. 14 (December 1975):8–9.

11. Bernard Berelson, "Romania's 1966 anti-abortion decree: The demographic experience of the first decade," *Population Studies* 33, no. 2 (1979):209–222.

12. Alan Guttmacher Institute, *Abortion and the Poor: Private Morality, Public Responsibility* (New York: 1979).

13. In addition, there have been a number of serious proposals for incentives in recent years that have not been effectuated to our knowledge, e.g.: insurance policy on sons in families of three or fewer children, as social security for parents, reported under consideration in Pakistan (Herz); incentives to delay marriage, through dowry payments or training programs (Herz); incentives to delay first birth or space out later ones (Herz); vasectomy bond, cashable as social security (Herz); community incentives for desired fertility performance in the form of roads, schools, agricultural improvements, health services, land pooling (Kangas); large awards in Rupees to districts with best records (Landman); group incentives for various professions or occupations under consideration in India according to the 1976 policy statement, including small-family requirement for employment and promotion in civil service, as models for population at large (Lee); and a variety of such incentive and tax and welfare schemes proposed in the past (Berelson). Also, see community incentives schemes currently under consideration, e.g., in Indonesia (Freedman). See Barbara K. Herz, "Socio-economic policies to encourage smaller families," IGCC Report on *Reducing Fertility Through Beyond Family Planning Measures*, January 1978, pp. 23ff; Lenni Kangas, "Integrated incentives for fertility control," *Science* 69 (25 September 1970): 278–283, which also includes examples and discussions of various other incentive schemes; Lynn C. Landman, "Birth control in India: The carrot and the rod?" *Family Planning Perspectives* 9, no. 3 (May/June 1977):103; Luke T. Lee, "Human rights aspects of

'beyond family planning measures,'" IGCC, cited above, p. 31; Bernard Berelson, "Beyond family planning," *Studies in Family Planning* 1, no. 38 (February 1969); and Ronald Freedman, "Evaluation and research on family planning, fertility and population in Indonesia," May 1978, pp. 24–26.

14. For examples, see Bernard Berelson, ed., *Population Policy in Developed Countries* (New York: McGraw-Hill, 1974); and Jason L. Finkle and Alison McIntosh, "Policy responses to population stagnation in developed societies," Center for Population Planning, University of Michigan, July 1977. As Thomas J. Espenshade recently pointed out in "Zero population growth and the economies of developed nations" [*Population and Development Review* 4, no. 4 (December 1978):645], the well known British economist Roy Harrod sought a democratic solution to the Great Depression "by urging child allowances on a 'generous, even lavish, scale,' " in 1939. That suggestion must be put alongside David Glass's wry observation that "however urgently governments may have declared their desire to increase the supply of births, they have nevertheless persistently tried to buy babies at bargain prices" (from his *Population Policies and Movements in Europe*, 1940, p. 371).

15. For examples, see Berelson et al., cited in note 1; and Robert J. McIntyre, "Pronatalist programmes in Eastern Europe," *Soviet Studies* 27, no. 3 (July 1975):366–380. Reuters reported that "Romania has transferred money from its military budget to pay increased family allowances" in the amount of $41.5 million, enabling monthly allowances to be raised by 83 cents a child. *New York Times* (4 March 1979).

16. Pravin Visaria and Anrudh K. Jain, "India," *Country Profiles* (New York: The Population Council, 1976), p. 33. In the April 1976 policy statement, since repudiated, the Health Minister announced a graduated fee system of "monetary compensation for sterilization (both male and female)" of Rs. 150 for a parent with two or fewer living children, Rs. 100 for three children, and Rs. 70 for four or more. *National Population Policy*, Statement of Dr. Karan Singh, Minister of Health and Family Planning, New Delhi, April 1976. A poignant comment on the situation is made by a small "feasibility study" conducted in a Bombay hospital that showed how difficult it would be to determine size of family under such conditions: ". . . even an enquiry about family size (at the time of confinement) created apprehension amongst multiparae of forced permanent contraception so that if they fail in the attempt to avoid discussion of sterilization by understating the size of their families, they seek registration for delivery at other centres." From P. V. Mehta and K. B. Pathack, "Some problems of compulsion in family planning," *Journal of Biosocial Science* 9 (1977):275.

17. Berelson et al., cited in note 1, p. 25.

18. Berelson et al., cited in note 1. For an analysis of recent developments in Czechoslovakia, their costs and their impact, see Tomas Frejka, "Fertility related population policies and trends: Czechoslovakia in the 1970s," unpublished manuscript, April 1979.

19. Oliver D. Finnigan III and T. H. Sun, "Planning, starting, and operating an educational incentives project," *Studies in Family Planning* 3, no. 1 (January 1972); C. M. Wang and S. Y. Chen, "Evaluation of the first year of the educational savings program in Taiwan," *Studies in Family Planning* 4, no. 7 (July 1973):157–161.

20. Ronald Ridker, "Savings accounts for family planning: An illustration from the tea estates of India," *Studies in Family Planning* 2, no. 7 (July 1971): 150–152.

21. Margaret S. Wolfson, *Serving the People: Some Impressions of Social Development in China*. Report of a Study Mission to the People's Republic of China, November 1975, p. 12.

22. *Singapore. Country Paper in Reducing Fertility Through Beyond Family Planning Measures*, Inter Governmental Coordinating Committee (IGCC), Southeast Asia Regional Cooperation in Family and Population Planning, A Report on the Regional Workshop, January 1978, pp. 107–116. See also Janet Salaff and Aline K. Wong, "Are disincentives coercive? The view from Singapore," *International Family Planning Perspectives and Digest* 4, no. 2 (Summer 1978):50–55. For a review of the effectiveness of these policies, see S. B. Tan et al., "Effects of social disincentive policies on fertility behavior in Singapore," *American Journal of Public Health* 68, no. 2 (February 1978):119–124.

23. Here too there have been a number of proposals, not taken up. (We do not include here certain irresponsible proposals, like sterilants in the water supply, or marketable licenses to have children, or random contraceptive injections to a fixed quota, or temporary sterilization of all girls with government approval required for reversibility; for specifics, see Berelson, cited in note 13.) Some of the following, indeed, border on the unrealistic and/or unreasonable:

On aid to developing countries: "Insofar as villages are organized to make public improvements in such things as the water supply, education, irrigation and public health, the same group in charge of these activities could also take charge of the assignment of reproductive rights—that is, it could see that a communal decision is reached concerning who will have the privilege of conceiving a child in a given year. If there is a public works program, employment in it could be restricted to single men and women. . . . The United States could use its aid, whatever its form, as an incentive—an incentive leading less developed countries to initiate population policies with teeth in them." (Davis)

From India during the Emergency: "We are of the view that where a State legislature, in the exercise of its own powers, decides that the time is ripe and it is necessary to pass legislation for compulsory sterilization, it may do so. Our advice to the States in such cases will be to bring in the limitation after three children." (Singh)

In order "to produce a desirable population *composition*" between Jews and Arabs in Israel, "consider the possibility of using legislation to *guarantee* the maintenance of at least a three-quarters Jewish majority. . . . It is not yet time for such '75 percent Jewish law' . . . but should the Israeli Arabs' 'will to power' be too strong to be countered by a process fostering voluntary reproductive control, there would be only one alternative: *involuntarism*. . . . The likeliest means for implementing an involuntary population policy, in Israel or elsewhere, would be mandatory sterilization following the birth of a certain number of children." (Lenski)

And, from Bangladesh: "No civilized measure would be too drastic to keep the population of Bangladesh on the smaller side of 15 crores (150 million) for sheer ecological viability of the nation. For this the nation has to be mobilised, and early. . . . We must consider the imposition of progressively increasing punitive measures against additional children after the second child on all couples. Once the programme gets well under way it may be worthwhile, for example, (i) to restrict ration cards in statutory and modified rationing areas to a maximum of two children, (ii) to debar couples from enjoying the benefit of fair price shops for more than two children per family. All couples should be required by law to register with family planning organization. The first phase of launching a major educational and motivational drive, if successful, should, at least, create a climate where the possibility of more drastic measures, such as, compulsory sterilization of either husband or wife after the second child, legalization of abortion and establishment of abortion clinics for performing abortion free of cost, social measures to bring about women's emancipation etc. may be considered." (Bangladesh Planning Commission)

See Kingsley Davis, "World population growth and United States foreign aid," prepared for Hearings before the Committee on Appropriations of the House of Representatives, March 1977; Singh, cited in note 16, paragraph 15, p. 4; Robert G. Lenski, "An Israeli dilemma," *The Mankind Quarterly* 18, no. 2 (October-December 1977):98, 111–114; Bangladesh Planning Commission, *The First Five Year Plan 1973–78*, November 1973, chapter 16, pp. 538–539.

24. Luke T. Lee, in IGCC, cited in note 13, pp. 29–30.

25. Wolfson, cited in note 21, p. 11.

26. "Minimum age at marriage: 20 years of legal reform," a *People* fact sheet, c. 1978.

27. John S. Aird, "Fertility decline and birth control in the People's Republic of China," *Population and Development Review* 4, no. 2 (June 1978):225–254.

28. Terence H. Hull, Valerie J. Hull, and Masri Singarimbun, "Indonesia's family planning story: Success and challenge," *Population Bulletin* 32, no. 8 (November 1977): 25–30. A softer version of the experience, seen as an appropriate community-based effort in which the responsibility is well placed in the "educational and social pressure emanating from the *banjar*," is presented in Nancy and David Piet, *Family Planning and the Banjars of Bali*, Cycle Publications, n.d.

29. The closest is Davidson R. Gwatkin, "Political will and family planning: The implications of India's Emergency experience," *Population and Development Review* 5, no. 1 (March 1979):29–60. See also Landman, cited in note 13, pp. 101–103.

30. Though such measures have been proposed, see note 26, plus further examples from Ehrlich, Boulding, Ketchel, Shockley, and Davis, as listed in Berelson, cited in note 13. As special cases, we do not consider here the issues of compulsory sterilization on criminal or genetic grounds (e.g., Justice Holmes' famous judgment that three generations of imbeciles are enough), since we are exclusively concerned with demographic matters.

31. For example, see Salaff and Wong, cited in note 22, who conclude that the actual effects are limited but that "they work by creating an image of comprehensiveness and stringency. . . . The majority of the respondents have come to accept the role of the government as a 'moral arbitrator' or as an external 'educating force' to mold family life in the interest of the society as a whole" (pp. 52,55).

32. This is as appropriate a point as any to note that these issues, when they arise, affect large numbers of people indeed—not that ethical proprieties could ever rest on discommoding a minority, even a tiny one, for the benefit of the majority (e.g., the famous Benthamite example that one tortured man, unseen and unheard, would not justify the welfare of a large community). Anyway, as for fertility reduction in the poorer countries, something like 40 percent of all births are of 4th order or higher, and 30 percent of 5th order or higher, so that a major part of the community is involved. For example, see Anrudh K. Jain, "Identification of the target group for vasectomy," *Demography India* 5 (1976); confirmed by recent World Fertility Survey data kindly supplied by colleagues Richard Monteverde and W. Parker Mauldin.

33. The argument over paternalism goes back to J. S. Mill, *On Liberty* (London: 1864). See further Gerald Dworkin, "Paternalism," in *Morality and The Law*, ed. Richard A. Wasserstrom (Belmont: Wadsworth Publications, 1971), and the controversy over Millian principles, in H. L. A. Hart, *Law, Liberty, and Morality*

(Stanford University Press: 1963), and Patrick Devlin, *The Enforcement of Morals* (London: Oxford University Press, 1965). The question is whether the state can properly legislate to protect the citizen against himself, or only against others (though the line is often difficult to draw—smoking? social security?). See also Veil, cited in note 4, p. 320, and Rawls's first principle in J. Rawls, *A Theory of Justice* (Cambridge, Mass.: Harvard University Press, 1971).

34. In this respect, Veil, cited in note 4, makes a distinction between pronatalist and antinatalist incentives: "the act of giving a certain sum of money to a couple because they have a child and the act of giving them the same sum because they do not have one or will not have any more are two very different measures: The first increases real choice, the second limits it" (p. 320). Why the latter is any more limiting than the former escapes us; might it be that her country, France, simply has had much more experience with the former, and is once again debating the issues of population "stagnation"?

35. Can any unethically discriminatory aspects of incentive programs be reduced by attempting to scale incentives so that offers are of nearly equal attractiveness to rich and poor? There are tremendous economic and administrative difficulties with such a proposal, not to mention the ludicrous outcome of providing larger incentives to the already better off. See R. M. Veatch, "Governmental population incentives: Ethical issues at stake," *Studies in Family Planning* 8, no. 4 (April 1977):100–108; and Frederick S. Jaffe, "Alarums, excursions, and delusions of grandeur: Implicit assumptions of group efforts to alter differential fertility trends," in *Zero Population Growth—For Whom?*, ed. Milton Himmelfarb and Victor Baras (Greenwood Press: 1978), pp. 26–40.

36. Or, some say, Singapore. See *World Population: Myths and Realities*, cited in note 6.

37. McNicoll would add a more specific quid pro quo: "How should we judge sterner measures—not the draconian but typically short-lived excesses occasionally seen but the policies routinely pursued in, say, China or Indonesia? I think an argument can be made, not wholly persuasive, that this policy direction can be justified provided that people for whom children are essentially the only instrument to attain a degree of security are given some alternative support" (as Chinese villages and Balinese hamlets). From Geoffrey McNicoll, "On fertility policy research," *Population and Development Review* 4, no. 4 (December 1978):689–690. In this view, some ethical value is traded off for some social security—but not without some doubts.

38. But not to Bernardo Colombo, ["Human rights, ideology, and population policies," in *Proceedings of the International Population Conference, Mexico 1977* (Liège, Belgium: IUSSP, 1978)], who seems to prefer direct coercion from the center: "This constant checking by neighbours (small local groups of an autonomous community responsibility)...on most intimate decisions and relationships seems to me to be a form of coercion which is incompatible with safeguarding human rights, and is also less psychologically tolerable than a rough plan directly imposed by the central power, with which it would probably ultimately end in agreement on sanctions concerning the deviants from the system" (p. 40).

39. Here we agree with Sissela Bok, *Lying: Moral Choice in Public Life* (New York: Pantheon, 1978): "Many have labored to erect such systems; to find a method by which to judge moral choice, or some single principle from which judgments can be derived, or some hierarchy among principles so as to resolve conflicts.... These structures are often elegant in operation, noble in design. They refine our moral perception (etc. etc.).... But when we have to make difficult concrete moral choices, they give us little help" (p. 56).

40. See Rawls, cited in note 33, sec. 9, 87.

41. This is a common theme in John Dewey. See his *Theory of the Moral Life* (New York: Irvington Press, 1960).

42. William K. Frankena, *Ethics* (Englewood Cliffs, N.J.: Prentice-Hall, 1963), p. 98.

43. This is essentially the distinction in Dworkin, cited in note 33, between secondary and primary values, respectively.

44. This is the underlying defect in Nozick's book. R. Dworkin, in his *Taking Rights Seriously* (Cambridge, Mass.: Harvard University Press, 1978), has a more sophisticated view. And note that Rawls, cited in note 40, in an unappreciated passage, also predicates the value upon first attaining "a certain level of wealth," i.e., removal from dire poverty (paragraph 82).

45. So some room for "choice" is already there. By effective choice, however, we mean something more: not only the information and knowledge to make the choice real, but also a genuine capacity or agency to express one's preferences. (See also Colombo, cited in note 38, p. 25.)

46. The discussion of the worth of liberties in J. Rawls, cited in note 33, concerns this point. See also N. Daniels, "Equal liberty and unequal worth of liberty," in Daniels, *Reading Rawls* (New York: Basic Books, 1976).

47. For still further discussions of "coercion," see R. Nozick, "Coercion," in *Philosophy, Science, and Method*, ed. Morgenbesser, Suppes, and White (New York: 1969), and references there to works by Bay,

Dahl, and Schelling. Also V. Held, "Coercion and coercive offers," *Nomos* 14, New York, 1972.

48. Essentially this point is as old as Locke, who claimed that all law or sanction involved appeal to coercion.

49. An enormous and interesting literature has been provoked by the problems posed by our so-called obligations to future generations, and the issue is too great for us to analyze here. Clearly, there are more or less just savings of resources and capital for future generations: to save nothing would be immoral, to save everything would be ludicrous. For a discussion, see Rawls, cited in note 33, section 44, and references therein. Another much discussed problem is one for utilitarianism, which in some versions recommends maximizing (expected) social utility; under certain conditions of population increase, a very low average well-being may follow: cf. Rawls, pp. 162–163. A third problem for all–utilitarians and nonutilitarians alike–concerns the analysis of our obligations to future but nonexistent persons: Since they are potential, but not actual, persons, can we have duties toward them at all? Is the idea of right or wrong action against a potential person at all coherent? Is it better to create future persons even if unhappy rather than none at all? For a variety of views, see the collection edited by R. I. Sikora and Brian Barry, *Obligations To Future Generations* (Philadelphia: Temple University Press, 1978), especially the essays by Narveson, Sikora, Summer, Kavka, and Barry; and the amusing yet telling argument by Nozick, first with regard to animals but then applied to humans, cited in note 4, pp. 38–39.

50. For a discussion, inter alia, see "Legal analysis and population control: The problem of coercion," *Harvard Law Review* 84 (1971): 1856–1911, specifically p. 1882. And see also Charles Fried, *Right and Wrong* (Cambridge, Mass.: Harvard University Press, 1978), p. 194.

51. See Rawls, cited in note 33, sec. 22. On the ethics of deliberation, an old issue, see Rawls, pp. 416ff.

52. Nor, indeed, are they at all benign. Consider "those rejection policies often encountered in African urban areas. Typically, migrants are either encouraged to 'return to the land' or forcibly removed and transported back to home communities. . . . In some cases, the forcible rejection policy can take on violent forms, as, for example, in the periodic burning-down or leveling of squatter settlements on the periphery of cities like Nairobi, Lagos, or Kampala. Clearly there are better and more humane ways to deal with problems of explosive urban population growth than forcible expulsion. In any case, such expulsion rarely works." (Michael Todaro, "Internal migration, urban population growth, and unemployment in developing countries: Issues and controversies," Working Paper, Center for Population Studies, Population Council, December 1978, p. 20).

53. As Veil, cited in note 4, puts it: "We have therefore arrived at a curious reversal of things: Out of liberty is born obligation, and the exercise of a right is rendered essentially compulsory (as with compulsory education). Similarly, the right to good health implies various constraints from compulsory vaccination to mandatory membership in a social security system. In this case it is particularly clear that to affirm the right to good health is meaningless unless the state adopts concrete, even restrictive measures" (p. 317). Participants in the UN Symposium, cited in note 4, took a different position with regard to "coercion," as summarized in paragraph 132.

54. Bernard Berelson, "An evaluation of the effects of population control programmes," in *Population and Its Problems: A Plain Man's Guide*, ed. H. B. Parry (Oxford: Clarendon Press, The Wolfson College Lectures, 1973), pp. 162–163.

55. For one illustration of such a continuum, see Figure 1, p. 5, in ESCAP, *Report of the Expert Group Meeting on Socio-Economic Measures Affecting Fertility Behaviour with Special Emphasis on Actionable Programmes*, Asian Population Studies Series, no. 41, 1978. That meeting went moderately far, especially for one held under United Nations auspices, in legitimating "coercion" in this field, as in the sections on "Legal and ethical considerations," pp. 18–19, and "Legal and ethical acceptability," pp. 24–25, concluding inter alia that "the use of coercive measures to further human rights is not necessarily incompatible with human rights principles" (p. 18). For a further discussion along the same line, see Luke T. Lee, "Compulsory sterilization and human rights," *Populi* 3, no. 4 (1976).

56. In the tension between the family's and the community's interest in children, who knows better? According to Kingsley Davis, "By stressing the right of parents to have the number of children they want, it [family planning] evades the basic question of population policy which is how to give societies the number of children they need" ["Population policy: Will current programs succeed?," *Science* (November 1967):738]. To a philosopher like Jacques Maritain, the very issue falls away: "Nothing is more illusory than to pose the problem of the person and the common good in terms of opposition. In reality, it is posed in terms of reciprocal subordination and mutual implication. . . . Man, a part of society, should be ordained to the common good and the common work. . . . Social life should impose numerous restraints and sacrifices upon his life as a person, considered as a part of the whole. . . . In the measure that

these sacrifices and restraints are required and accepted in the name of justice and amity, they raise higher the spiritual level of the person" [*The Person and the Common Good* (University of Notre Dame Press: 1966), pp. 65–66].

57. Kenneth J. Arrow, *Social Choice and Individual Values* (New Haven: Yale University Press, 1951), chapter 5.

58. We have speculated, but only that, about the relative "control" the ordinary citizens of the world have over life decisions considered important by them: childbearing in an Indonesian village, for example, as against restraint on nuclear energy plants in the United States, gasoline availability, or the progressive income tax.

Part VIII – Specialized Investigations

13
A Study in Fertility Control

Written with Ronald Freedman

Can modern concepts of family planning have a significant impact in the underdeveloped countries? A study in Taiwan suggests that fertility can indeed be changed substantially by a planned program.

It is widely recognized that in many parts of the world there is a "population problem": the high rate of increase in population makes social and economic development difficult if not impossible. Can anything be done about the problem? Practical means of fertility control are available to individual couples, but can the control of fertility actually be implemented on a large scale in the developing areas? This article will describe an experiment designed to find out what can be done in one of the world's most densely populated places: the island of Taiwan off the coast of mainland China.

Large-scale efforts to control fertility are, to be sure, not unknown. A number of governments have assumed the responsibility of providing their people with information and services on family planning, and some countries have organized major national programs. Lowering a birthrate is a novel objective for a government, however, and no country has yet managed to achieve widespread family limitation through a planned social effort. Current programs are therefore handicapped by a lack of information on attitudes toward fertility control and by a lack of experience with programs to implement family planning.

Since any change in birthrate depends on individual decisions by large numbers of husbands and wives, it is essential to know first of all how the people concerned feel about family size and limitation. Do they need to be motivated toward family planning? If they are so motivated, how can they best be helped to accomplish their aim? To investigate these questions the Taiwan study was inaugurated a year and a half ago under the sponsorship of the provincial health department of Taiwan with the support of The Population Council, a U.S. foundation that advances scientific training and study in population matters. The most significant preliminary finding is that the people do not need to be motivated. They want to plan their families, but they need to know how. Teaching them how—implementing a family planning program—has proved to be feasible.

Taiwan has a population of about 12 million in an area of 14,000 square miles, and its population is increasing rapidly. In recent years mortality has fallen almost to Western levels: life expectancy is more than 60 years and the death rate is less than eight per 1,000 of population per year. The birthrate is about 37 per 1,000, so the rate of increase is almost 3 percent per year, or enough to double the population in 25 years. Nevertheless, compared with other parts of Asia, Taiwan provides a favorable situation for the diffusion of family planning. The island is relatively urbanized and industrialized, the farmers are oriented toward a market economy, literacy and popular education are fairly widespread, there is a good transportation and communication system and a solid network of medical facilities. The standard of living is high for a population of this size in Asia outside of Japan. The society is highly organized. Women are not sharply subordinated and there are few religious or ideological objections to contraception.

The birthrate in Taiwan has been falling slowly since 1958. When fertility rates are analyzed by

---

Reprinted with permission from *Scientific American* 1964;21(5):29–37, ©1964 by Scientific American, Inc.

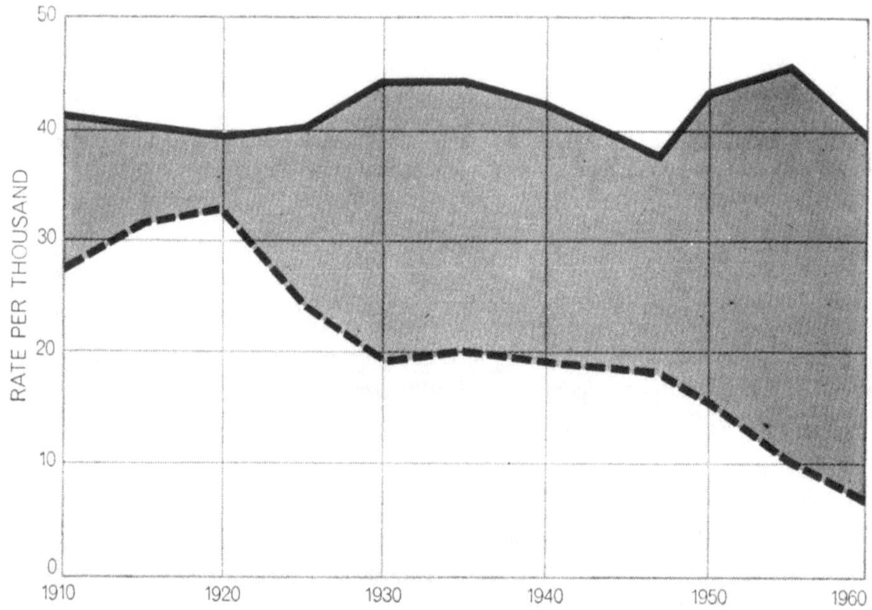

FIGURE 13.1. Rate of increase in Taiwan's population *(shaded area)* has grown because the birthrate *(solid line)* has remained high while the death rate *(broken line)* has fallen. From A Study in Fertility Control, by Bernard Berelson and Ronald Freedman. ©1964 by Scientific American, Inc. All rights reserved.

age group [*see* Fig. 13.2], it becomes apparent that they have decreased first and most for the older women of the childbearing population. This is exactly what one would expect if many women wanted to have a moderate number of children, had them with low mortality by the age of 30 and then tried to limit the size of their families in some way. The same pattern was observed earlier in a number of Western countries at the beginning of the declines in fertility that have tended to follow declines in mortality.

Although the situation in Taiwan was quite favorable for family planning and the birthrate trend had been downward, this was not to say that it would be a simple matter to accelerate the decline in fertility. As a first step in that effort the population studies centers in Taiwan and at the University of Michigan undertook a survey that would serve as a base line and also as a guide for a program of action. Between October, 1962, and January, 1963, public health nurses interviewed nearly 2,500 married women of the city of Taichung in the prime reproductive age group (ages 20 to 39) as to their attitudes toward family planning, their information about it and what they did about it. The survey made it clear that these women as a group wanted to have a moderate number of children, were having more children than they wanted, approved of the idea of family limitation and were trying–ineffectively–to limit the size of their families.

The number of children most of the women wanted was four, and women who had already borne more than that number acknowledged that they would have preferred fewer children [*see* Fig. 13.3]. More than 90 percent of Taichung's wives (and their husbands too, according to the wives) were favorably inclined toward limiting family size. They had few objections in principle, they saw the value of such limitation for the economic welfare of their families and they did not believe that the number of children should be left to "fate" or "providence." In this regard (and the same has been found to be true in other countries) their attitudes are more advanced than some officials believe them to be.

The women were in general poorly informed about family planning methods and indeed about the physiology of reproduction. About a fourth of them had employed some means of contraception, but in most cases only after four or five pregnancies and in many cases without success. The

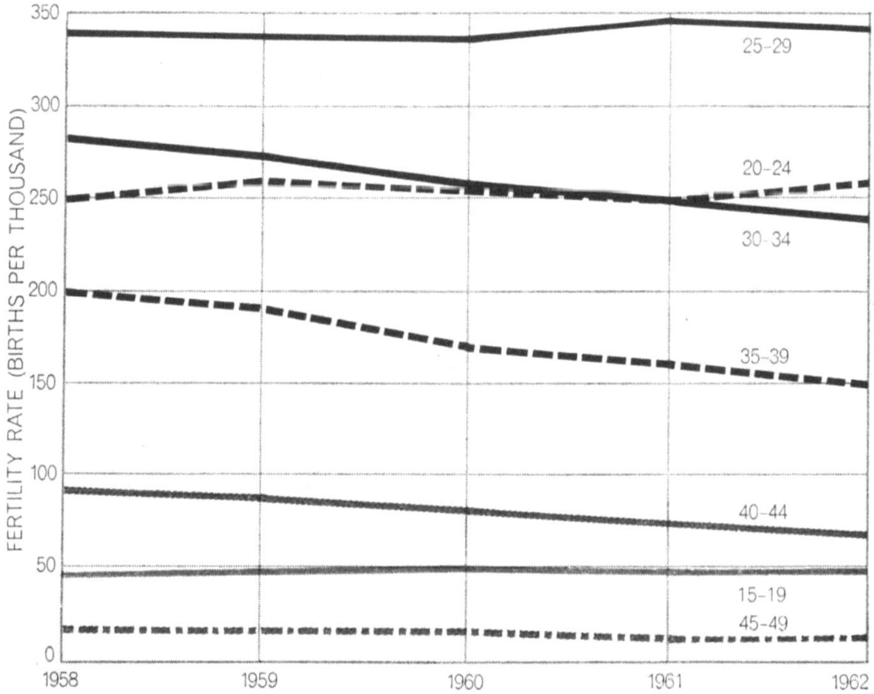

FIGURE 13.2. Fertility rates, shown here for Taiwan women in seven age groups *(figures at right)*, have fallen since 1958 in the case of the older women, presumably because they are trying to limit their families. The rates are birthrates per 1,000 women of the relevant age groups. From A Study in Fertility Control, by Bernard Berelson and Ronald Freedman.

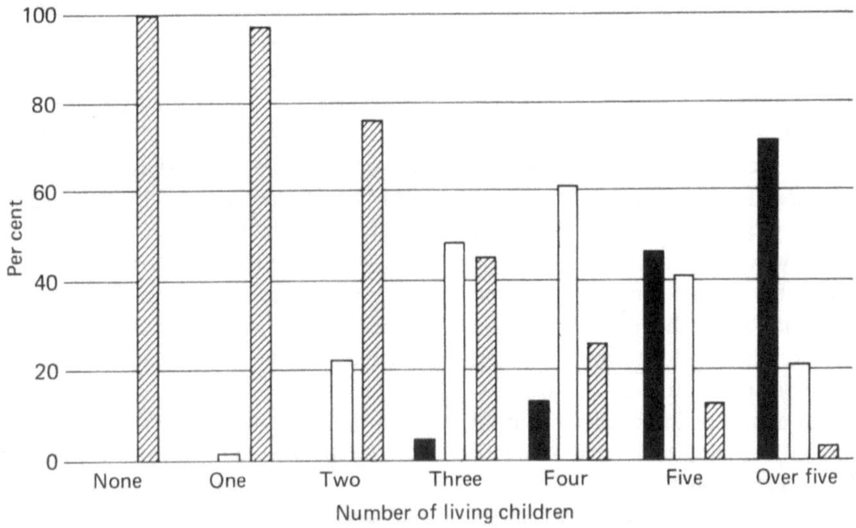

FIGURE 13.3. Family-size preferences are charted for Taichung wives according to the number of children they have. The chart shows the per cent of wives in each group who said they would have preferred fewer children *(solid bars)* or more children *(hatched bars)* than they had or were satisfied with the number of children they had *(clear bars)*. From A Study in Fertility Control, by Bernard Berelson and Ronald Freedman.

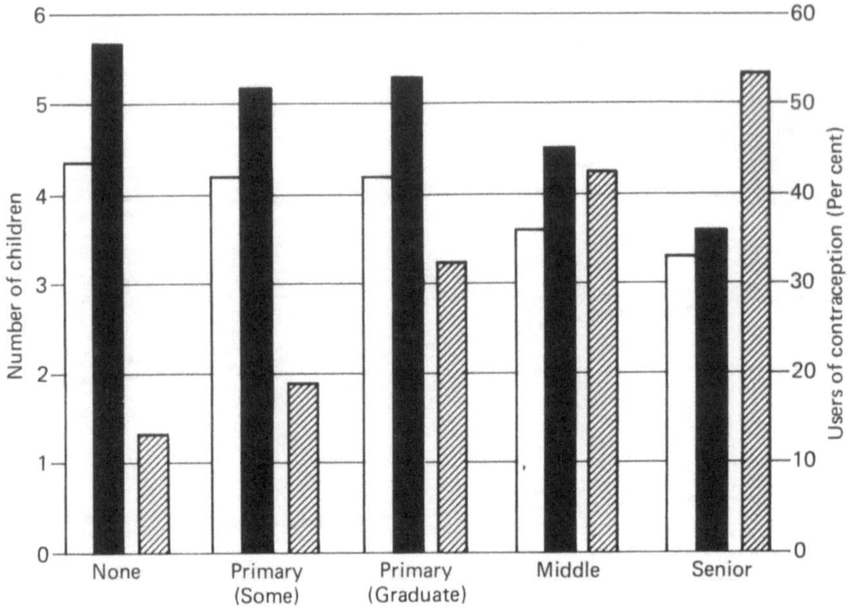

FIGURE 13.4. Education affects family size and the use of contraceptives. The chart groups women 35 to 39 years old according to the level of schooling they had reached. The bars show the average number of children they said they had wanted *(clear bars)* and the number they had borne *(solid bars)*, and the per cent of each group practicing contraception *(hatched bars)*. From A Study in Fertility Control, by Bernard Berelson and Ronald Freedman. ©1964 by Scientific American, Inc. All rights reserved.

women expressed strong interest in learning and adopting better methods. And in their own minds family planning did not conflict with their traditional feelings about the Chinese family or its central role in their lives.

Experience with contraception or other methods of limiting family size was naturally most common in the "modernized" sectors of the population: the best-educated women, the most literate and those with an urban background. The women's actual and desired fertility were also related to these characteristics [*see* Fig. 13.4], but we found that on every educational level the average woman between 35 and 39, when childbearing is not yet over, had borne more children than she wanted. This was true even of groups in which substantial numbers of women had tried to limit the size of their families: contraception had arrived on the scene too late and was too ineffective to enable such women to attain their goals.

The survey data made it clear that the women had become aware of the decline of infant mortality in their community. This is an important perception, and one that does not follow automatically on the event. (Other surveys have shown that women sometimes perceive a decrease in infant mortality as an increase in births.) Because they recognized that more children were surviving, the women appreciated that, unlike their parents, they did not need to have five to seven children in order to see three or four survive to adulthood.

The salient message of the survey was that in Taichung people have more children than they want. There are indications that the same thing is true in many similar societies. It seems clear that if throughout the world unwanted children were not conceived, a large part of the "population problem" would disappear.

The next task was to facilitate the matching of behavior to attitude—to implement family planning. Several things were required beyond the mere wish to limit the number of children: information and knowledge, supplies and services, public acceptance and social support. To study how best to enable the people of Taiwan to do what they themselves said they wanted to do, the provincial health authorities undertook to develop a program of action to make the practice of family planning more readily available in the city of Taichung. This effort, we think, is one of the most extensive and elaborate social science experiments ever carried out in a natural setting.

Taichung has a population of about 300,000, including about 36,000 married women from 20 to 39 years old, of whom 60 per cent have had three or more children. Most of the people live in a central region of shops, offices and residences, but there are also rural areas within the city's administrative limits. A number of government health stations and hospital clinics provide focal points for the action program.

The city as a whole was exposed to only two aspects of the program: a general distribution of posters pointing out the advantages of family planning and a series of meetings with community leaders to inform them about the program, get their advice and enlist their support. That was the extent of the community-wide effort; the remainder of the program was designed as a differentiated experiment involving various kinds and degrees of effort. The objective was to learn how much family planning could be achieved at how much cost in money, personnel and time. To this end the local health authorities and a cooperating team from the U.S. devised four different "treatments," and applied one of them to each of the 2,389 *lin's*, or neighborhoods of 20 to 30 families, into which Taichung is divided. In order of increasing effort, the treatments were designated "Nothing," "Mail," "Everything (wives only)" and "Everything (wives and husbands)."

In the "Nothing" *lin's* there was no activity beyond the distribution of posters and the meetings with leaders. In the "Mail" *lin's* there was a direct-mail campaign addressed to two groups: newlywed couples and parents with two or more children. It was in the "Everything" neighborhoods that the major effort was made to increase family planning. The primary procedure was a personal visit to the home of every married woman from 20 to 39 years old by a specially trained staff of nurse-midwives. The fieldworkers made appointments for people at the health stations, provided contraceptive supplies, answered questions and did whatever else was necessary to satisfy a couple's desire for family planning guidance. In half of the "Everything" *lin's* the visits were made to wives only; in the other half the visits were extended to both husbands and wives, who were seen either separately or together.

TABLE 13.1.

Treatment	Heavy (13,908)	Medium (11,154)	Light (11,326)	Total (36,388)
Nothing	232	243	292	767
Mail	232	244	292	768
Everything				
(wives only)	232	122	73	427
(wives and husbands)	232	122	73	427
Total *lin's*	928	731	730	2,389

Matrix shows the allocation of various "treatments" among the *lin's* in the three density sectors. The figures in parentheses give the total number of women 20 to 39 years old. From A Study in Fertility Control, by Bernard Berelson and Ronald Freedman.

Rather than apply each of these treatments to a different part of the city, the investigators decided to arrange matters so as to test a central economic issue: How much "circulation effect" can one expect in a program of this kind? To what extent can one depend on the population itself to spread the desired innovation, and how large an initial effort is required to prime the process? There has been substantial testimony that word-of-mouth diffusion played a large role in spreading ideas about family planning in the West and Japan; any such effect would clearly be of major importance to national efforts in the underdeveloped countries, which must influence large numbers of people and do so with limited resources.

In order to investigate this question of "spread" it seemed advisable to apply the four treatments in different concentrations in different parts of the city. Taichung was divided into three sectors roughly equivalent in urban-rural distribution, socioeconomic status and fertility, and designated as areas of heavy, medium and light "density." In the heavy-density sector the two "Everything" treatments were administered to half of the *lin's*, in the medium sector to a third of them and in the light sector to a fifth. In each sector the remaining *lin's* were assigned equally to the "Nothing" and the "Mail" treatment groups [*see* Table 13.1]. The *lin's* were assigned at random, although always in the proper proportion, and those designated for a particular treatment received exactly the same program regardless of their location in the city. They differed only in their environment; in the heavy-density sector, for example, "Nothing" *lin's* were much more closely surrounded by "Everything" *lin's* than were the "Nothing" neighborhoods in the two lighter-density sectors.

The program got under way in mid-February of 1963: the posters went up, meetings were held, 18 fieldworkers fanned out through the "Everything" *lin's* and the health stations prepared to receive inquiries. A set of educational materials was prepared for group and individual discussion, primarily visual aids dealing with the elementary facts about the physiology of reproduction, the reasons for practicing family planning and the major methods of contraception. The fieldworkers offered a wide choice of methods, encouraging couples to select whichever seemed most suitable: jelly, foam tablet, diaphragm, condom, rhythm, withdrawal, the oral pill and the new intra-uterine device. (The last is a recent development that holds great promise for mass programs to reduce fertility because it does not require continued supply, sustained motivation or repeated actions on the part of the user. A plastic ring or coil is inserted in the uterus by a physician and remains there; it is extremely effective as a contraceptive, although its mode of action is still unclear.) Contraceptive supplies were provided at or below cost, or free if necessary; the pills sold for the equivalent of 75 cents for a cycle of 20. The same charge was made for the insertion of an intra-uterine device.

By the end of June fieldworkers had visited each of the nearly 12,000 designated homes at least once and more than 500 neighborhood meetings had been held. Between then and the middle of October follow-up visits were made to women or couples who had indicated interest and to women who had been pregnant or had been nursing infants earlier in the year. A final phase began in late October and is still continuing; direct action has been terminated, but services and supplies are still available at the health stations, and the momentum of the program is continuing to have effect as of this writing.

There are three ways in which the effectiveness of the whole program will be measured. One is through case records kept for all couples who were visited in their homes or came to clinics as a result of the action program. The second is a before-and-after survey of a random sample of 2,432 women of childbearing age. The final story will be told in fertility statistics to be compiled eventually from the official register.

So far one result has emerged from the before-and-after survey, and it is a key measure of the outcome: at the end of 1962, 14.2 per cent of the women in the sample were pregnant, and at the end of 1963, 11.4 per cent were pregnant, a decline of about a fifth.

Aside from this one statistic, only the case records are available. Even for the people directly involved it is too early to measure the effect of the program on fertility; an immediate effect would take at least nine months to begin to show up! A presumptive effect, however, can be gauged from the record of "acceptances," defined as the insertion of an intra-uterine device or the receipt of instructions and the purchase of supplies for other methods, together with expressed intent to practice contraception. In the 13 months ending in mid-March of this year the action program was responsible for a total of 5,297 acceptances of family planning, 4,007 of which were from women living within Taichung proper. (The remainder came from outside the city even though no direct action was carried on there.)

How good is that record? There are different ways to appraise the figure of 4,000-odd acceptances within the city. First, the acceptors constitute 11 per cent of the married women from 20 to 39. Not all the women in that age group, however, were "eligible" to accept family planning as a result of this program. About 16 per cent were already practicing contraception to their own satisfaction. Another 16 per cent had been sterilized or were believed to be sterile. Nine per cent were pregnant, 3 per cent lactating and 1 per cent experiencing menstrual irregularities of one kind or another. If these women are eliminated, only about 55 per cent of the 36,000 in the age group were "eligible." Of these 20,000 or so women, the program secured about 20 per cent as family planners. Included in that definition of eligibility, however, are women who actively want another child—young wives who have not completed their families or those who want a son. If they are considered not really eligible for contraception at this time, the "currently eligible" category is reduced to some 10,000 women, and those who have taken up contracep-

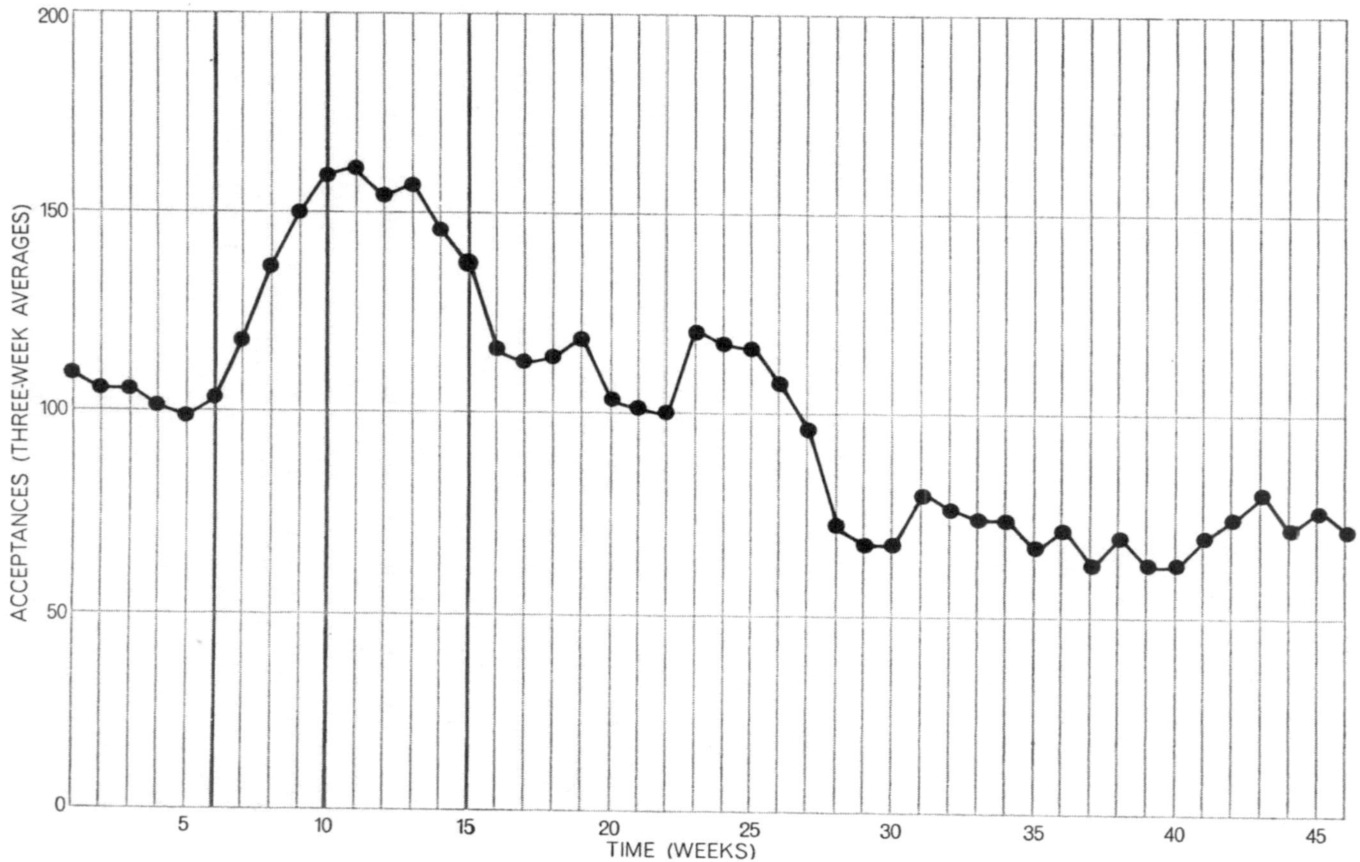

FIGURE 13.5. Progress of action program is traced by a curve showing the trend of "acceptances" of contraception in Taichung each week from the end of February 1963 to mid-January 1964. The three heavy vertical grid lines show *(left to right)* the points at which 40 per cent, 62 per cent, and 85 per cent of the home visits had been completed. The program reached a peak, then leveled off. From A Study in Fertility Control, by Bernard Berelson and Ronald Freedman.

tion in the first 13 months come to about 40 per cent of this truly eligible population.

This arithmetic helps to define a "success" in the spread of family planning in the underdeveloped countries. At any given time somewhere between half and three-fourths of the target population is simply out of bounds for the purpose. If a program can get as many as a half—or even a third or a fourth—of the remaining group to begin practicing contraception within a few years, it has probably achieved a good deal. In this kind of work, then, having an impact on 10 per cent of the target population in a year or so is not a disappointing failure but a substantial success; one should report "Fully 10 per cent," not "Only 10 per cent"! Another way to appraise the Taichung results to date is to recognize that whereas in February, 1963, about 16 per cent of the married women from 20 to 39 were practicing contraception, by March of this year about 27 per cent were doing so, an increase of nearly 70 per cent.

The impact of such a program is not felt immediately or at one time or evenly. At the outset the acceptance rate was remarkably constant, but after some seven weeks, when 40 per cent of the home visits had been made and word-of-mouth reports of the program were well established, the curve began to climb steadily [*see* Fig. 13.5]. It hit a plateau in about four weeks and stayed there for about a month before declining. This was the height of the program, when two-thirds of the home visits had been completed and interest was strong. By the beginning of June, when nearly all the visits had been made, the cream had been skimmed: the women who were strongly motivated toward family planning had heard of the program and had decided what they would do about it. By the end of the summer follow-up visits were reaching less motivated women and the curve returned to its starting point. In the fall, when home visits ended but supplies and services were still available, the acceptances settled to a lower but steady rate.

A program of this kind, then, apparently starts off reasonably well, builds up quite rapidly and achieves roughly half of its first year's return within the first four months. The important thing is to develop a "critical mass" that can generate enough personal motivation and social support to carry on without further home visits. A poor country simply cannot afford visits to the entire population, so any realistic plan must rely heavily on personal and informal contacts from trusted sources; it may be that the job will have to be done by relatives, neighbors and friends or not at all. The task of a planned program will thus be to develop enough knowledgeable and convinced users of contraceptives to start a movement that reaches out to the ill-informed and unconvinced.

TABLE 13.2.

Treatment	Heavy	Medium	Light	Total
Nothing	7	5	5	5
Mail	7	5	6	6
Everything				
(wives only)	16	13	11	14
(wives and husbands)	18	10	12	15
All treatments	12	7	7	9

Results of the program are given as of the end of last December. The figures show the acceptors as a per cent of the married women aged 20 to 39, by "treatment" and density sector. From A Study in Fertility Control, by Bernard Berelson and Ronald Freedman.

The indirect effects were extremely important in Taichung. The most dramatic indication is the fact that by the end of 1963 some 20 per cent of the acceptances had come from women who did not even live in the city. (That figure has since risen to almost 25 per cent.) Within the city about 60 per cent of the acceptances were from "Everything" *lin's*; the other 40 per cent were divided about equally between the "Nothing" and the "Mail" *lin's*. Even in the "Everything" neighborhoods about a sixth of those who accepted contraceptives actually came forward before their scheduled home visits had been made. Direct home visits, in other words, accounted for only some 40 per cent of the acceptances by the end of December.

As for the effectiveness of various concentrations of effort, the proportion of those who accepted contraceptives was indeed higher in the heavy-density sector, but this effect was almost completely within the "Everything" *lin's* themselves [*see* Table 13.2]. The indirect effect—the "rub-off" from the home-visit areas to the "Nothing" and "Mail" *lin's*—was remarkably constant in

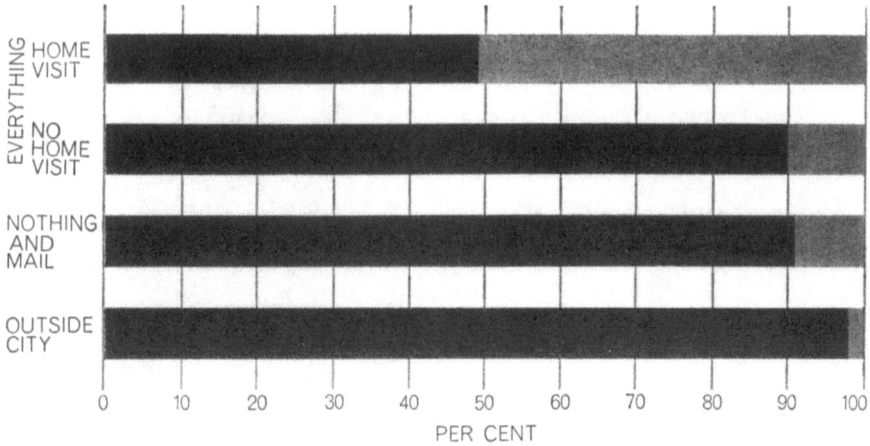

FIGURE 13.6. Indirect diffusion of family planning was particularly marked in the case of the intra-uterine device. Almost all women who accepted contraception without home visits chose this device *(dark segments of bars)* rather than a traditional method *(light segments)*. From A Study in Fertility Control, by Bernard Berelson and Ronald Freedman.

the three sectors. Our tentative conclusion is that the maximum return for minimum expenditure can be obtained with something less than the heavy-sector degree of concentration. Finally, the added effect of visiting husbands as well as wives was not worth the expense, perhaps because in this program the preferred contraceptive method was one involving the wife alone.

The nature of the contraceptive method, as a matter of fact, has more of an effect on the success of a program than may have been generally recognized. A "one-time" method requires far less field effort over a long term than a method dependent on resupply and sustained motivation. In Taichung the choice turned out to be overwhelmingly for the intra-uterine devices, which were preferred by 78 per cent of those who accepted contraceptives; 20 per cent selected one of the more traditional methods (mainly foam tablets or condoms) and 2 per cent chose the oral pill (which was, to be sure, the most expensive method). The women themselves, in other words, elected the "one-time" method. This was particularly significant in view of the method's high effectiveness and what might be called its "accountability" through scheduled medical follow-ups. The six-month checkup shows that only some 20 per cent of the devices have been removed or involuntarily expelled, whereas about 30 per cent of the women who chose the traditional methods are no longer practicing contraception regularly.

The Taichung study revealed another significant advantage of the intra-uterine device: a striking tendency for information about it to be disseminated indirectly by word-of-mouth, obviating much of the task of communication and persuasion. Nearly 75 per cent of the new devices were accepted without the necessity of a home visit, compared with only 15 per cent in the case of the traditional methods. The intra-uterine devices "sold" themselves; what the home visits did, in effect, was to secure acceptance of the traditional methods [*see* Fig. 13.6]. Since last October, when the action program proper was terminated, more than half of those who have accepted contraceptives have come from a widening circle around the city, and almost all of these women have chosen the new devices. This is presumably what happens when word of the method reaches women who are ready for family planning but want an easier and "better" way than they have heard of before.

Family planning does not, of course, diffuse evenly among the different kinds of people in a community. Acceptance varies with education and age and—in Taichung at least—above all with number of children and number of sons. When couples

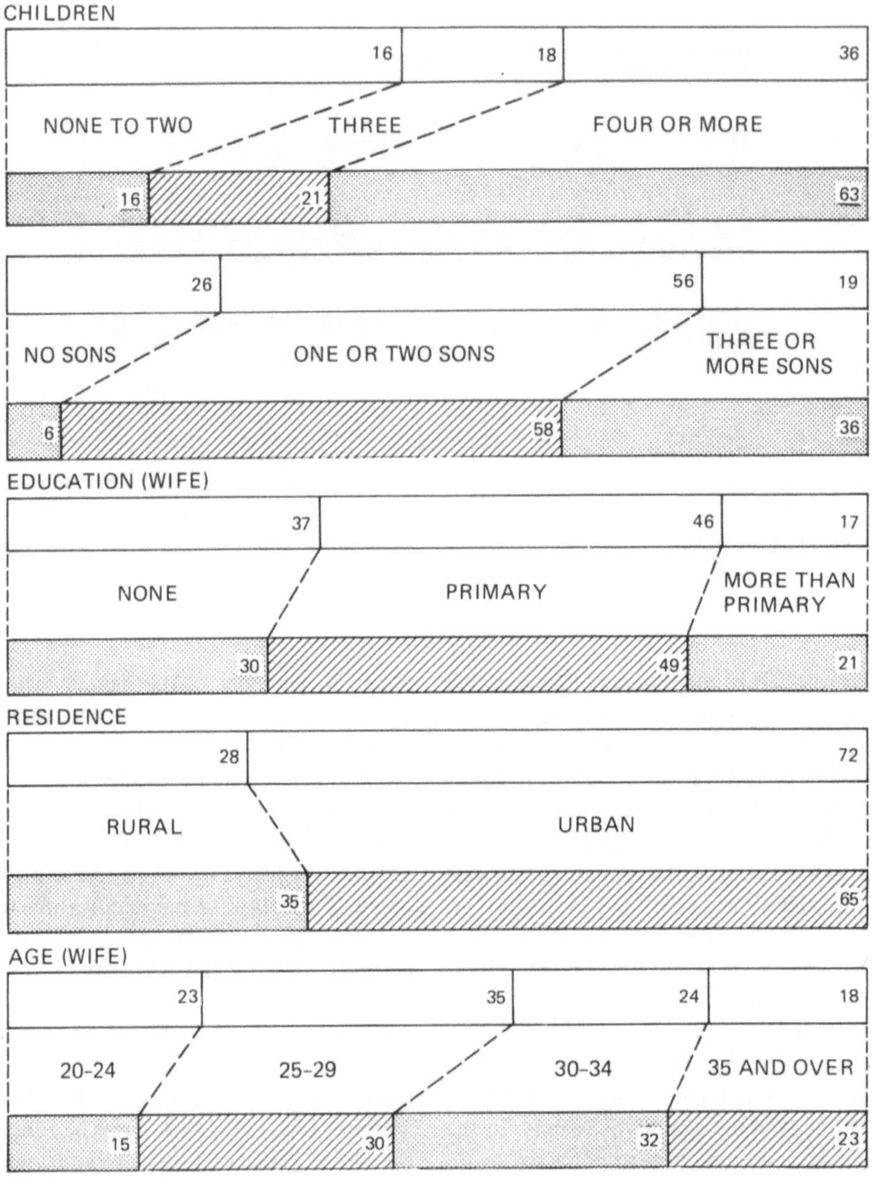

FIGURE 13.7. Acceptance of family planning varied in different groups. In this chart, the women are categorized according to various characteristics. The clear bars show the per cent of the "currently eligible" women who fell into each category. The dotted and hatched bars show the per cent of the new acceptors of contraception who fell into the same categories as of the end of 1963. From A Study in Fertility Control, by Bernard Berelson and Ronald Freedman.

in Taiwan have four children, they have all they want and they are ready to do something about it—if there is something available that is reasonably effective, inexpensive and easy to use. The evidence here is that whereas the slow long-term "natural" spread of contraception through a population reaches the better-educated people first, a deliberate and accelerated effort like the Taichung program can quickly have a major impact on the families that already have large numbers of children.

Taiwan is one of many low-income countries where rapid increases in population thwart economic development and threaten to slow further improvements in the standard of living. In the long run, to be sure, it seems likely that economic and social pressures combined with personal aspirations will lead individuals to limit their families. The underdeveloped countries, however, cannot wait for a long-term solution to their present crisis. The program in Taichung suggests that fertility control can be spread by a planned effort—not so easily or so fast as death control, but nevertheless substantially, in a short period of time and economically. (The cost of each acceptance was between $4 and $8, far below the eventual economic value of each prevented birth, which has been estimated as being between one and two times the annual per capita income.)

A good deal of the story in Taiwan remains to be told, of course, including the results of the sample survey and the critical check of official birth statistics over the next months and years. Health agencies in Taiwan are now extending the program to a larger segment of the population, testing the Taichung results and trying out new approaches in the slum areas of cities and in poor fishing and mining villages. At this point one can at least say that fertility in Taiwan is changing and can be changed—changing over the long run as the result of unplanned social processes but, most significantly, changeable in the short run as the result of a planned effort to help people have the number of children they really want.

Acknowledgments. The authors wish to acknowledge the valuable contributions of their colleagues on the Taiwan project: S.C. Hsu of the Joint Commission on Rural Reconstruction in Taiwan; T.C. Hsu, Commissioner of Health; C.L. Chen and J.Y. Peng of the Maternal and Child Health Institute, and John Takeshita of the University of Michigan.

Bibliography

Colonial Development and Population in Taiwan. George W. Barclay. Princeton University Press, 1954.

The Growth of World Population. Publication 1091, National Academy of Sciences—National Research Council, 1963.

The Population Dilemma. Edited by Philip M. Hauser. Prentice-Hall, Inc., 1963.

Research in Family Planning. Edited by Clyde V. Kiser. Princeton University Press, 1962.

14

Prospects and Programs for Fertility Reduction: What? Where?

The task is to discern the prospects for fertility reduction in the developing world and the programs required to bring it about: the probable course of fertility in the developing world for the remainder of the twentieth century and, on that basis, the policy interventions that present themselves for remedial action where needed and desired.

Despite all the scientific and professional effort that has recently been applied to this field, the double task is difficult to say the least: forecasting what will happen to fertility levels is risky, and finding policy interventions that will work is, if anything, harder still. Yet the enterprise is of such importance that the effort continues, and the following analysis is offered as one way of taking hold of the problem and trying to see it through to the end. As such, it is meant as a contribution to the ongoing debate, certainly not as a definitive answer to the questions posed in the title—which of course the field will answer by its actions over time, one way or another.

For the purpose of this exercise, I start from the proposition that rapid population growth in the developing world not only is undesirable for development ("modernization") and all that implies for human welfare (education and literacy, health and nutrition, income and income distribution, status of women, human rights), but that it is undesirable enough to warrant intervention by public policy, within reason (meaning limited investment of resources and use of acceptable measures).[1] That is, reduction of the growth rate through reduction of fertility is beneficial, though not necessarily the first item on a list of national priorities. I posit this simply as a concise restatement of "the population problem" that energized international action in the 1960s and, in the view underlying this paper, is still valid today.

In order to focus the exercise, I stipulate two targets. The substantive target is to reach a crude birth rate of 20 per thousand population per year (CBR 20) for the developing world by the year 2000—or, more precisely, to maximize the probability of reaching that target and/or minimize the shortfall. As we shall see, different countries will end up nearer to or farther from that target, but such a numerical specification of both magnitude and time forces us to focus on the problem in a way that generalized goals do not. CBR 20—under these conditions, roughly a 2.5-child family on average—is taken as the touchstone in order to achieve a rate of natural increase (NI) of close to 1 percent in the year 2000, based on the UN projections of a crude death rate between 8 and 10 per thousand population per year (CDR 8–10).[2] The procedural target is to identify a sensible strategy of intervention for the next 5–10 years, on the ground that future strategies can take care of themselves in this fast-changing field. This does not mean that current strategies cannot last longer than 5–10 years or

Reprinted with permission from *Population and Development Review* 1978;4(4):579–616, The Population Council, New York, NY.

cannot have consequences beyond that period—most would—but that optimal policies for the coming years must be decided now, and they can (and should) be reviewed and revised at appropriate intervals later.

In the following appraisals and forecasts, I rely upon current findings of demographic and social science research as applied to current data on demographic states and trends, socioeconomic settings and changes, and program efforts in this field—all as detailed below: what the record shows about the momentum of fertility trends, which fertility determinants appear to be influential, what the socioeconomic "thresholds" for fertility decline might be, where family planning programs seem to fit in. I seek to draw the fullest possible inferences from the present state of relevant scientific knowledge; in a way, I suppose, I squeeze today's wisdom for all it is worth—perhaps for slightly more. Yet despite its gaps, which will always be present in some form and degree, that is the best starting point we have. What does current knowledge indicate to the involved policymaker? What is likely to happen to the birth rate of developing countries between now and 2000? Then, in order to reach or approach the designated target, what is to be done beyond present practice, and where?

Given these stipulations, how does the task break down? The 1975 population of the developing world is estimated at 2.9 billion[3] in about 120 countries. Actually, 90 percent of that population lives in the 35 countries that have over 10 million inhabitants. I begin with these 35 countries, which have the following estimated populations (in millions) as of 1975 as shown on the right.[4] By a current appraisal, six of these countries are not accessible on this issue in this period because of local political conditions: Vietnam, Burma, North Korea, Ethiopia, Uganda, Iraq. Accordingly, they are excluded from further consideration (although they are reintroduced in note 8 to show where they would fit in the analysis).

That leaves 29 countries, with 85 percent of the population of the developing world. On the basis of present knowledge, plus reasonable and minimal assumptions about continuing trends, what are their prospects for reaching CBR 20 in the next 20–25 years? And then, what are the policy implications of such prospects?

Asia		Latin America		Middle East and North Africa		Sub-Saharan Africa	
China	830	Brazil	108	Turkey	39	Nigeria	63
India	598	Mexico	60	Egypt	37	Ethiopia	28
Indonesia	132	Colombia	25	Iran	34	Zaire	25
Bangladesh	79	Peru	16	Morocco	17	Sudan	18
Pakistan	70	Venezuela	12	Algeria	17	Tanzania	15
Vietnam[a]	44	Chile	10	Iraq	12	Kenya	13
Philippines	42					Uganda	12
Thailand	42						
South Korea	35						
Burma	31						
Afghanistan	19						
Taiwan	16						
North Korea	16						
Sri Lanka	14						
Nepal	13						
Malaysia	11						

[a]In 1975, Democratic Republic of Vietnam, 24 million; Republic of Vietnam, 20 million.

Prospects

In looking to the demographic future, we can be certain only of uncertainty: demography has its share of scars on that score. But policy is meant to change the future, and hence rests on some vision of that future—a vision of conditions to be expedited, slowed, or altered in some regard. In reviewing policy it is well to make that vision explicit so that proposals can be judged in context. Some forecast is needed to set the policy process in motion—the likelier the better. Accordingly, I examine first what chances the 29 countries have to reach CBR 20 by the century's end by looking at (1) their present demographic rates and trends; (2) their social setting—that is, their standing with respect to socioeconomic factors and values ("thresholds") believed to be associated with fertility decline.[5] The so-called thresholds used here, and taken as rough approximations of socioeconomic values that help to achieve a fertility decline, are as follows:

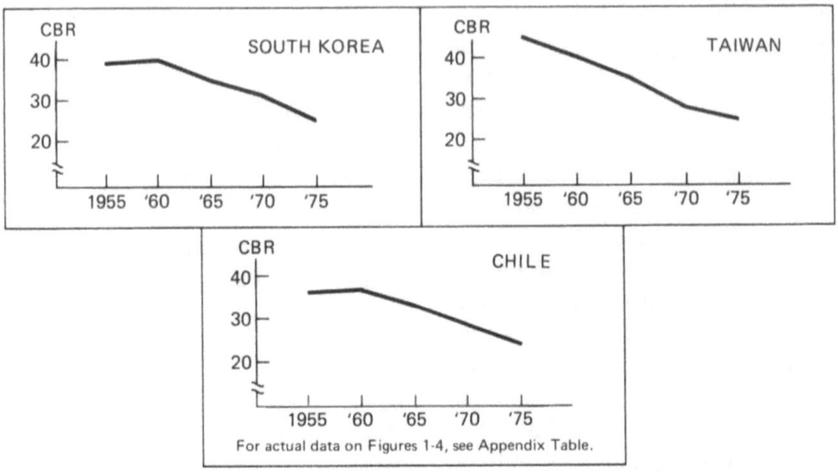

FIGURE 14.1. CBR trends, 1955–75, for countries in the Certain category.

Factor	Threshold value for CBR 35	Threshold value for CBR 20
Adult literacy (lit)	70%	93%
School enrollment, age 5–19 (enr)	55%	69%
Life expectancy (exp)	60 years	69 years
Infant mortality rate (IMR)	65	32
Nonagricultural labor force (nonagr)	55%	80%
Per capita GNP (GNP)	$450	$1,080
Females 15–19 never married (fem)	80%	–

Exact precision in this regard is not possible, warranted, or needed, and even the analysts of thresholds consider them tentative, preliminary, questionable. I do not take these thresholds literally, in the sense that only these values of only these variables will do the trick, but rather as rough indicators of a socioeconomic setting congenial to fertility reduction—markers or surrogates, if not controlling in their own right. This notion is further confirmed for the present case by detailed analysis in Mauldin and Berelson (see note 5), which concludes that no particular set heralds a fertility transition (although some appear to be more influential than others) and that three or four such factors correlate about as well with fertility decline as a larger number, as indicative of the whole. Finally (3) their family planning program effort is examined. Data on all three matters are shown in Table 14.1.

With regard to attaining the indicated target, the countries fall into four groups—the Certain, the Probable, the Possible, and the Unlikely. Naturally, some countries are borderline, and I shall point them out as we go.[6]

The Certain

South Korea, Taiwan, Chile

With as much certainty as such sociodemographic events can be predicted, these three countries should reach CBR 20 well before the end of the century: their CBRs are in the low 20s now; they have low mortality and infant mortality rates; they already have favorable social settings, with improvements continuing; they are beyond the (presumed) CBR 35 thresholds for fertility reduction on several factors; they have no major retarding effect from ethnic traditions; they have the requisite family planning program effort; they are riding a substantial downward trend in fertility of at least 15 years' duration (see Table 14.1 and Figure 14.1). If their fertility in 1975–85 declines merely by the percentage it did in 1965–75, they will already have CBRs well below 20.

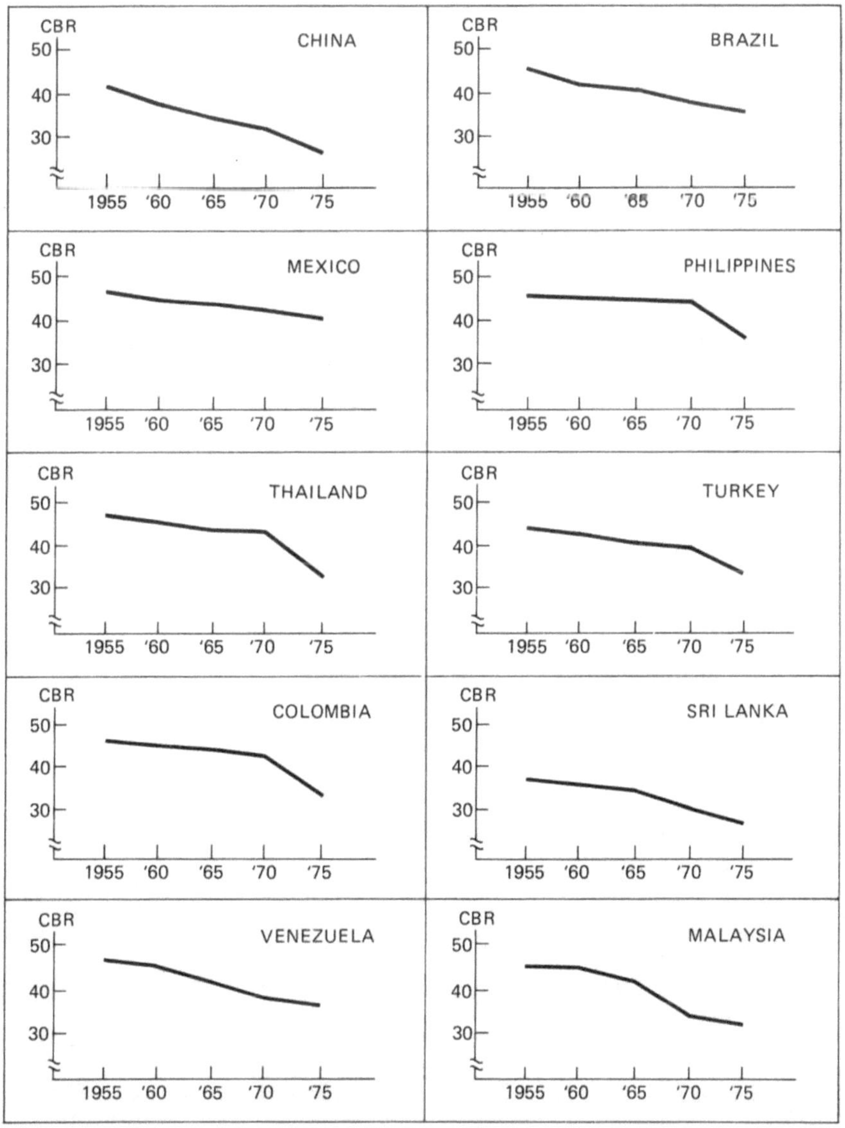

FIGURE 14.2. CBR trends, 1955–75, for countries in the Probable category.

TABLE 14.1. Relevant data on present state and trend for 29 developing countries, classified by prospect of attaining CBR 20 by 2000

Category and country	Demographic data: Population, 1975 (millions) (1)	Natural increase rate, 1975 (2)	Crude death rate, 1975 (3)	Crude birth rate, 1975 (4)	CBR decline, 1955–75: Points (5)	CBR decline, 1955–75: Percent (6)	CBR decline, 1965–75: Points (7)	CBR decline, 1965–75: Percent (8)	Social data: Social setting: c.1970 (9)	Social setting: Change, 1960–70 (10)	Ethnicity (11)	Thresholds met (12)	Program data: Family planning program effort 1965–75 (13)
The Certain													
South Korea	35	1.7	7	24	16	40	11	32	Hi	Hi	Chinese	lit, enr, exp, IMR, fem	Str
Taiwan	16	1.8	5	23	21	48	10	30	Hi	Hi	Chinese	lit, enr, exp, IMR, non-agr, GNP, fem	Str
Chile	10	1.6	8	23	13	36	10	29	Hi	Hi	Catholic	lit, enr, exp, nonagr, GNP, fem	Mod
The Probable													
China	830	1.4	10	26	9	25	8	24	UpMid	- UpMid	Chinese	exp	Str
Brazil	108	2.8	10	38	3	7	4	10	Hi	UpMid	Catholic	lit, enr, exp, GNP, fem	Wk
Mexico	60	3.0	8	40	6	13	4	9	Hi	Hi	Catholic	lit, enr, exp, IMR, GNP, fem	Wk
Philippines	42	2.6	11	36	9	20	8	19	UpMid	Hi	Catholic	lit, enr, exp, GNP, fem	Mod
Thailand	42	2.8	9	34	13	28	10	23	UpMid	UpMid	Chinese	lit, enr, exp, fem	Mod
Turkey	39	2.3	11	34	11	24	7	16	UpMid	Hi	Moslem	enr, exp, GNP, fem	Wk
Colombia	25	2.2	9	33	13	28	11	25	Hi	UpMid	Catholic	lit, enr, exp, GNP, fem	Mod
Sri Lanka	14	1.9	9	27	11	28	6	18	UpMid	Lo	Other	lit, enr, exp, IMR, fem	Mod

Venezuela	12	2.9	7	37	9	20	5	11	Hi	UpMid	Catholic	lit, enr, exp, IMR, non-agr, GNP, fem	Wk
Malaysia	11	2.4	6	31	15	31	11	26	UpMid	UpMid	Other	enr, exp, IMR, GNP, fem	Mod
The Possible													
India	598	1.9	16	36	7	17	7	16	LoMid	LoMid	Other		Mod
Indonesia	132	2.3	20	40	6	13	6	13	LoMid	Hi	Moslem		Mod
Egypt	37	2.3	12	35	9	22	7	17	UpMid	Lo	Moslem	enr	Wk
Peru	16	3.0	13	42	3	5	1	2	Hi	LoMid	Catholic	lit, enr, GNP, fem	Wk
The Unlikely													
Bangladesh	79	2.8	18	49	1	1	1	2	Lo	Lo	Moslem		Wk
Pakistan	70	2.8	15	47	2	5	1	1	LoMid	LoMid	Moslem		Wk
Nigeria	63	2.7	23	49	0	0	1	1	LoMid	Hi	African		Wk
Iran	34	2.9	14	45	2	6	1	2	UpMid	Hi	Moslem	enr, GNP	Mod
Zaire	25	2.3	21	44	3	7	3	6	UpMid	LoMid	African	enr	Wk
Afghanistan	19	2.5	24	49	0	0	0	+2	Lo	LoMid	Moslem		Wk
Sudan	18	3.0	18	49	2	2	0	0	Lo	Lo	Moslem		Wk
Morocco	17	3.0	16	48	2	5	1	2	UpMid	LoMid	Moslem		Wk
Algeria	17	3.3	15	48	3	6	2	4	UpMid	LoMid	Moslem	GNP	Wk
Tanzania	15	2.5	19	48	3	7	3	5	Lo	LoMid	African		Wk
Kenya	13	3.3	16	50	+2	+4	0	0	LoMid	UpMid	African		Wk
Nepal	13	2.2	21	45	1	2	+1	+1	Lo	Lo	Moslem		Wk

Sources: Cols. 1–3: From Fact Book, 8th and 9th eds. (cited in note 1).
Cols. 4, 7, 8, 9, 11, 13: From Mauldin and Berelson, cited in note 5.
Cols. 5, 6, 10: From Population Council data bank utilized for Mauldin and Berelson, cited in note 5.
Col. 12: From Table 14.4. Abbreviations are as specified in table, page 192.

So these countries will surely reach the target. But this group, as of now, has only 2 percent of the population of the developing world.

The Probable

China, Brazil, Mexico, Philippines, Thailand, Turkey, Colombia, Sri Lanka, Venezuela, Malaysia

These countries have a strong chance to achieve the target: they now have CBRs in the 30s or below (with the possible exception of Mexico, though it too is reported to be under 40 by now); the crude death rates are in the 6–11 range; they have favorable social settings, with advances in progress (except for Sri Lanka); they meet several threshold requirements (except China, which is questionable because of insufficient data); only one (Moslem Turkey) has a high-fertility ethnic tradition, and that country is rapidly modernizing with a sharp fertility reduction in recent years; only six have the requisite family planning program effort, but another (Mexico) is now vitalizing its effort and the other three (Brazil, Turkey, Venezuela) have the administrative potential; use of fertility control is in the 30–40 percent range in countries with programs of some duration (e.g., Thailand, Malaysia); they all appear to be on a downward trend, which in some cases is quite sharp, although their recency leaves them somewhat suspect (see Table 14.1 and Figure 14.2). Again, if 1975–85 repeats 1965–75, all but three will have CBRs in the 20s by 1985, and those three (Brazil, Mexico, Venezuela) will be in the transitional mid-30s and with favorable developments (e.g., improved social setting, strong threshold positions).

As designated, this group has 42 percent of the total developing population. Actually, for four countries the chances of reaching the target might be considered even better than probable—China, Colombia, Sri Lanka, Malaysia—in that another decade of decline like 1965–75 would put them all in the low 20s (assuming that the data and reports on China are reasonably accurate);[7] and three others (Philippines, Thailand, Turkey) would be in the 20s. Still, the large countries of Brazil and Mexico remain somewhat problematic. At the least, it seems fair to say that the countries of the Probable category will come close to the target, or could if they would.

The Possible

India, Indonesia, Egypt, Peru

These countries present a mixed picture. On the one hand, two are now in the transitional mid-30s (India, Egypt); three have impressive recent fertility declines (India, Indonesia, Egypt); and two

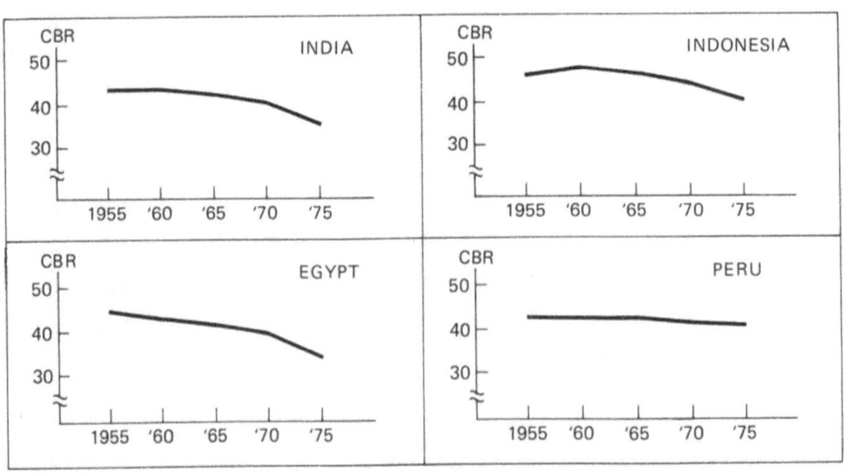

FIGURE 14.3. CBR trends, 1955–75, for countries in the Possible category.

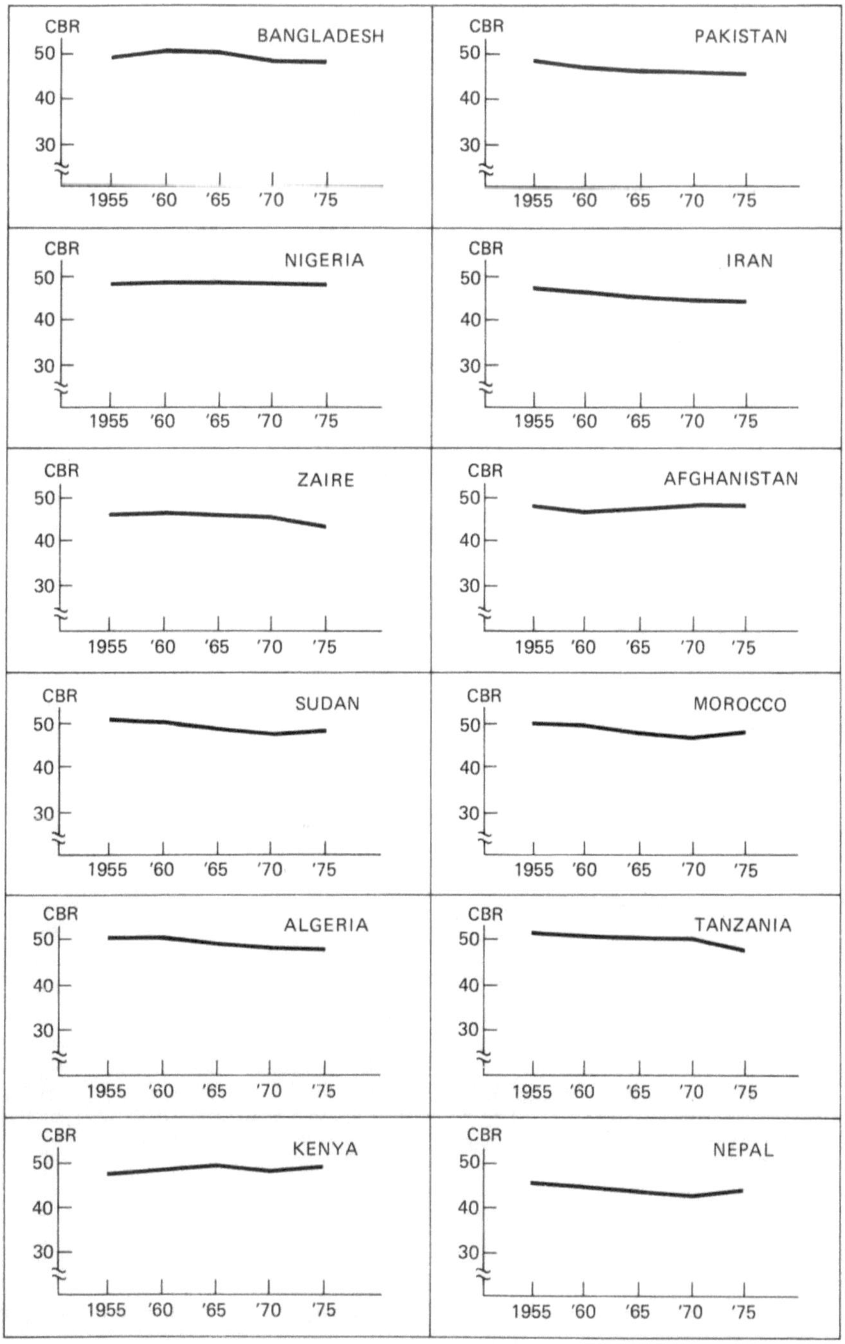

FIGURE 14.4. CBR trends, 1955–75, for countries in the Unlikely category.

TABLE 14.2. Assumed projections of CBR, 1975–2000

Category and country	Percent decline, 1955–75	Percent decline, 1965–75	CBR, 1975	CBR by 2000 if: Percent decline = 1955–75	CBR by 2000 if: Percent decline = double 1965–75	UN projections of CBR, 1995–2000: Medium variant	UN projections of CBR, 1995–2000: Low variant
The Certain							
South Korea	40	32	24	15[b]	15[b]	19.6	17.6
Taiwan	48	30	23	15[b]	15[b]	—[c]	—[c]
Chile	36	29	23	15[b]	15[b]	19.8	17.6
The Probable							
China	25	24	26	19	15[b]	18.3	17.1
Brazil	7	10	38	35	30	29.4	22.7
Mexico	13	9	40	35	33	35.2	32.1
Philippines	20	19	36	29	23	28.6	25.1
Thailand	28	23	34	25	18	29.1	27.4
Turkey	24	16	34	26	23	26.5	21.4
Colombia	28	25	33	24	16	26.9	21.6
Sri Lanka	28	18	27	20	18	18.7	17.6
Venezuela	20	11	37	30	29	26.4	22.6
Malaysia	31	26	31	22	15	22.6	20.2
The Possible							
India	17	16	36	30	25	26.3	24.1
Indonesia	13	13	40	35	30	26.7	25.4
Egypt	22	17	35	27	23	28.3	24.8
Peru	5	2	42	39	40	31.4	25.2
The Unlikely							
Bangladesh	1	2	49	48	47	36.4	33.8
Pakistan	5	1	47	45	46	32.5	30.6
Nigeria	0	1	49	49	48	44.8	40.0
Iran	6	2	45	43	43	31.0	29.1
Zaire	7	6	44	41	39	40.6	37.4
Afghanistan	0	+2[a]	49	50	51	36.5	34.8
Sudan	2	0	49	47	49	35.8	33.1
Morocco	5	2	48	46	46	32.0	28.3
Algeria	6	4	48	45	44	33.1	29.6
Tanzania	7	5	48	45	43	42.2	33.6
Kenya	+4[a]	0	50	52	50	41.8	33.3
Nepal	2	+1[a]	45	44	46	33.4	31.7

Data for UN projections as cited in note 11.
[a]Considered as zero change in extrapolation.
[b]Arbitrary floor at CBR 15.
[c]Taiwan not included in UN documents.

(India, Indonesia) have had good family planning program efforts for their settings, although the program of the former is now (1978) in a relapsed position from which it may not soon recover. On the other hand, death rates are still on the high side; social factors are mixed to unfavorable for the three large countries; only Peru has a favorable threshold position; and two countries (and a substantial proportion of a third) are Moslem (see Table 14.1 and Figure 14.3). If 1975–85 repeats 1965–75, India and Egypt will be at about CBR 30, Indonesia at 35, and Peru still at 40.

This group has 28 percent of the population of the developing world. They have a chance at reaching the target, but it will take some doing; and given the difficulties in the two large countries, a CBR of 25 would be a signal achievement.

The Unlikely

Bangladesh, Pakistan, Nigeria, Iran, Zaire, Afghanistan, Sudan, Morocco, Algeria, Tanzania, Kenya, Nepal

In these countries, all the indicators are unfavorable: birth rates from the mid-40s up and stable, so that the initial break in fertility is still to come; death rates still high; an unfavorable and only slowly changing socioeconomic setting; thresholds unmet; Moslem and/or Sub-Saharan African high-fertility traditions; no real family planning effort in recent years (see Table 14.1 and Figure 14.4). The fertility decline for 1965–75, if any, is barely measurable.

This group, with 13 percent of the developing population, has no discernible chance to achieve the stipulated target under expectable circumstances. And it is even difficult to see a country bordering on the Possible category (if pressed, maybe Iran, with two threshold levels met and relatively rapid improvement in socioeconomic setting, but with political turbulence and opposition). By present indications, these countries would do well to reach CBR 30, or even 35, by the indicated date—that is, 10–15 points off in the next 25 years.

So that is one prospect for this 85 percent of the developing world.[8] Now let us see what would happen if recent fertility trends continued for the remainder of the century. With that scenario, how close will the sector as a whole come to the stipulated target by 2000?

The rate of decline in the near future will surely differ among categories of countries, as well as within the same country at different times.[9] But as a start, assume that fertility decline for the rest of the century will (1) equal that for the past 20 years (i.e., 1955–75), country by country, or (2) double that for the past decade (1965–75), a more recent and more rapid measure. And note that, by way of a safety margin, there are an extra five years in the projected period—that is, 25 years from 1975, not just 20.

A continued decline approximating that of the past two decades, as depicted in the Appendix Table, would bring this portion of the developing sector to CBR 30 under the first assumption and CBR 26 under the second, as shown in these CBR projections for 1975–2000 (weighted by population size; country details in Table 14.2).

Country category	CBR, 1975	CBR by 2000 if: Decline = 1955–75	Decline = double 1965–75
The Certain	24	15	15
The Probable	29	24	19
The Possible	37	31	26
The Unlikely	48	47	46
Total	34	30	26

Note: None of the projections was taken below CBR 15; the three cases with slight increases in the 1955–65–75 data were considered as no change.

It would obviously take a much faster downward trend to reach CBR 20—on the order of a 40 percent decline over that period, not the 15–25 percent calculated here.[10] If even the 1955–75 rates are too optimistic—an unlikely prospect—then the CBR in 2000 will be correspondingly higher, though probably not by much: after all, it is already about 34.

The comparable CBRs for the year 2000, from the latest UN projections that take age structure into account,[11] are these (weighted by population size):

Country category	Medium variant	Low variant
The Certain*	19.6	17.6
The Probable	21.5	19.4
The Possible	26.6	24.4
The Unlikely	36.8	33.6
Total, these countries	25.6	23.2
Total, developing world	27.8	25.0

*Taiwan not included in UN documents.

The total values are quite similar, but that is accounted for by greater declines in the UN projections for the Possible (about 5 points) and the Unlikely (10–13 points) and less decline in the Certain (3–5 points), with the Probable about the same, as can be seen in the country-by-country comparisons in Table 14.2.

Of particular importance in this connection, fertility in several of the countries will have fallen somewhat faster than the CBR by the century's end—in the sense that the changing age structure will work against a CBR decline. In the first 10–15 years after a fertility decline begins, the difference between CBR and total fertility rate (the number of births a woman would have if she were to bear children at the age-specific fertility rates prevailing in the year to which the rate refers throughout her reproductive span) in percentage decline is quite small, but after that it begins to build up to the order of a 10–15 percent differential in favor of the total fertility rate (which is independent of age structure). Thus the CBRs for 2000, influenced by changes in age structure, will be relatively high in those countries where a fertility decline has occurred or will soon occur (before 1985). That is, as fertility measures, CBRs are indeed "crude": they reflect not only actual fertility declines but also any changes in age structure. The total fertility rates, on the other hand, reflect fertility trends per se and will show a steeper decline than the CBRs. What this means, in short, is that even now in those countries where fertility began to decline a decade or more ago, and will do so increasingly in the next decades, any CBR decline will be pushing against the age structural residuals from earlier declines (which, in effect, leave a higher percentage of women in the reproductive ages),[12] and in their absence would be lower by 2-4 points depending upon time, duration, level, and speed of the decline.

For perspective on such prospects, recall by way of comparative standard that the CBR decline for the latest available decade (1965–75) was 5.5 points and that the world's record for the modern era—Japan's dramatic decline from 1947 to 1957—was 17 points.[13] The declines projected for our four categories in Table 14.2 range from 2 points off for the Unlikely to 6–11 points off for the others, with an overall decline of 6–10 points below the 1975 CBR. That would seem to bracket the possibilities and to suggest that substantial declines are definitely reachable,[14] though at this rate not enough to achieve the designated target.

I have used CBR 35 and its associated thresholds inasmuch as they may signal a transition downward. Let us look at a possible future of fertility decline by taking off from a notable analysis of the "years historically and currently required for countries to reduce annual crude birth rates from 35 to 20."[15] Dudley Kirk found an acceleration through time in the rate at which countries move through that transition, culminating in a mean of 15 years for countries beginning in the period 1950–, a median of 14, and a range of 10-26. But Kirk's data, for only six countries, ended around 1969, and we now have additional information to work with, both in time and in numbers. What does it show?

With later data and hence less extrapolation, the six countries in Kirk's analysis now appear to be taking longer to decline from CBR 35 to CBR 20 than he estimated: 21–22 years rather than 14–15, although the range has not changed much (see Table 14.3). Actually, two countries have reached CBR 20 by now, the special cases of the city-states. In addition, 16 countries can now be identified that reached the gateway of CBR 35 in this period, most of them since Kirk's cutoff date. None of them has yet reached CBR 20 but a few are close. The similarity in time required between Kirk's original six and the additional 16 is remarkable:

	Years required	
Measure	Kirk's 6 (rev.)	Additional 16
Mean	21	23
Median	22	21
Range	11-33	15-40

And of these 22 countries, all but three reach CBR 20 by the year 2000, and those three (Albania, Turkey, and Egypt) miss that target by only five years.

That list, which includes smaller countries as well, has 11 in our size class with 38 percent of the population of the (now) developing world. Moreover, with another decade of decline like that of 1965–75, all the countries in the Probable and Possible categories (except Peru) would be within the transition border of CBR 35 by 1985 and hence "destined" to complete the transition by 2000 or shortly thereafter. And if that were to happen, with the countries in the Unlikely category still at CBR 40 and the excluded and smaller countries at CBR 30—both conservative assumptions—the CBR of the developing world, as currently defined, would then be 24.[16]

Finally, an even more compressed view of the situation focuses on the largest countries—say, the

TABLE 14.3. Prospects for reaching CBR 20 in countries reaching CBR 35 after 1950

Country	Year reached CBR 35 (1)	Year reached CBR 20 (2)	CBR, 1975 (3)	Percent decline in CBR, 1965–75 (4)	Percent decline, col. 4, extrapolated to CBR 20 (in yrs.) (5)	Approximate years from CBR 35 to 20 (6)
The Kirk Group						
Chile*	1952		23.2	29	5 = 1980	28
Puerto Rico	1955		23.1	20	6 = 1981	26
Hong Kong	1960	1972				12
Ceylon* (Sri Lanka)	1961		27.2	18	15 = 1990	29
Singapore	1962	1973				11
Taiwan*	1963		23.0	30	5 = 1980	17
Additions						
China*	1954		26.0	24	9 = 1984	30
Trinidad and Tobago	1963		23.0	29	4 = 1979	16
South Korea*	1965		24.0	32	5 = 1980	15
Albania	1965		33.3	15[a]	30 = 2005	40
Mauritius	1966		25.6	29	8 = 1983	17
Fiji	1966		28.0	22	13 = 1988	22
Malaysia*	1969		31.4	26	15 = 1990	21
Jamaica	1970		30.3	21	18 = 1993	23
Costa Rica	1970		29.3	29	11 = 1986	16
Panama	1972		31.0	22	18 = 1993	21
Thailand*	1974		34.0	23	20 = 1995	21
Turkey*	1974		34.0	16	30 = 2005	31
Colombia*	1974		33.0	25	18 = 1993	19
North Vietnam*	1974		32.0	23	18 = 1993	19
Tunisia	1974		33.9	24	19 = 1994	20
Egypt*	1975		34.8	17	30 = 2005	30

* = Countries with a population of 10 million or more, included in general analysis.
[a]Interpolated from percent decline 1960–75.

eight with 50 million or more population that together total nearly 70 percent of the developing sector:

Certain	Probable	Possible	Unlikely
	China	India	Bangladesh
	Brazil	Indonesia	Pakistan
	Mexico		Nigeria

Given the stipulations, that is where the core of the problem is, in magnitude, and where effort might be concentrated to the extent that it would promise reasonable results. The task is varied, but difficult at best: China we pretty much have to take on faith at the moment; Brazil and Mexico could probably make the most impact most easily, if they genuinely wished to; India and Indonesia have shown important results from impressive family planning efforts, but it remains to be seen whether such gains can be sustained in the absence of supporting socioeconomic trends and/or firm determination on program; the other three have dim prospects on all counts. It may well be (in the absence of an absolutely ideal means of fertility control suited to each culture, and maybe not even then) that, except for China, Brazil, and Mexico,[17] these countries cannot reach or closely approach the target without some use of "harder" measures —said by way of analysis not recommendation.

The next six countries in size, from 35 to 50 million with 8 percent of the total population (or over

75 percent if added to the largest eight), have a much better chance, as documented above:

Certain	Probable	Possible	Unlikely
South Korea	Philippines Thailand Turkey	Egypt	Iran

The three East Asian countries are well on the way, and the three Middle Eastern countries (Moslem) might succeed with a strong family planning effort (perhaps even Iran, given its improving position with regard to thresholds and discounting political obstacles).

Programs

So even the continuation of recent fertility declines, themselves unprecedented for the developing sector, will fall short of the stipulated target of CBR 20 and a growth rate of 1 percent by the year 2000. But the continuation of present trends is by no means "destined" to occur in what might be termed the natural course of events. Public policy will also have an impact. To the extent that this analysis and prognosis is roughly correct, or at least points to a useful direction for consideration, then what is to be done, and where, by those professionally interested in achieving fertility declines approaching the stipulated or similar target, with realistic means—in the countries themselves and in the donor community?

For this purpose, consider a range of strategic interventions that are presently used or proposed: (1) family planning programs, traditional or integrated with health services, limited or augmented with sterilization, abortion, or a new method—all in order to extend the supply of fertility control means; (2) development generally or "integrated," "selective," or "restructured" development—for example, efforts to improve popular education, infant mortality rates, women's status, income redistribution—in order to increase the demand or motivation for fertility control (i.e., what might be termed the Bucharest prescription);[18] (3) procedural, administrative, and organizational rearrangements at the community level, in order to internalize costs, minimize the negative externalities of individual fertility behavior, and rationalize (reverse) the social signals that govern such behavior;[19] and (4) official incentives, pressures, or sanctions against undesired fertility behavior or for desired behavior (as, for example, the monetary fees for sterilization in India, the reported organized pressures in China, or a legal and enforced rise in age at marriage), in order to attack the problem directly. There are several lists of such interventions[20] and several other ways of classifying such policies, but the preceding probably cover what is currently pursued or proposed and will suffice for the present purpose.

As we look back over the categories of countries and their prospects, how might such possible interventions, realistically considered, improve the chances for realizing or approaching a crude birth rate around 20?

The Certain

There is no problem here: the socioeconomic background and trends are favorable, the program effort is satisfactory or better, the practice of fertility control is already established. These countries seem safe for the stipulated target, and even below it.

The Probable

There are problems, hence opportunities, here. From recent analyses it would appear that improved family planning efforts could make a marked difference in fertility decline under the favorable socioeconomic conditions of Brazil, Mexico, and Venezuela[21] and a substantial difference in the Philippines, Sri Lanka, and Turkey. The other four—China, Thailand, Colombia, and Malaysia—are already close to the maximum effect to be expected from such efforts,[22] unless the latter two were to stress sterilization and/or abortion, unrealistic given local sentiments (the same could be said for the other Latin American countries in this category as well). The developmental situation is moderately satisfactory, and the continuation of current improvements may well suffice. The current state in this regard is favorable relative to the CBR 35 thresholds (see Table 14.4, including the Certain as well). Of the 87 available cases in the two categories (13 countries × 7 factors = 91 minus 4 no-data instances for China), fully 64, or

TABLE 14.4. Present state of seven factors compared to CBR 35 threshold values for major socioeconomic factors circa 1970 (values in parentheses)

Category and country	Life expectancy (60 yrs.)	Infant mortality rate (65)	Adult literacy (70%)	School enrollment (55%)	Nonagri-cultural labor force (55%)	Per capita GNP ($450)	Females 15–19 never married (80%)	Number of thresholds met (est. 1975)
The Certain								
South Korea	59 yrs.	60	88%	76%	45%	$344	97%	5
Taiwan	68	19	81	78	65	623	94	7
Chile	62	79	88	83	57	811	91	6
Median (app.)	62	60	85	78	57	623	94	6
The Probable								
China	60	–	–	–	34	170	–	?
Brazil	61	109	66	58	41	680	87	4
Mexico	62	68	74	69	42	996	79	6
Philippines	57	82	83	87	33	289	89	4
Thailand	57	80	79	58	21	269	81	4
Turkey	56	145	51	69	38	612	80	4
Colombia	60	76	76	63	44	432	86	5
Sri Lanka	67	50	81	73	41	129	89	5
Venezuela	57	49	82	75	57	1,837	84	7
Malaysia	58	41	58	62	42	555	84	5
Median (app.)	60	75	75	70	40	360	85	5
The Possible								
India	48	130	33	40	32	140	43	0
Indonesia	46	140	60	43	29	146	63	0
Egypt	51	120	35	52	38	266	70	1
Peru	55	135	74	75	41	659	83	5
Median (app.)	50	130	50	50	35	175	65	1
The Unlikely								
Bangladesh	40	140	22	33	14	119	11	0
Pakistan	49	136	22	27	37	131	69	0
Nigeria	40	157	25	21	31	219	28	0
Iran	50	140	29	54	43	882	54	2
Zaire	43	115	35	68	30	134	–	1
Afghanistan	39	190	8	14	18	102	49	0
Sudan	47	145	20	21	17	139	–	0
Morocco	52	133	21	32	35	378	66	0
Algeria	52	145	26	45	33	655	54	1
Tanzania	43	167	37	22	17	156	29	0
Kenya	49	126	35	42	21	178	64	0
Nepal	42	200	13	19	8	102	39	0
Median (app.)	45	145	25	30	25	150	50	0

– = data not available.

Source: Threshold values are as shown above. First six factors from Mauldin and Berelson (note 5), Table 6, pp. 100–101; column on females 15–19 never married from Population Council data bank. Values within a few points of the threshold in 1970 are given the benefit of improvement to threshold status by 1975.

74 percent, were already quite close to, at, or above the threshold value in 1970; and of the remainder only the following countries would *not* reach the specified threshold levels by 1990, assuming continuation of 1960–70 trends in each instance:

Nonagricultural labor force	Per capita GNP
China	(China, n.d.)
Brazil	Philippines
Mexico	Sri Lanka
Philippines	
Thailand	
Sri Lanka	
Malaysia	

That is, no country in the Certain category would be below any threshold, and none in the Probable group would be below on any other factor—and given the heightened pace of industrialization and urbanization, some of these cases will probably reach the labor force threshold too. Moreover, the median country in these categories is already at or near the corresponding threshold values for CBR 20 in half of the six available measures[23] (not to imply that all are necessary; indeed that is almost certainly not the case):

Factor	Correspondence value for CBR 20	Medians		Countries at or near threshold
		Certain	Probable	
Life expectancy	69 years	62 years	60 years	Sri Lanka
Infant mortality rate	32	60	75	Taiwan
Adult literacy	93%	85%	75%	South Korea, Chile
School enrollment	69%	78%	70%	South Korea, Taiwan, Chile, Mexico, Turkey, Sri Lanka, Venezuela
Nonagricultural labor force	80%	57%	40%	None
Per capita GNP	$1,080	$623	$360	Venezuela

Note: Data on females 15–19 never married not available.

As for pressure and/or sanction, that is reportedly already being applied in perhaps the only country in this group that would tolerate it for this end.

Thus countries in the Probable category can likely rely on improved program effort, particularly in the larger countries after China (i.e., Brazil, Mexico, Philippines, Thailand, Turkey). With the exception of Brazil and perhaps Turkey, they all genuinely accept that policy, such programs are administratively feasible in their settings, and the programs have such other-than-demographic rationales and consequences that support them as maternal health. For this group, it would appear that if there is the will, there is a way.

The Possible

The same is probably not true for this group. Except for Peru, the threshold position is weak and is likely to remain so for some time. The two large countries, India and Indonesia, have made major family planning efforts against heavy social-setting odds; like China, they require a particularly strong program in order to overcome the drag on fertility decline from the traditional socioeconomic background. Indeed, some observers believe that in these three largest developing countries, even the current achievements have depended in significant degree upon the application of official pressure to back up the family planning program—and the recent Indian turn-around demonstrates the fragility of that approach in an open state.[24]

In any case, with or without pressure, such efforts in such settings probably require continuous and/or certain methods (i.e., sterilization in India, abortion in China) to have a significant demographic impact.[25] As for Egypt and Peru, a stronger family planning effort should make a substantial difference in the latter (although it may be starting too far back to reach the target) and a smaller one in the former,[26] even though there too the more effective methods are probably unacceptable—and official pressure is certainly so.

Beyond program and "pressure," what else presents itself to the policymaker? Given the current socioeconomic situation and trend, improvements to or near CBR 35 threshold levels may be expected in the next two decades on life expectancy in India and Egypt, adult literacy in Indonesia, and school enrollment in all three, but not on any other factors. These societies are still far from the thresholds, and advancing rather slowly.

Two more decades of improvement equivalent to 1960–70 would bring countries in the Possible and the Unlikely categories to the designated thresholds for CBR 35 in 1990 in these cases:

Country category	Life expectancy	Infant mortality rate	Adult literacy	School enrollment	Nonagricultural labor force	Per capita GNP	Females 15–19 never married
The Possible	India Egypt Peru		Indonesia Peru*	India Indonesia Egypt Peru*		Peru*	Peru*
The Unlikely	Pakistan Iran Morocco Algeria Kenya	Iran		Iran Zaire* Algeria Kenya	Iran	Iran* Morocco* Algeria	Pakistan Morocco

*Already at or above threshold.

For example, if India or Iran were to experience two more decades of advance in school enrollment like that of 1960–70, they would reach the threshold level of 55 percent, which Peru and Zaire already exceed. For detailed data, see Table 14.5.

Here lies a central challenge for population policy, specifically for those advocating the Bucharest redefinition: How is development in India, Indonesia, or Egypt[27] to be realistically "restructured" in order to expedite fertility decline—not through mere advocacy of the goals (more education, lower infant mortality, better income and more equal distribution, higher status for women) but through specific and concrete measures capable of realization in reasonable time and adoptable on demographic grounds? And the same challenge exists for advocates of community-level reorganization to this end, with recognition of the potential political dangers as well as benefits.

The Unlikely

Here the picture is even darker, on all scores. Half the countries have family planning programs for *non*demographic reasons, a less effective version (as against fewer than a quarter in the first three categories). Strong programs can be administered in these countries only with great difficulty, if at all: there is only one moderate program in the entire array (Iran, still mainly information—not service-oriented), despite years of trying in some countries. Moreover, such efforts might not have much demographic impact without the continuous and/or certain methods (sterilization and abortion) that are not approved in most of these societies. Neither are the hard measures of pressure and sanction, although Bangladesh has talked of them and several countries have used them in other matters; but when push comes to shove, that cure is usually considered worse than the disease. As for development, general or "restructured," the situation is even more discouraging than with the countries in the Possible category, both with regard to present state (see Table 14.4) and in the 20-year extrapolation relative to CBR 35 thresholds (table above and Table 14.5), where only Iran does well, and perhaps the North African countries. So the challenge to "restructured" development and to community reorganization as demographic instruments is even sharper with this group than with the Possible.[28]

Proximate Determinants

Finally, whether and whatever the approach via the so-called basic determinants, in order to affect fertility they need to operate through intermediate factors—what my colleague John Bongaarts calls proximate determinants[29] and defines as "the biological and behavioral factors through which

TABLE 14.5. Points under threshold (u) in 1970 and points improved (i), 1960–70

Category and country	Life expectancy		Infant mortality rate		Adult literacy		School enrollment		Nonagri-cultural labor force		Per capita GNP		Females 15–19 never married	
	(u)	(i)	(u)	(i)	(u)	(i)	(u)	(i)	(u)	(i)	(u)	(i)	(u)	(i)
The Possible														
India	12	5	65	9	37	5	15	13	23	4	310	21	37	14
Indonesia	14	5	75	26	10	21	12	8	26	7	304	25	17	3
Egypt	9	5	55	0	35	6	3	9	17	2	184	44	10	3
Peru	5	5	70	−43[a]	over	13	over	17	14	4	over	138	over	−1
Median (app.)	10	5	65	5	25	10	8	10	20	5	250	35	15	5
The Unlikely														
Bangladesh	20	0	75	7	48	0	22	8	41	1	331	14	69	3
Pakistan	11	6	71	6	48	6	28	5	18	0	319	45	11	22
Nigeria	20	5	92	6	45	–	34	0	24	5	231	53	52	–
Iran	10	4	75	60	41	12	1	25	12	5	over	366	26	–
Zaire	17	3	50	−11[a]	35	–	over	20[b]	25	5	316	29	–	–
Afghanistan	21	5	135	–	62	5	41	9	37	3	348	0	31	–
Sudan	13	5	80	–	50	8	34	10	38	4	311	−15	–	–
Morocco	8	5	68	16	49	7	23	7	20	5	72	49	14	21
Algeria	8	5	80	34	44	–	10	17	22	4	over	−118	26	–
Tanzania	17	5	102	23	33	9	33	7	38	4	294	35	51	–
Kenya	11	5	61	–	35	7	13	13	34	4	272	26	16	6
Nepal	18	5	135	–	57	4	36	11	47	1	348	7	41	13
Median (app.)	15	5	80	10	45	7	25	9	30	4	300	28	30	10

– = Data not available.
over = At or beyond threshold in 1970.
[a]Probably a measurement artifact, particularly in Peru.
[b]Data for 1960 not available; estimated from 18-point improvement 1965–70.

socioeconomic, cultural, and environmental variables affect fertility" (p. 105). In that study he finds that "variations in four factors—marriage, contraception, lactation, and induced abortion—are the primary proximate causes of fertility differences among populations" (p. 125). What are the implications for the present analysis? More specifically, what would be needed by way of contraceptive practice or, more broadly, the practice of fertility control?[30]

First, here are the approximate levels of the four factors in populations with CBRs of 45, 35, and 25—corresponding to those in our categories of countries:

Crude birth rate	Proportion of reproductive years (15–45) spent in marriage*	Proportion of married women of reproductive age (MWRA) currently using contraception	Duration of lactation (months)	Total induced abortion rate
45	0.80	0.05	26	0
35	0.70	0.30	15	0.5
25	0.65	0.50	8	1.0

Note: The reported use of family planning methods for several countries contained in the Fact Book, Table 23, roughly approximates these model figures, by category of countries.
*An echo of this factor can be seen in Table 14.4 in the column "Females 15–19 Never Married," where the medians for the four country categories are 94, 85, 65, and 50 percent.

Now let us determine the proportions that would be required to use contraception in order to reach CBR 20, assuming reasonable levels for the other three factors. That is, what would the proportions need to be in a society with, say, long duration of lactation, low abortion, and high marriage rates (or any other such combination, in order to establish some limits)? Here are the approximate percentages of married women of reproductive age currently using contraception for a CBR of 20, given the conditions as stipulated:

Duration of lactation		12 Months		3 Months	
Total induced abortion rate		1.5	0.5	1.5	0.5
Proportion of reproductive years (15–45) spent in marriage	0.7	54%	62%	63%	69%
	0.8	62%	69%	69%	74%

There are several important points to be made about this tabulation: (1) under these conditions, contraceptive use must be quite high in order to achieve CBR 20; (2) the range in such usage is 54–74 percent, but six of the eight values fall within 65 percent, plus or minus 4 points; (3) at the designated levels, reasonably empirical in each case and selected to this end, the three factors make about the same difference in their contraceptive requirements (an average of about 7 points)—that is, a difference of 10 percentage points in proportion in marriage equals nine months of lactation equals one abortion per lifetime so far as contraceptive use is concerned; and (4) under average conditions in these regards, the required increase in contraceptive use in countries in the Certain category needs to be only about 15 points (from the 50 percent in the first table to, say, an average of 65 percent in the second), whereas in the Probable and the Possible, with average CBRs of about 35, it needs to more than double (from 30 percent to 65 percent), and for the Unlikely to increase well over tenfold.

Should conditions shift in all three respects in such a manner as to reduce substantially the need for contraceptive use—to lactation of 24 months, three abortions per lifetime, and proportion married of 0.6—the average required contraceptive use drops to an average of about 35 percent, with a range of 18–54 percent. Here is the table, with the indicated comparisons.

Duration of lactation		24 Months		12 Months	
Total induced abortion rate		3	1.5	3	1.5
Proportion of reproductive years spent in marriage	0.6	18%	29%	29%	43%
	0.7	29%	42%	43%	54%

Moreover, in that case each of the three conditions by itself accounts for about the same decrease in contraceptive use, or 12–13 points: 1.5 more abortions equals an additional year of lactation equals a 10 point decline in the proportion married at that level (which in turn, other things being equal, means a rise in average age at marriage of about three years).

Summary and Conclusion

Where does that leave us with regard to the questions posed in the title? Let me summarize to this point.

Here is a reminder of the present state of the country categories with regard to major fertility-related matters:

Country category	Demographic data: Rate of natural increase, 1975	Crude death rate, 1975	Crude birth rate, 1975	Percent CBR decline, 1965–75	Selected socioeconomic factors, circa 1970 (and threshold values for CBR 35): Life expectancy (60 yrs.)	Nonagricultural labor force (55%)	Per capita GNP ($450)	Females 15–19 never married (80%)	Number of thresholds met (of 7)	Family planning program effort
The Certain (3 for 2%)*	1.7	7	23	30	62 yrs.	57%	$625	94%	6	Str
The Probable (10 for 42%)	2.5	9	34	18	60	40	360	85	5	Mod
The Possible (4 for 28%)	2.3	14	36	15	50	35	175	65	1	Mod/Wk
The Unlikely (12 for 13%)	2.8	18	48	2	45	25	150	50	0	Wk

Note: The entries are approximate medians. The first three socioeconomic factors are the most powerful in the Mauldin and Berelson analysis (cited in note 5, Table 9), and together account for almost as much variance as the entire seven. I add the female measure not only as the best available index of women's status but even more as an indicator of the important factor of age at marriage.
*Number of countries and percent of total population in developing countries.

The major disparities are strikingly evident:

–The top row is uniformly favorable–on present indications, countries in this category seem sure to achieve CBR 20 by century's end.
–The crude death rate reduction still lags in the bottom two categories, particularly important if it is generally true that "declines in birth rate come . . . at about the time the death-rate decline has largely spent itself."[31]
–The two middle categories, with most of the population, are at the CBR 35 transition level, with substantial declines in the 1965–75 decade.
–The socioeconomic base presumably "required" or at least favorable for fertility reduction is absent in the bottom two categories.
–Program effort is good at the top, poor at the bottom, and mixed in between.

That is where things now stand.

And here is a similar reminder of what seems to emerge as indicated prescriptions for population policy:

Country category	Family planning	Development	Community organization	Incentive, pressure, sanction
The Certain	Present situation and trends satisfactory; continue them, with perhaps some program strengthening.		Not needed.	Not needed.
The Probable	Strengthened efforts in several countries, as specified in text.	Moderately satisfactory; continuation of present trends will probably suffice.	Not particularly needed beyond present practice, and probably infeasible.	Not needed or wanted, beyond present practice.
The Possible	Maintain, extend, and intensify current efforts; to extent feasible, stress certain and/or continuous methods.	Proponents need to specify the concrete measures feasible under the circumstances, either in design for population policy itself or as redesign of general development policy.		Would have an impact to the extent feasible, but not wanted beyond present practice.

Country category	Family planning	Development	Community organization	Incentive, pressure, sanction
The Unlikely	Program improvement administratively limited in most countries, and program impact likely to be small. Stress on certain and/or continuous methods especially important, but unacceptable in most settings.	Improvements needed here, even more strongly. But probably more difficult on two grounds: initial socioeconomic positions and interest in population policy both significantly lower in most places.		Not only unacceptable, but administratively infeasible as well.

With regard to the family planning intervention, it is necessary from the demographic standpoint to stress the importance of sterilization and/or abortion (or a new method that has not only acceptability and effectiveness but also long continuation, like a vaccine), particularly in the most problematic situations. With regard to incentives and "pressure," as noted above, experience has shown that they are effective though sometimes difficult-to-dangerous in operation, but perhaps required to reach low-fertility targets in the least developed societies within a reasonable time—again offered as empirical finding, not normative prescription (which is of course the proper province of the societies themselves, as is the choice of fertility control methods). That leaves us with the larger matters of basic changes in socioeconomic factors (development) and/or social or community structure, both typically requiring long-term realization whether by incremental or revolutionary approach. That, coupled perhaps with size-of-country considerations for special attention, summarizes the current state-of-play: problems and opportunities.

In this context, the challenge to "the Bucharest prescription" is clear. A central recommendation of the World Population Plan of Action was contained in paragraph 31: "that countries wishing to affect fertility levels give priority to implementing development programmes and educational and health strategies which, while contributing to economic growth and higher standards of living, have a decisive impact upon demographic trends, including fertility." That was then spelled out in paragraph 32 to include, *inter alia*, the reduction of infant and child mortality through improved nutrition, sanitation, and maternal health; the full integration of women through educational and employment opportunities; more equitable distribution of income and land; promotion of education for both sexes; and the establishment of social security benefits. Such goals in themselves are obviously beyond the reach of population-designated funds, estimated to be about 2 percent of all development-designated funds, so they presumably constitute a claim upon the other 98 percent.

What can be done in the name of population policy, with population- or development-designated funds, to improve the position of critical countries on such matters—using policies that are politically realistic, administratively feasible, economically viable? That question needs to be addressed further, unless the approach through "integrated" or "restructured" development is simply a way of dismissing the importance of fertility reduction and lowered population growth as a contribution to human welfare, or of reinforcing a political position attached to "the new international economic order." But if the initial demographic stipulations are granted, then these remain serious questions to which answers, in the fifth post-Bucharest year, are overdue from those subscribing to that position. So far, at least, actual efforts in the field do not appear to have been much affected along this line.

More specifically, for example, what can be done from this standpoint in the critical countries (on size grounds) of India, Indonesia, Bangladesh, Pakistan, and Nigeria, with over 80 percent of the population in the Possible and Unlikely categories (or in those five plus Egypt and Iran, for 87 percent), to advance the present situation with regard to such illustrative targets and shortfalls as these, as of circa 1970 (and note, again, that these are threshold values corresponding to CBR 35 not 20, or the difference between a 5-child and a 2.5-child family; for socioeconomic differences in threshold values, see text above):

Country	Life expectancy (60 yrs.)	Nonagricultural labor force (55%)	Per capita GNP ($450)	Females 15–19 never married (80%)
India	48 yrs.	32%	$140	43%
Indonesia	46	29	146	63
Bangladesh	40	14	119	11
Pakistan	49	37	131	69
Nigeria	40	31	219	28
Egypt	51	38	266	70
Iran	50	43	Met	54

Where and how is the timely leverage to be exerted, with regard to these "requirements," or some comparable set of presumed socioeconomic determinants? Similarly, how is the "community approach" to be applied in these settings? If the position is that "harder" measures are undesirable or unacceptable and that family planning "has failed" or "will fail," then the problem is essentially here, in subject and in site. Remedial prescriptions for "restructuring" development to such ends need to be addressed that have a decent chance of being applied and realized in the field, and without begging the question of reducing fertility thereby. That is, the objective of the whole exercise is to expedite that reduction in order to hasten development; so recommending the latter as a way to achieve the former rather misses the point.

We are now in a better position to discern what is required in the most problematic countries—those in which achievement of this target is only Possible or Unlikely; and, more than that, to approximate the efficiencies and the tradeoffs. For example, in the typical such country, which of the so-called thresholds in socioeconomic factors can most readily be achieved by 1980 (in order to leave 20 years or so for their working-out in fertility reduction from CBR 35 to CBR 20), as against the indicated increases in abortion, lactation, nonmarriage, and contraceptive use? Or, as in the real world, what combinations of these basic and proximate determinants are most efficient in given settings?[32]

To illustrate, let us take the median examples from the two categories at issue, the Possible and the Unlikely. With regard to the so-called basic determinants (Table 14.4), they would have to increase life expectancy by 10–15 years, lower infant mortality rates by half or more, increase adult literacy by 20–45 percentage points, increase school enrollment by 5–30 points, increase the nonagricultural labor force by 20–30 points, increase per capita GNP by 2.5–3 times, or some selected combination thereof, in order to reach the average of CBR 35 taken to represent the start of a 20-to-25-year transition to CBR 20—and, of course, would have to achieve substantially greater social improvements to reach corresponding points for CBR 20, as listed above.

With regard to proximate determinants, while the empirical data are somewhat sparse, we can estimate with some assurance that lactation in such countries is long (say, 24 months), induced abortion is low (e.g., 0.05 reported for India, itself a major recent increase), and the proportion married is high (0.7–0.9). Under those three conditions, contraceptive use would have to be nearly 65 percent in order to achieve CBR 20. The contraceptive requirements for CBR 35 are not quite half that under the same conditions, as indicated in this set of equivalent data for contraceptive use for CBR 35:

Duration of lactation		24 Months			12 Months			3 Months		
Total induced abortion rate		3	1.5	0.5	3	1.5	0.5	3	1.5	0.5
Proportion of	0.6	–	–	–	–	8%	16%	13%	25%	32%
reproductive years	0.7	–	7%	15%	15%	25%	32%	29%	38%	44%
spent in marriage	0.8	16%	24%	31%	31%	39%	44%	43%	50%	55%

– = no contraceptive use needed under such conditions.

In general, the countries in the Possible category seem to be approaching this standard of CBR 35, but the Unlikely group is still some distance away, with little sign of significant downward movement. For them, the requirements for CBR 35, in basic and/or proximate determinants, may be appropriate targets for the remainder of the century, and the relative feasibilities and efficiencies of achieving even that target may be the determining considerations.

That seems a useful way to look at the nature of the problem, especially when applied to the individual case. Which of these basic and proximate determinants are most efficiently achieved in the various categories of countries by the indicated requirements, equivalencies, and tradeoffs, alone or in combinations? What is easier, what harder to realize? Where should investment and effort be best placed? What is to be done, and where?

To conclude: there is no magic to the target of CBR 20 in the developing world for the year 2000. That target is arbitrary, as any other would be—although it may be appropriate as a gauge of what is desirable on the one hand and what may be possible on the other. In any case, the analysis suggests what would be needed for a higher or a lower target, or one to be met earlier or later, or one more differentiated. Nor is there any finality attached to the particular group of "threshold" factors or values used here; yet so interrelated are the so-called basic determinants of a social-structural character that any similarly plausible set would yield essentially the same results.

The shorthand forecast for our four groups of countries is *will*, *can*, *might*, and *won't*;[33] and their CBR targets could be set or projected accordingly. For example, if the Certain and the Probable were to average CBR 20 by the end of the century, the Possible CBR 25, the Unlikely CBR 35 (to the border of transition), and the politically excluded and smaller countries CBR 30, then the CBR for the (now) developing world would then be CBR 25. That is not the stipulated target but it is close, and with favorable trend.[34]

The rate of natural increase for the developing sector in 1975–80 is estimated by the Population Council Fact Book at 2.4 percent. If the crude death rate is in the 8–10 range in 2000 (as in UN estimates), then the natural increase rate in 2000 would be 1.5 percent or slightly above—substantially above 1 percent but still a major achievement by historic standards. If some current observers are correct that death rates will decline more slowly in the next decades,[35] then the growth rate will be correspondingly lower. By present indications, more could not be expected without heroic efforts.

What does all this mean for the policy path ahead? At the risk of repetition, but by way of summary emphasis, what could be done beyond traditional family planning to further reduce fertility? In this context, there appear to be three options, each with its own deficiencies: (1) more sterilization and abortion within the family planning program (or a surrogate in the form of a suitable new method)—but these methods, especially abortion, are not acceptable where most needed, and the new method is not yet available; furthermore, even if all

Appendix Table 14.6. CBRs, 1955–75

Category and country	1955	1960	1965	1970	1975
The Certain					
South Korea	39.7	40.6	35.1	30.1	24.0
Taiwan	44.1	39.4	33.1	26.8	23.0
Chile	36.3	36.6	32.8	28.9	23.2
The Probable					
China	42.0	38.0	35.0	32.0	26.0
Brazil	45.3	43.3	41.4	38.6	36.2
Mexico	46.1	45.1	43.7	42.4	40.0
Philippines	45.1	44.5	44.2	44.0	36.0
Thailand	47.1	46.1	44.3	43.6	34.0
Turkey	44.8	42.9	40.6	39.7	34.0
Colombia	46.1	45.3	44.2	42.1	33.0
Sri Lanka	37.6	35.7	33.1	30.0	27.2
Venezuela	46.4	45.5	42.1	37.8	37.3
Malaysia	45.5	45.0	42.2	33.9	31.4
The Possible					
India	43.2	44.0	42.6	40.6	36.0
Indonesia	46.0	46.9	45.9	43.9	40.0
Egypt	44.5	43.6	42.1	39.4	34.8
Peru	44.4	43.7	42.9	42.0	41.8
The Unlikely					
Bangladesh	49.8	50.5	50.2	49.6	49.2
Pakistan	49.2	48.4	47.6	47.3	47.0
Nigeria	49.3	49.7	49.8	49.4	49.2
Iran	47.5	46.8	45.9	45.3	45.1
Zaire	47.3	47.0	46.8	46.0	44.0
Afghanistan	49.0	48.0	48.7	49.5	49.5
Sudan	50.7	50.4	48.9	48.1	48.9
Morocco	50.4	50.2	49.1	47.2	48.0
Algeria	50.9	50.6	50.0	49.1	48.0
Tanzania	51.5	50.9	50.5	50.4	48.0
Kenya	48.5	48.9	50.0	48.8	50.0
Nepal	46.3	45.8	44.7	43.6	45.0

Source: From the Population Council data bank, cited in note 5. Brazil interpolated from other years.

three were available and approved, the medical infrastructure would have some difficulty in delivering them; (2) some form(s) of pressure or sanction—also generally unacceptable for this purpose and thus a hard decision even for governments faced with and peoples used to hard decisions; for example, the relatively mild yet effective sanction bearing on age at marriage would require not simply the issuance of a decree or the passage of a law, but at the least the strongly convinced support of national and community leadership and probably certain supporting socioeconomic developments as well; and (3) "restructured" development of some kind—that is, the Bucharest prescription, of which few instances exist as yet in realizable form.

Thus, under current considerations and expectations, it would appear that CBR 20 and a growth rate of 1 percent seem out of reach by 2000 for the developing sector. In any case, a much larger population size is ahead for these countries as a whole under the best circumstances—on the order of 60 percent more than in 1975.

Those appear to be the prospects and the programs. Are they reasonable targets and projections? Will population policy contribute significantly to achieving that much? Can it achieve more? How? In this attempt I have tried to say *what* the problem is, *where* it is, and *how* it is being and might be addressed. What *else* is to be done, and where?

Notes

1. This is not the place for the supporting argument. Suffice it here simply to note that countries with nearly 80 percent of the population of the developing world now have an "official policy to reduce the population growth rate." Dorothy L. Nortman and Ellen Hofstatter, *Population and Family Planning Programs*, A Population Council Fact Book, 9th ed. (New York: The Population Council, 1978), Table 5, p. 18. Hereafter referred to as the Fact Book.

2. The comparative figures for 1975–80, from the Fact Book (cited in note 1), Table 1, col. 3, are NI 2.4 percent, CDR 12.8 and CBR 36.4.

3. Fact Book, cited in note 1, Table 1.

4. This exercise could be carried out for all 120 countries, or for the 91 with one million plus, or the 54 with 5 million plus, or even the 18 with 25 million plus (and about 80 percent of the total). But the 10 million cutoff seems reasonable in manageable numbers as well as in magnitude of population. The population figures are taken from the Fact Book (cited in note 1) except for a few cases.

5. They are based on the literature review but mainly the UNRISD "correspondence points analysis" as reported in W. Parker Mauldin and Bernard Berelson, "Conditions of fertility decline in developing countries, 1965–1975," *Studies in Family Planning* 9, no. 5 (May 1978): Table 1 and paragraph 4, pp. 92–93, and Table 11 and text, pp. 108–109. For actual values, see Table 14.4. I have taken the liberty of rounding the values and occasionally extrapolating 1–3 points for 1970–75 advances when countries were that close to a threshold value in the earlier year (to which the data apply, taken from the Population Council data bank). The last factor is used as the best available indicator of female status in a society, from the Mauldin and Berelson analysis.

6. The characterizations themselves are shorthand designations for convenience of presentation. A more circumspect description might be Certain to Probable, Probable to Possible, Possible to Unlikely, and Unlikely to Impossible.

7. For an elaboration, see Mauldin and Berelson (cited in note 5), footnote 15, p. 130.

8. If the six developing countries that qualify on size but were excluded on accessibility were to be included in this analysis, they would be classified as follows, in conformity with the above rationale:

Certain	Probable	Possible	Unlikely
None	Vietnam	Burma	Ethiopia
	North Korea		Uganda
			Iraq

Their addition would make only a 1 or 2 percentage point increase in the population segments per category.

9. These data, and those in all tables and figures, are taken from the Population Council data bank, courtesy of Parker Mauldin and Richard Monteverde, to whom sincere thanks. The time series on CBRs, as depicted in Figures 14.1–14.4, is contained in the Appendix Table.

10. Actually, considerations omitted on both sides of these rough calculations perhaps balance out. On the one hand, as noted in the text, the period has an extra five years to run, so these CBRs might be a point or two lower. On the other hand, the more difficult countries will be increasing faster over this period, and a few of the least difficult will "graduate" from developing status, so the former will count for relatively more in the total than they now do. But that, too, is unlikely to make much difference in these estimates.

11. "Selected world demographic indicators by countries, 1950–2000," UN Population Division, May 1975.

12. Information and instruction courtesy of my colleagues Tomas Frejka and Parker Mauldin. The UN projections estimate that the proportion of women aged 15–49 in the developing world will be about 10 percent greater in 2000 than in 1975 (i.e., 51–53 percent of all females in the medium and low variants, as against 47 percent now).

13. But note that Japan's record runs from peak to trough, not for an arbitrarily designated decade, and that it is somewhat exaggerated, at least by a few points, in that the CBR was elevated above the secular trend at the outset, as a postwar phenomenon. Incidentally, the sharp decline was in large degree occasioned by a family planning measure—namely, the increased availability of induced abortion.

14. Large declines by individual countries are illustrative (points off the CBR):

1955–75		1965–75	
Taiwan	21	South Korea,	
South Korea	16	Colombia,	
Malaysia	15	Malaysia	11
Thailand,		Taiwan,	
Colombia,		Chile,	
Chile	13	Thailand	10
Turkey	11		
Sri Lanka	10		

Actually, even larger declines were posted for smaller countries: Singapore, 25 points off, 1955–75; Cuba and Costa Rica, 13 and 12 points off, 1965–75.

15. Dudley Kirk, "A new demographic transition?," in *Rapid Population Growth: Consequences and Policy Implications*, prepared by the National Academy of Sciences (Baltimore: The Johns Hopkins Press, 1971), p. 132. Kirk's data presumably derive from his Table 1, mine from the Population Council data bank series used above (see note 5). Kirk linearly extrapolated the average annual percent reduction for the period subsequent to reaching CBR 35; I did so for longer time periods where appropriate and based on the latest available decade—that is, 1965–75. He used three-year averages; I did not. He included only countries over one million with a continuous decline initiated before 1960 and at least five years of CBR 35 or less; I obviously did not (but even the six countries starting in 1974–75 have essentially the same averages and range). Thus, the conformity of data and method is not precise, but for present policy purposes close enough.

Naturally, there is nothing immutable about the CBR 35 to 20 transition. There can be reversals in the trend downward, though there have been few exceptions in the past: once a country gets to CBR 35 it is usually on the way. On the other side of the coin, this analysis does not assume a further acceleration of the rate, although Kirk found a consistent increase in average decline every 25-year period since 1875, from 48 years (mean) to 38 to 31 to 15 (as here revised, just over 20); nor does it take into account the recent emergence of active governmental efforts to reduce fertility rates.

16. Note this interesting comparison with the latest UN projections (cited in note 11):

Countries with 1 million or more population in 2000 that reach CBR 35 between 1950 and 1980 and . . .

. . . Reach CBR 20 by 2000

	By medium variant	
Country	Period	No. of years
Hong Kong	1959–71	12
Mauritius	1961–75	14
Singapore	1966–83	17
Trinidad and Tobago	1963–87	24
Puerto Rico	1955–82	27
Guyana	1970–98	28
Sri Lanka	1962–92	30
South Korea	1966–97	31
China	1955–87	32
Chile	1963–97	34
Mean		25
Median		27.5
	By low variant	
Hong Kong	1960–70	10
Mauritius	1965–76	11
Singapore	1960–73	13
Malaysia	1980–97	17
Haiti	1980–97	17
Trinidad and Tobago	1964–85	21
Puerto Rico	1955–78	23
South Korea	1965–90	25
China	1955–82	27
Guyana	1968–95	27
Jamaica	1970–98	28
Chile	1963–93	30
Albania	1966–96	30
Sri Lanka	1960–90	30
Mean		22
Median		24

. . . Do not reach CBR 20 by 2000

	By medium variant	
Country	Year reach CBR 35	CBR in 1995–2000
Costa Rica	1962	26.4
Albania	1967	21.5

Jamaica	1970	22.7
Polynesia	1970	23.3
North Korea	1973	24.4
Egypt	1978	28.3
Panama	1978	29.2
Venezuela	1980	26.4
Unweighted mean		25.3
	By low variant	
Polynesia	1969	21.8
Costa Rica	1970	26.1
North Korea	1972	22.1
Panama	1974	22.4
Venezuela	1974	22.6
Egypt	1974	24.8
Brazil	1975	22.7
Mongolia	1975	23.7
Colombia	1980	21.6
India	1980	24.1
Peru	1980	25.2
Unweighted mean		23.4

The means for those countries completing the transition to CBR 20 by 2000 are roughly similar to those reported above, and precisely so for the low variant, as are the ranges. If an additional 10 years is allowed on average for those not yet reaching CBR 20 under the medium variant and an additional five years for the low variant, the total means for both sets of countries become 31 and 26 years, respectively.

17. For recent cautions on China, see John S. Aird, "Fertility decline and birth control in the People's Republic of China," and Leo F. Goodstadt, "Official targets, data, and policies for China's population growth: An assessment," *Population and Development Review* 4, no. 2 (June 1978): 225–254 and 254–275, respectively. Mexico now genuinely wishes to make an impact, as evidenced by its intensified family planning program of the past five years or so; and Brazil is beginning to move in that direction, though much more slowly. See Morvan de Mello Moreira, Léa Melo da Silva, and Robert McLaughlin, "Brazil," *Country Profiles* (New York: The Population Council, 1978), pp. 16ff.

18. This appears to be the currently fashionable prescription for policy—although specific and concrete programmatic proposals are fewer in evidence than general exhortations as to the goodness of the ends or their potential effectiveness in impact. In practice such programs would have their own problems of realization, as is only too evident from development experience; the cost-effectiveness of such efforts for fertility purposes would appear to be unfavorable; the practicability of "restructuring" such large efforts on fertility or demographic grounds is yet to be demonstrated, even via priority to certain sectors believed to be particularly fertility-relevant; and perhaps most elementary of all, the policy represents a bizarre inversion of ends and means, of what the problem is supposed to be: *from* reduce-growth (fertility)-in-order-to-promote-development *to* promote-development-in-order-to-reduce-growth (fertility). For a revealing review of what has happened in this connection, see Margaret Wolfson, "Population programmes, post-Bucharest," Joint Development Centre/IBRD Study, OECD, April 1978.

19. For example: Geoffrey McNicoll, "Community-level population policy: An exploration," *Population and Development Review* 1, no. 1 (September 1975): 1–21; Geoffrey McNicoll, "Population and development: Outlines for a structuralist approach," *Journal of Development Studies* 14, no. 4 (July 1978); and Paul Demeny, "Observations on population policy and population program in Bangladesh," *Population and Development Review* 1, no. 2 (December 1975): 307–321.

20. For example, Bernard Berelson, "Paths to fertility reduction: 'The policy cube'," *Family Planning Perspectives* 9, no. 5 (September/October 1977):214–219. The specific case of increased age of marriage, often proposed as an instrument of fertility reduction, is included there as a legal sanction, although the extent to which it is insufficient in itself and requires major social change of the kind envisaged in the second intervention above is documented in C. Stephen Baldwin, "Policies and realities of delayed marriage," *PRB Report* 3, no. 4 (September 1977), summarizing a monograph by M. Badrud Duza and Baldwin entitled *Nuptiality and Population Policy* (New York: The Population Council, 1977).

21. See Mauldin and Berelson (cited in note 5), p. 111, paragraph 4, and the Sykes analysis therein.

22. See Mauldin and Berelson (cited in note 5), Table 12, p. 110.

23. The only similar countries in the Possible and Unlikely categories are Peru and Zaire in school enrollment.

24. With the result that the program, without stress on sterilization, fell into insignificance. In May 1978 the Prime Minister announced that "the Centre has decided to establish a linkage between the performance in respect of family planning work in the States and the release of Central plan assistance to them—that 8 percent of the Central plan assistance to each state will be released on the basis of the evaluation of their performance" (*Indian Express*, 13 May 1978), but more recent reports continue to tell of a demoralized and weakened effort. Meanwhile, in order to meet the upward-revised target of CBR 30 by 1983, the need has been calculated for 6–8 million

acceptors per year – a goal reached, indeed exceeded, only in the "pressured" FY 1975 and 1976, and far, far from realization under current circumstances – in Dorothy Nortman, "India's new birth rate target: An analysis," *Population and Development Review* 4, no. 2 (June 1978): 277–312.

25. As argued in Bernard Berelson, "Demographic requirements of fertility control technology: 15 propositions," PIACT Papers, Program for the Introduction and Adaptation of Contraceptive Technology, 1978, particularly paragraph 13c. There can be little question about the importance of sterilization and/or abortion in difficult settings – in the absence of a critically improved technology, most likely an acceptable vaccine. At present only India has made sterilization its major programmatic method, but in a few other countries it now accounts for 20–30 percent of the acceptances (South Korea, Sri Lanka, Thailand). Leaving aside China, abortions are programmatically significant only in Singapore and Tunisia. Data from Fact Book, cited in note 1, Table 16.

26. Mauldin and Berelson, cited in note 5, Table 12 and related text.

27. For one such plan, see Aziz Bindary, "Egypt studies a new plan of action," *Studies in Family Planning* 3, no. 8 (August 1972): 193–194. After an extended period of discussion, some such effort has been informally reported to be in experimental operation, but to my knowledge the details and the outcomes have not yet appeared in the literature.

28. The difficulties are ably illustrated in W. Brian Arthur and Geoffrey McNicoll, "An analytical survey of population and development in Bangladesh," *Population and Development Review* 4, no. 1 (March 1978): 23–80. They conclude that "the country's present problems are less the result of not having some 'right' combination of national policies than they are the consequence of a local societal structure that the government cannot quite reach. . . . The type of 'intermediate level' strategy – directed at a level between the national government and the individual – that we see as essential to tackle the problems of Bangladesh is more a matter of structural change than of programmatic policy. . . . It would be no short-term task" (pp. 65, 67). The models they consider include Java and China – neither without questions, as they acknowledge.

29. John Bongaarts, "A framework for analyzing the proximate determinants of fertility," *Population and Development Review* 4, no. 1 (March 1978): 105–132. The data presented here were especially developed by him for this purpose, based on the procedures described in his article, and I am much indebted for his gracious cooperation. The key definitions are: *Contraception* – any deliberate parity-dependent practice, including abstention and sterilization, undertaken to reduce the risk of conception. Contraceptors are all assumed to be fecund, and contraceptive use-effectiveness was assumed to be 0.85. *Lactation* – following a pregnancy a woman remains infecundable (i.e., unable to conceive) until the normal pattern of ovulation and menstruation is restored. The duration of the period of infecundity is a function of the duration and intensity of lactation (and approaches nearly one-half the period of lactation at the high end). *Total induced abortion rate* – the average number of induced abortions per woman at the end of the reproductive period.

30. With Dr. Bongaarts' kind collaboration, the broad requirements for reaching CBR 20 under various combinations of these four proximate determinants are presented.

31. Frank Wm. Oechsli and Dudley Kirk, "Modernization and demographic transition in Latin America and the Caribbean," *Economic Development and Cultural Change* 23 (April 1975): 408. Note that this conclusion is based on a limited geographical area.

32. Note that improvements in development tend to go along with at least two proximate determinants – contraception and lowered marital rate – but to run counter to the needed increase in lactation (which is typically lower in more developed societies). According to the UN *Demographic Yearbook*, the median marital rate for the available countries of the Certain and Probable categories (a total of ten) is already about 68 percent, as compared with the United States at 66 percent and the record low of 53 percent in Ireland; whereas the median for the ten countries available in the Possible and Unlikely categories is about 80 percent, with a range from 73 percent (Indonesia) to 91 percent (Bangladesh).

33. Such designations often shift with the mood of the times. In 1978, for example, the mood is up on Indonesia and down on India, whereas only a few years ago it was the other way around. But whatever the shifting mood (assuming that the current reportage on China turns out to be correct), these two are key swing states for the record of the developing world as a whole by 2000. For an account of a "success story probably unrivaled in family planning history" on Java and Bali, where typical threshold values of a socioeconomic character are still low, see Terence H. Hull et al., "Indonesia's family planning story: Success and challenge," *Population Bulletin* 32, no. 6 (November 1977).

34. Actually, the projected CBR would be slightly higher then because the high-fertility countries would contribute slightly more population in the weighting process than they do now. The latest UN projections distribute the 2000 population of these countries (medium

variant) to our four categories as 2 percent, 38 percent, 28 percent, and 16 percent of the total developing world, respectively, as against 2 percent, 42 percent, 28 percent, and 13 percent in 1975.

35. For example, R. H. Cassen, "Current trends in population change and their causes," *Population and Development Review* 4, no. 2 (June 1978): 331–353; and Davidson R. Gwatkin, "The end of an era: A review of the literature and data concerning third world mortality trends" (Unpublished manuscript, Overseas Development Council, July 1978). At the same time, the changes in age structure that follow upon a fertility decline, as noted above, tend to lower the CDR while they tend to increase the CBR.

15
Conditions of Fertility Decline in Developing Countries, 1965–75

Written with W. Parker Mauldin

This paper is a macro-analysis of the correlates of fertility decline in developing countries for the period 1965–75, during which there was substantial fertility decline in Asia, quite a bit in the Americas, some in North Africa, and almost none in black Africa. The analysis focuses on how much of the fertility decline is associated with such socioeconomic variables as health, education, economic status, and urbanization, or with "modernization" as a whole, and how much with population policies and programs, primarily family planning programs, designed to reduce rates of growth.

The data are examined in a variety of ways: simple correlations among the variables; multiple regression analyses using both 1970 values of socioeconomic variables and, for the alternative lag theory, 1960 values; change in the socioeconomic variables over time; a special form of regression analysis called path analysis in which program effort is considered to be partly a function of socioeconomic level; a relatively new type of analysis called exploratory data analysis; relation of socioeconomic level and program efforts to both absolute and percentage declines in fertility; and cross-tabulations of program effort with an index of socioeconomic variables.

Such data and analyses show that the level of "modernization" as reflected by seven socioeconomic factors has a substantial relationship to fertility decline but also that family planning programs have a significant, independent effect over and above the effect of socioeconomic factors. The key finding probably is that the two–social setting and program effort–go together most effectively. Countries that rank well on socioeconomic variables *and also* make substantial program effort have on average much more fertility decline than do countries that have one or the other, and far more than those with neither. Finally, the relationship between predicted and observed CBR decline for the 94 developing countries over this period is illustrated for different combinations of factors; and an attempt is made to estimate the quantitative impact of the major conditions upon the intermediate variables traditionally assumed to account for CBR changes.

This paper analyzes conditions associated with fertility decline in developing countries in the recent past, thus addressing a major issue of contemporary population policy that remains controversial within the scientific community.

Did fertility decline in developing countries from 1965 to 1975? Clearly yes in a number of Asian and Latin American countries; clearly no in most of Africa; still uncertain for several countries. In the nature of the case, the facts are by no means fully determined, but there are various indications of fertility decline, as detailed below; for our purposes we assume that they are by and large valid. If fertility has declined, why? That is a consequential issue for population policy, since it is caught up in the current international dispute over the relative contributions of "development" and "family planning" in affecting fertility rates, and, importantly, the views of planners influence the allocation of priorities and resources to reduce rates of population growth in order to achieve development.

In this paper, we analyze a range of possible influences on fertility, by country, in order to discern their relative impact. If the several factors are studied simultaneously, what do they show about the conditions of fertility decline? As with any

Reprinted with permission in an abridged form from *Studies in Family Planning* 1978; 9(5)84–148, The Population Council, New York, NY. Deletions due to space limitations include a section entitled "Exploratory Data Analysis," written by Zenas Sykes.

analysis of such social complexity, there are pitfalls everywhere: in quality of data, in adequacy of statistical technique, in validity of interpretation. We shall try to identify such problems as we nevertheless proceed—"nevertheless," because of the importance of the matter for both scientific and policy purposes. In short, what conditions were associated with different magnitudes of fertility decline in developing countries over the decade 1965 to 1975?

Viewed from a broad perspective, fertility can be considered a function of both demand and supply factors: demand factors that affect the level of interest in or motivation for fertility control and supply factors that affect the availability of information and services for fertility control. Both are continua: that is, the demand for fertility control can range from absolute to nil and the supply of fertility control means can range from very high to zero—and in the real world, both do so range. By and large, the two sets of factors go together in the current era: for example, high demand and high supply in the well-off, industrialized countries; low demand and low supply in poor, agricultural countries. However, given the complexity of this fundamental aspect of human behavior and the recent introduction of policies to influence population growth in the developing countries, there are many countries in which demand and supply levels do not correspond.

Within the demographic community, it is accepted that very high demand for fertility control can result in very low fertility even in the absence of much modern supply; at any rate, there are several historical cases to that effect.[1] But it is probably also acknowledged that strong supply of modern means of fertility control (especially if sterilization and abortion are included) can affect the magnitude and the pace of fertility control under certain conditions of demand; and similarly, there are contemporary cases to that effect.[2] Demand and supply factors are interwoven in a complex matrix of influences upon fertility behavior such that it is extremely difficult, and at this stage perhaps technically impossible, to disentangle their effects upon fertility rates with a substantial degree of precision and validity. But there have been attempts to do so, and this paper can be considered another attempt in that direction: a systematic effort to measure the relative impact of both demand and supply factors on fertility change in the indicated period across virtually the entire range of developing countries.

Before proceeding, we wish to clear away some semantic underbrush, or try to. We use the terms "demand" and "supply" as convenient shorthand terms that have appropriate echoes on both policy and scientific grounds. As for policy, "demand" represents the effect of development and its component elements upon fertility; "supply" represents the effect of family planning programs. Thus the terms tap into a major current debate within the field, particularly post-Bucharest (where a major slogan was, "Development is the best contraceptive"). As for science, "demand" represents the basic determinants of fertility—the fundamental socioeconomic, cultural, social-structural factors that give rise to interest or motivation to limit family size; "supply" represents one of the proximate determinants or intermediate factors—a necessary mechanism or instrument through which demand gets expressed in actual behavior. (In our case, the term includes not only supply of services and means for fertility control but also supply of associated information covering its legitimacy, benefits, and use.) In this context, supply differences may or may not make an impact upon fertility decline beyond levels or changes in demand; that is an empirical question we address here. Any such impact is independent of the socioeconomic setting in that sense, though not in the sense that supply itself always operates within a social setting that conditions its prospects and its own viability.

In short, as has recently been said:

> Studies of the causes of fertility levels and their changes often seek directly to measure the impact of socioeconomic factors on fertility. Such a procedure may be useful for some purposes, but substantial insights can be gained if in addition the specific mechanisms through which the socioeconomic factors operate are identified.[3]

That is the effort undertaken here, centered specifically upon certain socioeconomic factors on the one hand (demand) and family planning program effort on the other (supply).

The paper is organized into the following sections: (1) review of recent scientific literature on the question; (2) presentation of the measures and data used in the study; (3) statistical analyses of relationships between CBR declines and the indicated demand and supply variables, singly and in various combinations, on a base of 94 developing countries with a 1975 population of 2.8 billion, or 98 percent of the total population in developing countries; (4) reanalysis by cross-tabulation of demand and supply factors as related to CBR decline for the individual countries; and (5) conclusions.

The Literature

Heightened interest in population problems has stimulated a marked increase in fertility studies in recent years. We review here only those macrostudies that, like ours, focus on the correlates or determinants of fertility, that include multiple correlating or determining factors, that deal with countries as units, and that make intercountry analyses. Even so, the literature is substantial: we include 24 English-language publications of some quality in the past 15 years. In addition, the historical literature contains a number of similar studies, and this genre can be considered to be among the traditional modes of demographic research.

The 24 studies are of varying character. But the salient points appear to be these:

Countries

Of the 24 studies, 18 include both developed and developing countries; only 6 are limited to developing countries. The mean and median number of countries included per study are both about 50.

Fertility Measures

Fifteen studies use the crude birth rate (CBR); 7, the fertility rate in some form; 4, the gross reproduction rate; 4, acceptor data; 2, the child-woman ratio; 1, change in birth rates; and 1, births prevented. Some studies, of course, use more than one such measure.

Demand Factors

These cover a wide range of variables—a total of 44 identifiable factors (and another 30–35 if every variation is counted separately by, for example, counting 3 different measures of educational attainment as 3 instead of 1). Here is the list of the identifiable factors by frequency of use in the 24 studies:

19 income per capita
14 literacy
13 infant mortality rate; agricultural and nonagricultural labor force
12 newspaper circulation
10 education; urbanization
8 population density
7 life expectancy
6 energy consumption
4 religion; radios; hospital beds
3 female labor force; income distribution; index of overall development; marriage rates by age; telephones
2 caloric/protein consumption; political system; social security; linguistic homogeneity; crude death rate; racial composition; medical personnel
1 dependency ratio; inside water supply; mail; male/female ratio; cinema attendance; child labor; family structure; modernized attitudes; strength of labor movement; administrative efficiency; social mobility; strength of traditional elite; nationalism; government's commitment to economic development; economic structure; social tension; achievement motivation; class structure; income from agriculture

As acknowledged in several of the studies, this list should be considered a compromise between what the researchers may have wanted and what they found available in acceptable data for a suitable number of countries. In any case, it reflects the current perceptions of what is important by way of demand factors.

Supply Factors

Only four[4] of the studies include supply considerations in their analyses (all four, incidentally, done with the participation of donor agencies directly concerned with policy issues). The others, of a more traditional academic character, presumably did not consider the conditions of supply sufficiently important to include as a possible determinant of fertility, even though the supply differentials are large across the developed and developing countries—surely as large as the socio-economic factors traditionally included. This point appears to have been neglected if not forgotten, although the field was reminded to the contrary by one eminent demographer some years ago:

> An illustration is the rather common view that the rate of population growth declines as the standard of living rises. From this the deduction is sometimes made that birth control plays no role. Actually, the generalization is not true in all cases, but the main point is that the only way that a rise in the standard of living can reduce the growth rate is by increasing the death rate, lessening the net immigration, or reducing the birth rate. Since it usually does not cause the first two eventualities but rather the opposite, its normal channel for reducing population growth is through lowering fertility. But a rising level of living lowers the birth rate by the instrumentality of birth control. Therefore, to speak of a rise in the standard of living as accomplishing its effect on population growth *without the use of birth control* is to speak in erroneous terms" (emphasis in original).[5]

Only recently another demographer wrote that the three "preconditions for sustained decline in marital fertility" are perceived legitimacy of fertility control, perceived advantage, and the availability of "effective techniques of fertility reduction."[6]

Modes of Analysis

They are mainly of two kinds: multiple and partial regression analysis (with various technical refinements) in 17 studies and correlational analysis (usually simple correlations) in 11 studies. Beyond them, cross-tabulations were used in 5 studies, factor analysis and path analysis in 2 studies, and correspondence analysis, cluster analysis and histogram analysis in 1 each.

Findings

These vary widely, and even more so when all the usual scholarly qualifications as to data, measures, samples, and so on, are taken into account. This is not the place for a detailed summary[7] but a few points deserve mention:

1. On the whole the studies find the expected associations between fertility and education, literacy, urbanization, infant mortality rate, female and agricultural labor force, and the generalized factor of "modernization" or "development," but some disputes remain with regard to such economic measures as per capita income,[8] income distribution, and social security.
2. Various studies claim that the demand variables explain 45–90 percent of the variance in fertility across developed and developing countries at a given point in time, but:
3. Much less explanatory value is found *within* developing countries as a category. In other words, the wider the range of socioeconomic conditions, the greater the explanatory power of such demographic variables. Explanatory correlations are harder to come by within more homogeneous categories.
4. Only three studies (United Nations, Kirk, and Srikantan)[9] venture to suggest quantitative "threshold" values that trigger fertility declines. The thresholds are not defined identically; the sampled countries and time periods are different; and the threshold factors are not the same ones or measured in the same way. Still there are some rough similarities, as shown in Table 15.1, which lists those factors approximately similar in more than one study. In that array of ten factors, there is reasonable agreement on all but three (income per capita, energy consumption per capita, and radio distribution). For the other seven, the approximate thresholds for fertility decline, rounded off and averaged, appear to be:

Variable	Threshold range
Population in cities of 20,000+	16–50 percent
Nonagricultural labor force	50–65 percent
Life expectancy	60–70 years
Female marriage before age 20	10–20 percent
Female literacy	60–75 percent
Hospital beds per 1,000 population	5
Newspaper circulation per 1,000 population	70–100

At the same time, it is necessary to stress that different definitions and measures are used in these few studies and that the studies them-

TABLE 15.1. Threshold values for fertility decline that are roughly similar in three studies

Factor	Threshold value		
	United Nations	Kirk	Srikantan
Income per capita	US $230–339		US $704–1,056
Energy consumption per capita	360–1,012 kg.		687–2,998 kg.
Population in cities of 20,000+	16–33 percent	16–47 percent	18–63 percent
Nonagricultural labor force	45–61 percent	58–63 percent	47–74 percent
Life expectancy	62–63 years	59–67 years	64–69 years
Female marriage before age 20	11–15 percent		11–22 percent
Female literacy	62–75 percent	74–85 percent	55–70 percent
Hospital beds per 1,000 population	5–6	4–5	3–5
Newspaper circulation per 1,000 population	80–89	63–109	68–122
Radio receivers per 1,000 population	87–88		41–279

Note: The included countries, the definitions of "threshold," and the specification of measures can be found in the cited studies. The following factors are also included in only one of the studies: infant mortality, movie attendance, number of telephones, school enrollment, and number of medical personnel (physicians, nurses, midwives). The threshold values are the minimum values for countries of low fertility and maximum values for those of high fertility. The United Nations figures exclude the top 10 percent of the high-fertility countries and the bottom 10 percent of the low-fertility countries for each indicator.
Sources: United Nations, Department of Economic and Social Affairs, *Population Bulletin, no. 7-1963, with special reference to conditions and trends of fertility in the world* (United Nations, 1965); Dudley Kirk, "A new demographic transition?" in *Rapid Population Growth: Consequences and Policy Implications* (published for the National Academy of Sciences by the Johns Hopkins University Press, 1971) pp. 138–145; K. S. Srikantan, *The Family Planning Program in the Socioeconomic Context* (New York: The Population Council, 1977).

selves warn about the tentative nature of their conclusions: Kirk, for example, wrote that "Efforts to identify 'thresholds' for the initiation of fertility reduction are at a preliminary stage and their predictive capacity . . . remains to be tested,"[10] and the United Nations study approached the concept of "the threshold hypothesis" carefully indeed ". . . assuming it to have some validity, although admittedly the degree of its validity is questionable. . . ."[11]

5. Another three studies—Gregory et al., World Bank, and Beaver[12]—contain explicit quantitative values of the fertility decline that would be produced by a specified change in the independent variables (Table 15.2), but unfortunately there is no certain common estimate for comparison. For example, if the fertility index of the World Bank study (roughly equivalent to the general fertility rate) is transformed into an approximate CBR by dividing by 5, then the comparative figure for an increase of 40 years in life expectancy becomes 14.9 points off the CBR, as against 21.9 in Beaver—hardly a close similarity.
6. The only four studies that take supply factors into account find that they have some independent explanatory power.
7. While several studies suggest policy implications, of the increase-education or lower-mortality type (i.e., based on the logic of finding a determinant and then realizing it), hardly any address the resource allocation or practicability issues involved in realistic policy decisions made to reduce fertility.

This then is a background in the scientific literature. Compared with that array our study includes: (1) a relatively *large number* of countries, (2) only *developing* countries, (3) fertility *change over time*, (4) a small number of the presumably *more important demand factors* (selected after analysis of a much larger set), also summarized into an index of developmental status, (5) *supply measures* as well as demand, and (6) the *most-utilized modes of analysis* plus a few innovations thereon.

The Measures and the Data

This study includes 94 developing countries: all those with populations of one million or more as of 1975, minus South Africa and Rhodesia as special cases and plus Barbados, Fiji, and Mauritius. (The latter three are included because The Population

TABLE 15.2. Fertility declines producible by specified changes in variables, as found in three studies

Study	This change in determinants . . .	. . . makes for this change in fertility
Gregory et al.	In developing countries, "a one percent reduction in the illiteracy rate	tends to reduce the birth rate by .19 percent" (pp. 237–238).
	In developed countries, a one percent reduction in the illiteracy rate	"generates a .22 percent reduction in the birth rate" (p. 238).
	In developed countries, "a one percent increase in the female participation rate" in the labor force	"generates a .14 percent reduction in the birth rate" (p. 238).
	In both sets of countries "a reduction in the rate of infant mortality weighted by the rural ratio of one percent	will cause a .19 percent reduction in the birth rate" (p. 238).
World Bank Appendix A	"Each additional percentage point of total income received by the poorest 40 percent	reduces the fertility index by 2.9 points" (pp. 147–148).
	"Each additional year of life expectancy at birth	reduces the fertility index by 1.86 points" (p. 148).
Beaver	A decline in the crude death rate of about 5 points over ten years	"would suggest a corresponding temporary increase of 2.7 in the CBR" (p. 128).
	"An improvement of forty years in e_0^o" [expectation of life at birth]	". . . would imply a decline of 21.9 [points] in the CBR" (p. 129).
	"A 20 percentage point increase in urban population	would lower the CBR 1.24 points" (p. 133).

Sources: Paul Gregory, John Campbell, and Benjamin Cheng, "Differences in fertility determinants: Developed and developing countries," *Journal of Development Studies* 9 (1972): 233–241; World Bank, *Population Policies and Economic Development*, a World Bank Staff Report, coordinating author, Timothy King (Johns Hopkins University Press, 1974); Steven E. Beaver, *Demographic Transition Theory Reinterpreted: An Application to Recent Natality Trends in Latin America* (Lexington Books, 1975).

Council's data bank included them at the time of this analysis. They are so small as to be insignificant in any data weighted by population size; they have similar classifications by social setting and program effort and do not affect the average for such countries. In short, this inclusion does not affect the conclusions of this study to any appreciable extent.) While much has been and can be learned about fertility determinants in other ways—for example, from intracountry studies utilizing survey data or registration data for regions or districts, or from in-depth microstudies of individual families—we deal with countries as units since they are the effective policy entities for the interplay of fertility determinants and attempted interventions.

In order to proceed with our analysis, we need three sets of data: (1) measures of fertility change, (2) measures of demand, and (3) measures of supply. As everyone knows who has ever tried, it is not possible at the present time to construct a completely satisfactory set of data for such measures: numbers are often incomplete, inappropriate, suspect, or missing altogether. We have made a diligent effort to construct a good set of data but in the end all we can claim is that they are, so far as we know, only the best available data (and despite the unfortunate acronym produced by that phrase!). Despite their deficiencies, in our judgment they are generally correct in order of magnitude; they do differentiate in a broad qualitative way, if not always in precise exactitude; and they are serviceable for our purpose. With that caveat, we now describe the nature and source of our data.

Measures of Fertility Change

The measures are crude birth rates (CBRs) for 1965 and 1975 taken mainly from United Nations sources and from vital statistics for individual countries,[13] and total fertility rates (TFRs).[14] For the period 1965–75 the total fertility rate declined slightly more than did the crude birth rate, an average of 1 or 2 percentage points per country. This indicates that, over the 10-year span, changes in the age composition affected fertility rates only slightly, and in such a way that changes in crude birth rates understate fertility decline slightly in comparison with the more technical and professionally preferred measure. Moreover, the two rates are so closely correlated ($R = 0.97$) as to

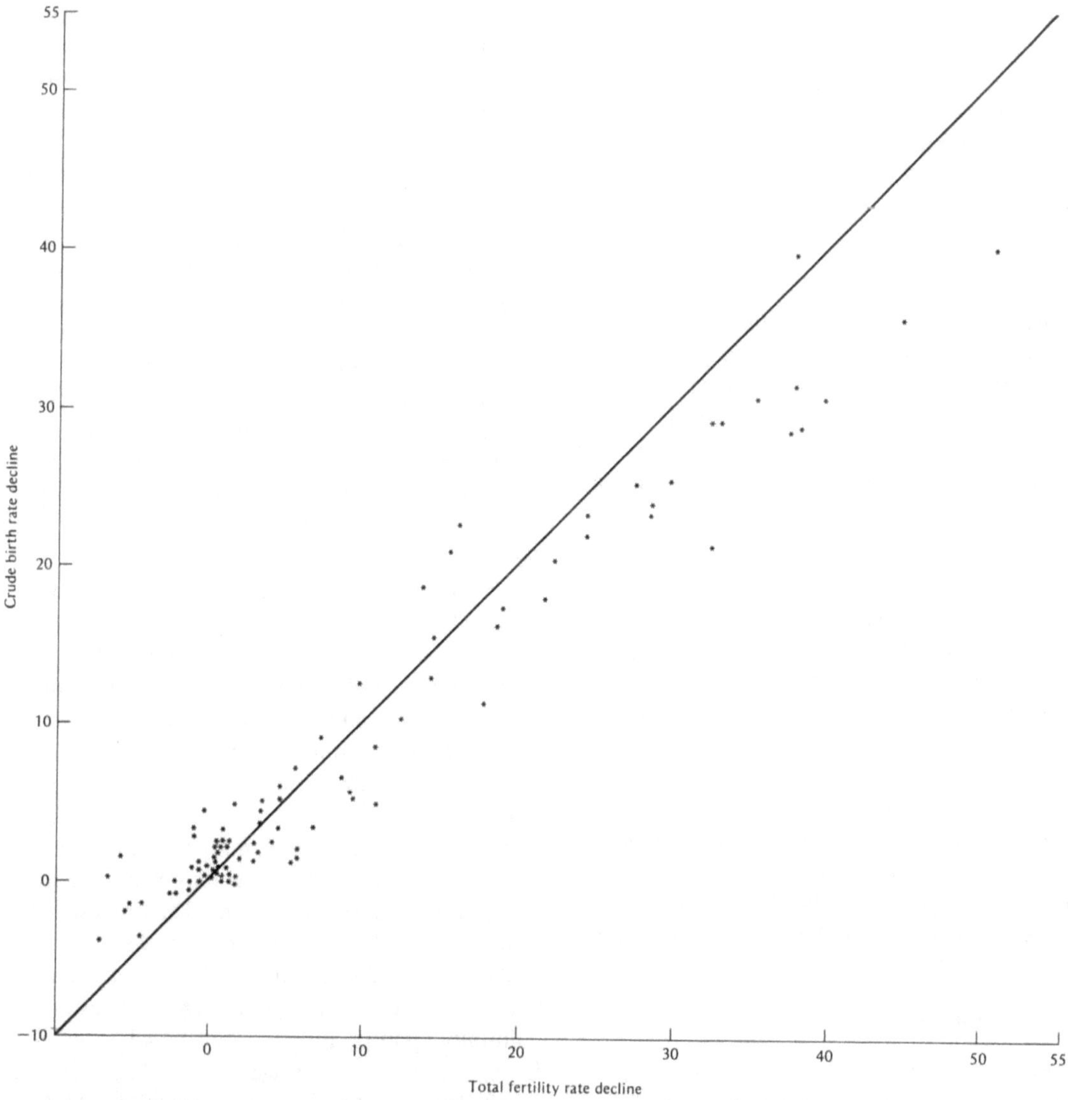

FIGURE 15.1. Percent 1965–75 crude birth rate declines, by decline in total fertility rate: 94 developing countries.

be virtually identical for practical purposes, and certainly for ours (Figure 15.1). (To be sure, there are exceptions to this generalization, principally countries with rapidly declining fertility in which the changing age structure tended to increase the number of births, and hence, total fertility rates declined somewhat more than crude birth rates.)

We use the crude birth rate in the tables that follow both because of its greater familiarity to the general reader and because of its availability. Because the crude birth rate, while reasonably available, is flawed by the normal technical difficulties of data collection in developing countries, reported CBR declines of less than 5 percent should be taken to indicate essentially no change, and declines of 5 to 10 percent merely suggest change.

The CBRs for 1965 and 1975 and the percentage decline from the earlier to the later year comprise our measure of fertility change for the 94 developing countries in this study. Overall, the CBR decline from 1965–75 in this sector of nearly 3 billion population was about 13 percent or 5.5 points—from a CBR of 41 to 35.5. However, that decline was unevenly distributed among countries of different size. The largest countries, with 35 million population or more – over 75 percent of the developing world – had the greatest declines in that decade, and crude birth rates appeared to be falling appreciably in most of them.[15] Among the smaller countries, the CBR declines were smaller and occurred in relatively fewer countries.

Components of Fertility Change

Changes in crude birth rates can be decomposed into three components: change brought about by the age structure, by marriage patterns (mainly age at marriage), and by marital fertility (using a broad definition of marriage and marital fertility in order to allow for consensual unions in Latin America).

Age Structure

High fertility countries tend to have relatively stable age structures; but when fertility begins to decline, the proportions in the youngest age groups decline. This leads to a slightly higher proportion in the reproductive ages, which tends to increase the crude birth rate. The examples given in Table 15.3 indicate that, for most of the countries listed, changes in age structure tended to increase the crude birth rate or to decrease the amount of decline in the crude birth rate (contributing perhaps – 5–10 percent of the change). That this is also true for countries without currently available data is uncertain.

Marriage Patterns

Changing marriage patterns have been an important component of the recent fertility decline in many developing countries. Data on this factor in Table 15.3 are limited to Asia and to one country in Africa because of the problems of defining and getting data on marriages in Latin America (where common law marriages are numerous) and because few countries in Africa have had significant fertility decline. All of the countries listed in the table had fertility declines of more than 10 percent, and seven of them had declines of more than 20 percent. Rising age at marriage accounted for about one-fourth of the change in three countries, for about one-half the change in three, and for less than one-quarter and for more than one-half in two each. Thus it is clear from these data that rising age at marriage has been a very important factor in fertility decline in many developing countries in recent years; and, as an order of magnitude, changing marriage patterns account for perhaps 35 to 40 percent of the total, but with great variation from country to country.

As illustrative of rapid change in age at marriage consider Tunisia. The proportions of females unmarried in the 15–19 age group were 58, 81, and 95 percent for 1956, 1966, and 1975, respectively. Comparable figures for the 20–24 age group were 20, 27, and 52 percent. Duza and Baldwin cite six factors that account for these rapid changes: sex-ratio imbalance in the usual marriage ages, socio-economic factors, change in marital values and orientation, legislation of minimum age at marriage, banning of polygyny, and the role played by a committed leadership, especially by President Bourguiba, in improving the status of women.[16] Their analysis indicates that the two major determinants of rising age at marriage were increases in education and employment of women. They also note that increased economic difficulties in Tunisia (as well as Sri Lanka, and particularly Malaysia), plus a drive to improve socioeconomic status, also appear to have contributed to the rising age at marriage.

In Malaysia, where age at marriage has also risen quite rapidly, the analysis is complicated by ethnic differences in marriage patterns. The Chinese have always had a higher age at marriage than the Malays and Indians. Caldwell[17] has noted that a "marriage squeeze" due to shortage of males in the culturally appropriate ages contributed to the rise in female age at marriage in the 1950s, as did increasing urbanization and education. Malays marry much earlier than do Chinese, but are also much more likely to divorce and remarry. Differentials in age at marriage are found both for the Chinese and the Malays by rural/urban residence and by level of education. These education and rural/urban differentials explain part of the ethnic differentials, since Malays are mostly rural and have the lowest levels of education and Chinese are mostly urban and have the highest education. But racial differences remain after standardizing for these factors.[18]

As these examples indicate, the causes of changes in marriage patterns are complex. Changes in socioeconomic status almost certainly play an important part. However, age at marriage has

TABLE 15.3. Components of crude birth rate declines: Selected developing countries, selected years, 1957–75

	Crude birth rate				Absolute change due to			Percent of decline due to		
Country and years	Beginning of period	End of period	Amount change	Percent change	Age structure	Marriage pattern	Marital fertility	Age structure	Marriage pattern	Marital fertility
Fiji, 1965/66–1974/75[a]	35.7	28.0	− 7.7	−22	1.6	− 2.2	− 7.1	−21	29	93
Hong Kong, 1961–71	35.5	19.7	−15.8	−45	−4.2	− 3.8	− 7.9	26	24	50
Korea, South, 1966–74	35.1	25.4	− 9.7	−28	0.0	− 0.9	− 8.8	0	9	91
Malaysia (West), 1960–69[b]	42.9	34.6	− 8.3	−19	−0.4	−5.6	− 2.3	5	67	28
Mauritius, 1962–72	38.0	24.4	−13.6	−36	3.4	− 7.2	− 9.9	−25	53	72
Singapore, 1957–70[c]	42.7	22.1	−20.6	−48	2.6	−10.9	−12.3	−13	53	60
Sri Lanka, 1963–71[d]	34.4	29.9	− 4.5	−13	1.9	− 4.0	− 2.4	−42	89	53
Taiwan, 1965–75[e]	32.1	23.0	− 9.1	−28	3.8	− 4.5	− 8.4	−42	49	93
Thailand, 1964/65–1974/75[f]	42.2	37.0	− 5.2	−12	1.2	− 1.0	− 5.4	−22	19	103
Turkey, 1960–75[g]	45	32	−13	−29	−1	− 3	− 9	8	23	69

Note: The crude birth rates shown in this table differ slightly in some instances from those shown in Table 3 of the original paper. We have not adjusted these figures because to do so would require an arbitrary adjustment of one or more of the components.

[a]There is evidence in the Fiji Fertility Survey, 1974, of the World Fertility Survey that birth registration has deteriorated for the Fijian population. For the purpose of this analysis, the age-specific fertility rates from 1965 and 1975 registration data were used with the 1966 and 1974 age structures and percent currently married, as given by the 1966 census and Fiji Fertility Survey, 1974. Therefore, marital fertility decline may be overestimated. The age-specific marital fertility rates were then adjusted to yield the CBRs given for 1965 and 1975.

[b]From Lee-Jay Cho and Robert D. Retherford, "Comparative analysis of recent fertility trends in East Asia," *International Population Conference, Liege, 1973*, vol. 2 (Liege: IUSSP, 1973) p. 167.

[c]Singapore calculations are based on data from Chen-Tung Chang, *Fertility Transition in Singapore* (Singapore University Press, 1974).

[d]Sri Lanka calculations are based on data from *Population of Sri Lanka*, ESCAP Country Monograph Series No. 4, 1976.

[e]Taiwan figures are based on data supplied by Ronald Freedman, University of Michigan.

[f]The 1964/65 age-structure and age-specific fertility rates were taken from the 1964/65 survey, which excluded Bangkok-Thonburi. The percents currently married in 1965 were interpolated from the 1960 and 1970 censuses.

[g]Ferhunde Ozbay, Frederic Shorter, and Samira Yener, "Accounting for the trend of fertility in Turkey," paper presented at *UN/UNFPA Expert Group Meeting on Demographic Transition and Socioeconomic Development, Istanbul, 27 April–4 May 1977.* The Kitagawa method was not used here.

changed more rapidly in a number of countries than have the presumed explanatory socioeconomic variables such as education, nonagricultural employment, husband's occupation, rural or urban residence, and income. The rapidity of change in marital patterns, as well as the factors mentioned in the Duza-Baldwin analysis referred to above, suggests that other factors are at work as well. It is possible that adoption of the concept of planning one's family contributes to the rise in age at marriage, in consonance with Knodel's analysis that:

> the spread of family limitation behaviour itself can serve as a catalyst to change fertility desires, especially within a context of general socio-cultural and economic change. Once the possibility of limiting family size is fully realized, and as other couples practising family limitation and experiencing benefits of reduced family size become available as examples for younger couples to follow, the

possibility of having even fewer children can appear much more realistic than before.... The important point is that family limitation behaviour may well influence fertility attitudes rather than just vice versa, and that this is consistent with a view of family limitation as innovative behaviour during the initial stages of the fertility transition.[19]

Nuptiality, or changing age at marriage and proportion married, is considered an intermediate variable rather than an explanatory variable. As we have indicated, the determinants of marriage patterns are not well known, and analysts have not yet found a satisfactory way of treating cultural determinants and, in particular, change in social norms relating to age at marriage. Nuptiality changes in themselves are partly attributable to the socioeconomic factors under consideration, to which we will turn in the next section.

Marital Fertility

Substantial declines in fertility are typically associated with declines in marital fertility. The demographic transition theory focuses on the shift from a large to a small number of children, and Coale describes this process as "the universality of the major decline in marital fertility in highly modernized societies."[20] Demeny writes that "Any reasonable description of fertility transition contains the idea that marital fertility is 'high' before transition, but 'low' after transition."[21] Ryder, writing of the Western transition toward low fertility, observes that "The primary demographic source of the fall in fertility was a decline in the mean completed parity of married women from the neighborhood of seven to a level below three."[22] Similarly, a study of demographic trends in Europe notes that the "decline in the average family size expected has been largely brought about by the virtual elimination of women expecting families of four or more children, and to the growing predominance of one- or two-child families."[23] Most studies of fertility trends and differentials are concerned with the average number of children born to married women.

Table 15.3 shows that for most countries marital fertility declines accounted for most of the crude birth rate decline; this is particularly true of countries having CBR declines of 20 percent or more. Indeed, if there are surprises in the figures shown in Table 15.3, they come from the extent to which changes in age structure and marital patterns influence fertility declines. These data suggest that a number of developing countries are well into the demographic transition and that the average number of children per married couple is decreasing.

Measures of Demand

Precisely what demand factors produce motivation for family limitation or account for fertility decline at different historical periods, in different societies, and in what magnitudes is uncertain. The one certainty is that numerous factors—social, economic, cultural, familial, religious, psychological, personal—have been discerned or proposed in the literature as having such an effect. These include education, mortality prospects especially for children, industrialization, urbanization and density, income and income distribution, status of women, nuptiality and age at marriage, religious and ethnic affiliation, "modernization," Westernization, nuclear family structure, old-age security, perception of familial advantages, perception of the costs and benefits of children, and reversal of intergenerational wealth flow from children-to-parents to parents-to-children.[24]

Again there are the twofold problems of data: what one might want is unavailable (e.g., on intergenerational wealth flows) and what is available is sometimes flawed. In what follows we mainly consider the major socioeconomic variables typically included in such studies summarized in a social setting index, plus a few additional qualitative factors of special interest.

With regard to social setting, we consider that as the values of the various socioeconomic variables increase (or improve) and as "modernization" advances, a larger proportion of couples want fewer children than was heretofore the case—with the desired number approaching the replacement level in highly modern countries (or societies or groups). That process results in growing motivation for planned control of family size, for "demand" for family planning information and services, and for actual practice of some form of family limitation.

We hypothesize that there are five categories of variables that lead toward demand for smaller families: namely, health, education, economic status, urbanization, and status of women. Working from this hypothesis, we initially put together a "data bank" of about 50 variables with presumed relevance as of 1970, the midpoint of our study period and thus reflecting order of magnitude for 1965–75, given the slowness with which such large matters change. We also examined the values for these variables for earlier periods, principally 1960, plus changes over time and male/female differences. Counting these derived measures, we examined well over 100 variables, the most important of which are listed below:

Education
Primary school enrollment: total, male, female
Secondary school enrollment: total, male, female
Primary and secondary school enrollment: total, male, female
Post-secondary school enrollment ratios: total, male, female
Vocational school enrollment

Health
Life expectancy at birth: total, male, female
Infant mortality rate
Physicians per 1,000 population
Hospital beds per 1,000 population
Crude death rate per 1,000 population
Calories consumed per person per day
Protein consumed per person per day

Economic status
Gross national product (GNP) per capita
Annual percentage growth in GNP per capita
Energy consumption per capita
Arable land per capita
Gini index of income distribution
Percentage of males aged 15–64 in agricultural labor force
Percentage of females aged 15–64 in agricultural labor force
Percentage of males aged 15–64 in nonagricultural labor force
Percentage of females aged 15–64 in nonagricultural labor force
Percentage economically active employed in specified industries
Savings as percentage of national income
Percentage dwellings with piped water
Percentage dwellings with electricity

Urbanization
Percentage of population urban, by local definition
Percentage living in cities of 100,000+

Status of women
Legal age of marriage
Percentage of females aged 15–19 never married
Percentage of females aged 20–24 never married
Some other indexes, as listed above, applied to women

After considerable preliminary analysis to eliminate redundancies and to identify major as against minor factors, and with consideration of the predominant scientific consensus on such a list, we retained the two variables in education, health, and economic status categories having the highest zero-order correlation with CBR decline, plus one with regard to urbanization. (We were not able to find satisfactory indexes of the status of women and therefore that is not included in the primary analysis of socioeconomic variables; it is dealt with separately in the Appendix.) We thus settled upon seven variables as simultaneously satisfying the two criteria of substantial relevance and substantial availability:

Education
Adult literacy (ages 15 and over)
Primary and secondary school enrollment as a percentage of the 5–19 age group

Health
Life expectancy at birth
Infant mortality rate[25]

Economy
Percentage of adult males in nonagricultural labor force
GNP per capita

Urbanization
Percentage of population living in cities of 100,000+

These seven variables serve as our major measure of social setting as it presumably affects motivation for fertility control. (Note that in this definition and selection, their association with CBR decline is being maximized.) Since all of them are considered a part of the general socioeconomic movement called development or modernization, it is only natural that they tend to hang together, or, to use the technical term, that they are characterized by multicollinearity, as shown in this table of intercorrelations:

Variable	Correlation						
	1	2	3	4	5	6	7
1. Adult literacy	1.00						
2. Primary and secondary school enrollment	.80	1.00					
3. Life expectancy	.87	.76	1.00				
4. Infant mortality rate	−.78	−.71	−.86	1.00			
5. Males aged 15–64 in nonagricultural labor force	.65	.73	.80	−.73	1.00		
6. GNP per capita	.23	.38	.40	−.37	.62	1.00	
7. Population in cities of 100,000+	.45	.58	.58	−.54	.78	.57	1.00

On average these factors correlate substantially with one another across the range of developing countries studied.

We do not mean to claim that these socioeconomic factors, or others like them, are necessarily *the* ones, and certainly not the *only* ones, that affect the demand for fertility control. There now appears to be some debate in the field as to whether such factors are only the surface and readily identifiable manifestations of some deeper or underlying structure of the decision process, which involves such factors as the perceived benefits and costs of children, the perceived legitimacy of fertility control, the intergenerational transfer of wealth, and the appreciation of negative externalities within the community (costs produced by individuals but borne by the community). It remains for the field to operationalize such concepts. At present, the "deeper structures" often get expressed in such measurable qualities as education, health, standard of living, urbanization, or the catch-alls of "development" or "modernization"; and, as we have seen, the literature is full of just such measures. In any case, there are plausible reasons why such factors do affect fertility decisions—for example, education, by increasing the economic value of children, heightening aspirations for children, inculcating modern attitudes in place of traditional ones, and making the future real; health, by reducing the number of children needed for a given number of survivors; economic modernization and urbanization, by changing the cost-benefit ratio of children, changing the status of women and traditional sex roles, and providing alternatives to early marriage, breaking down the traditional kinship networks and promoting the nuclear family.[26] Whether these factors are really determinants of fertility or only structural manifestations of some underlying theme or thesis we leave to current dispute and subsequent settlement. Their general association with fertility, however, despite contrary cases, is accepted in the demographic fraternity, whether as genuine cause or as causal surrogate. Moreover, these are the kinds of socioeconomic factors that are put forward as policy instruments in this field—prominently, for example, in the World Population Plan of Action—in connection with the development-*and*-family-planning or development-*versus*-family-planning debate. So we proceed on this basis without undue apology on the one hand or undue naivete on the other.

After considerable analysis we have concluded that for our purposes—that is, to distinguish among countries by their motivational readiness for fertility control—the use of additional socioeconomic variables does not increase correlations. Indeed, as we shall see, even fewer than these seven would yield essentially the same correlations with fertility decline. In short, without claiming that we have selected the single best set of socioeconomic factors for such an analysis, we do believe that we have a highly representative set of the major factors at work, which at the least reflect "deeper structures" if they are not instrumental in their own right, and that in multiple and cross-tabular analyses they yield essentially the same results as any equally qualified set.

In our correlational analyses we use [numerical values for crude birth rates, crude birth rate declines, population sizes, and the seven measures of social setting].* In our descriptive cross-tabulation we use an index constructed from the numerical values by ranking the countries on each of those variables from high to low (94 to 1), dividing each rank by the number of countries for which we had values, summing those ranks, dividing the sum by the number of variables for which a given country had numerical values, and multiplying the result by 100. Since no "natural" breaking points emerged, we divided the countries into four equal groups on what we term the "social setting" index– "high," "upper middle," "lower middle," and "low." While we do not claim precise discrimination point by point and the boundaries may tend to be fuzzy, we do think that this index differentiates broadly among developing countries by their 1970 level of development or modernization.

Measures of Supply

There is no single accepted index of the accessibility, at some adequate level of quality service, of modern means of fertility control (pill, IUD, condom, sterilization, abortion) that is available for a range of countries. As in the case of demand factors, in principle there are several ways to measure the concept of supply. It is difficult to settle upon an "ideal" measure, but it is useful, at least illustratively, to consider alternatives that, while not now available, may become so in the future. For example, consider this designation: how many people in the community have available to them the specified means of fertility control (or some locally approved selection thereof) at a specified level of quality service, at affordable cost, and within, say, 30 minutes travel time? In the industrialized countries that figure is probably around 80–90 percent; surely in some developing countries it is well under 10 percent (i.e., it is limited to some well-off urban dwellers).[27] Such a measure, while useful, requires data that are not presently available across the range of developing countries; thus we turn to another index of supply.

In view of concern with the impact of family planning programs, and in the absence of better data, we utilize as our major measure an index of program effort. By family planning programs we mean organized efforts, typically governmental, to extend the effective practice of modern fertility control without direct or major efforts to affect socioeconomic determinants or the structure of demand. Such programs range from vigorous and continuous efforts under skilled management to weak and spotty performance under indifferent administration, on down to no effort at all. It is a commonplace in the field that family planning programs vary widely in the effort with which they are pursued, from a paper policy with no actual implementation in some cases all the way to a highly efficient working organization in others. Our measure seeks to discern the will, energy, and capability of programmatic effort in order to distinguish among strong, moderate, and weak programs.

The measure was derived from the following 15 "programmatic criteria" ("procedures and supportive measures"), originally developed by Lapham and Mauldin,[28] intended to estimate family planning effort:

Fertility reduction included in official planning policy
Favorable public statements by political leaders
Contraception readily and easily available, publicly and commercially throughout the country
Customs and legal regulations allow importation of contraceptives not manufactured locally
Vigorous effort to provide family planning services to all MWRA (married women of reproductive age)
Adequate family planning administration structure
Training facilities available and utilized
Full-time home-visiting field workers
Postpartum information, education, and service program
Abortion services openly and legally available to all
Voluntary sterilization services (male and female) openly and legally available to all
Use of mass media on a substantial basis
Government provides substantial part of family planning budget from its own resources
Record keeping systems for clients at clinic level and for program service statistics
Serious and continuous evaluation effort

For each country, each criterion was scored yes–2

*Given in detail in Tables 3 and 6 of the original article.

points; qualified yes – 1 point; partially or no – 0 points. These ratings produced country scores ranging from 0 to 30, which are used in our correlational analysis. In our cross-tabulational analysis we use a fourfold classification of program effort: Strong – 20 points or more; Moderate – 10–19 points; Weak – 0–9 points; and None.[29]

The broad character of the classification is indicated by the following descriptions of prototypic programs:[30]

Strong: Programs with full political backing and energetic professional leadership as in South Korea, Taiwan, and reportedly North Vietnam and China (with its own brand of organized inducements); and programs in such relatively small and highly infrastructured societies as Singapore, Hong Kong, or Mauritius (where two programs were officially undertaken, one for the Catholic community).

Moderate: Programs with strong commitment and effort but confronted with overwhelming administrative and logistic difficulties, such as in India after the 1965 reorganization (before that it would have been classified as weak); programs that began slowly but had built up to considerable strength about midway in this period, as in Indonesia, the Philippines, or Thailand (which with a full decade of such effort would qualify as strong); programs that were pursued strongly in some parts of the country, typically the cities and towns, but less so elsewhere, as in Chile, Colombia, Iran, or Tunisia; and programs in smaller countries, in which they could be pursued moderately well through the existing health network and/or assigned to private agencies with government support, such as El Salvador, Trinidad and Tobago, or the Dominican Republic.

Weak: Programs with supporting formal policy but sparse implementation across the country as a whole, as in Egypt, Turkey, Pakistan, Bangladesh, Kenya, or Morocco; programs that became energized too late for impact on the period under review, as in Mexico; programs with less than full policy support and subsequent formal assignment to an understaffed existing bureaucracy or private agency, as in Venezuela, Honduras, Afghanistan, or Nigeria; and programs with both weak policy support and weak implementation, as in Algeria, Sudan, Tanzania, Haiti, or Uganda.

This measure of program effort may be a rough and approximate one, but we are satisfied on the basis of close and long observation that it correctly distinguishes stronger from weaker programs. With other measures of program effort, a few individual countries might be moved to an adjacent category, but it is highly unlikely that the overall distribution or analysis would be significantly affected. In any case, as will be seen later, the key empirical discrimination is between strong/moderate on the one hand and weak/none on the other, so the issue of borderline classification is narrower and less critical than it might appear here; and as will also be seen later, a classification by program duration alone yields essentially the same results.

We have now set forth the central measures on which this study proceeds: 1965–75 CBR declines, seven socioeconomic factors of a demand character, and program effort on the supply side. In the remainder of the paper, we utilize these measures to analyze the effect of the demand and the supply variables upon the specified declines. We do this first through correlational/regression analysis and then through cross-tabulational specification by individual countries.

Correlation and Regression Analysis[31]

Demand Factors

On the hypothesis that modernization leads to fertility reduction, we first examine the relationship of the 1965–75 decline in the crude birth rate to the socioeconomic demand factors, singly and together. First, the simple correlations:

Variable	Correlation coefficient with 1965–75 CBR decline
Life expectancy	.76
Infant mortality rate	–.71
Adult literacy	.70
Males in nonagricultural labor force	.61
Primary and secondary school enrollment	.60

Population in cities of 100,000+	.42
GNP per capita	.13

Among the traditional demand factors associated with fertility, in these data the health and literacy variables are most closely associated with fertility decline, with education and nonagricultural labor force not far behind, then urbanization, and the direct income measure clearly last.

But as we have noted, there is a considerable amount of intercorrelation among these factors, so we next analyze the combined effect of various sets of demand factors, by means of multiple correlations (R^2's) (see Table 15.4). For all seven factors, the R^2 is 0.66, or an "explanation" of about two-thirds of the observed decline. Actually, as indicated in the following data, that level of association is essentially reached with fewer of the demand variables (see regressions 1–6, Table 15.4); moreover, that level is about the plateau that would be reached by the addition of further demand factors from the original list, in view of the multicollinearity in the real world:

Variable	R^2's with 1965–75 CBR decline
Life expectancy	.58
That plus infant mortality rate	.59
Those plus adult literacy	.61
Those plus males in nonagricultural labor force	.61
Those plus primary and secondary school enrollment	.62

(*Continued on next page*)

TABLE 15.4. 1970 socioeconomic (demand) and program (supply) variables as predictors of crude birth rate declines: 94 developing countries, 1965–75

Item	Multiple regression											
	1	2	3	4	5	6	7	8	9	10	11	12
Multiple R	.81	.76	.80	.80	.81	.81	.91	.91	.91	.91	.91	.91
R^2	.66	.58	.64	.64	.66	.66	.83	.83	.83	.83	.83	.83
Socioeconomic (demand) variable	*Beta coefficients*											
Adults literate	.08				.04	.08	.04				.06	.03
Primary and secondary school enrollment	−.06					−.06	.04					.05
Life expectancy	.52	.77	.69	.57	.53	.52	.11	.20	.21	.16	.11	.11
Infant mortality rate	−.13			−.14	−.13	−.13	−.06			−.06	−.06	−.05
Percent males aged 15–64 in nonagricultural labor force	.28	−.01	.24	.24	.26	.28	.11	.09	.16	.14	.16	14
GNP per capita	−.28		−.29	−.29	−.28	−.28	−.10		−.10	−.09	−.09	−.09
Percent population in cities of 100,000+	.00						.04					
Program (supply) variable							.65	.70	.66	.66	.64	.65
Number of cases	89	94	92	91	89	89	89	94	92	91	89	89
Degrees of freedom	81	91	88	86	83	82	80	90	87	85	82	81
F-statistics	22.6	63.2	52.1	38.3	32.3	26.7	49.2	142.8	106.4	83.3	66.6	56.6
Significance level: P = <	.01	.01	.01	.01	.01	.01	.01	.01	.01	.01	.01	.01

Note: The figures shown for regression number 3, for example, indicate that three independent variables were used in the multiple correlation analysis. The multiple R was .80, and the multiple R^2 was .64. Beta values are given for the variables life expectancy, percent males aged 15–64 in nonagricultural labor force, and GNP per capita, thus indicating that those were the three variables used in computing the multiple correlation. The number of countries (cases) included in the analysis and three technical statistics relating to the significance of the regression are shown at the bottom of the table.

Those plus urbanization (population in cities of 100,000+)[32]	.62
Those plus GNP per capita, i.e., all 7 variables	.66

Or, to look at the same matter in another way, of the 35 separate combinations of four factors in our array, 28 have multiple R^2's between .58 and .64, 32 between .54 and .64, and all 35 between .52 and .66. Similarly, two factors (life expectancy, males in nonagricultural labor force) produce an R^2 of .58, and three factors (those plus GNP) an R^2 of .64. By such measures urbanization contributes nothing to the R^2 value, and literacy and enrollment not much (.016 each).

In short, these demand factors have a substantial association with CBR decline over the time span of a decade; they are themselves so interrelated (and thus reflective of the underlying general factor of modernization) that only a few of them (and virtually regardless of which ones) produce close to the maximum correlation; and as more and more socioeconomic factors are added to the multiple correlations (within our seven) they do not substantially increase its magnitude.

Demand Factors Plus Supply

That leads, then, to a consideration of what, if anything, is added by the supply factor of program effort. That is, we investigate the extended hypothesis that modernization combined with program effort leads to an increased reduction in fertility.

We note that just as the demand factors correlate with one another, so program effort correlates with them as well:

Variable	Correlation coefficient with program effort
Life expectancy	.70
Infant mortality rate	−.65
Adult literacy	.64
Males in nonagricultural labor force	.52
Primary and secondary school enrollment	.52
Population in cities of 100,000+	.32
GNP per capita	.07

These correlations are not as high as the intercorrelation among the demand factors but still they are substantial. So program effort, as measured, hangs together with the demand factors in the historical process of modernization, though not as closely as the socioeconomic factors do among themselves. But when it comes to the simple correlation of program effort with the 1965–75 CBR decline, where the demand factors range from .76 to .13, the figure for program effort is .89. And the multiple correlation (R^2) with CBR decline for all seven demand factors plus program effort is .83 (see regression number 7, Table 15.4) as compared with .66 for the demand factors alone.[33]

Thus it is clear that program effort adds substantially to the multiple R^2 of such factors, and in effect breaks through the plateau of small increments among these factors, presumably as "another kind" of influence (Figure 15.2).[34] Another demand factor that similarly extended the correlation would surely be considered a major influence on CBR decline.

Continuing the parallel analysis with the socioeconomic factors as above, we find that the Beta values are extremely high for program effort in combination with demand factors: .65–.70 for program effort as against .20 or less for each of the socioeconomic factors. And if they are combined into a single factor of "modernization," the corresponding Betas are still striking: .75 for program effort as against .22 for social setting.

In summarizing the effect of the different factors on CBR decline we get the following R^2 values (with the seven socioeconomic variables included as the original values):

Item	R^2
Socioeconomic factors	.66
Program effort	.78
Socioeconomic factors and program effort	.83

And when the appropriate subtractions are made from the total R^2 value, it is apparent that most of the association derives from the combination and only a small proportion from the net effect of a single factor—that is, by subtracting .66 from .83 for the net effect of program effort (.17) or by subtracting .78 from .83 for the net effect of socioeconomic factors (.05). This general picture is further elucidated using rank order on socioeconomic factors rather than the individual values of each vari-

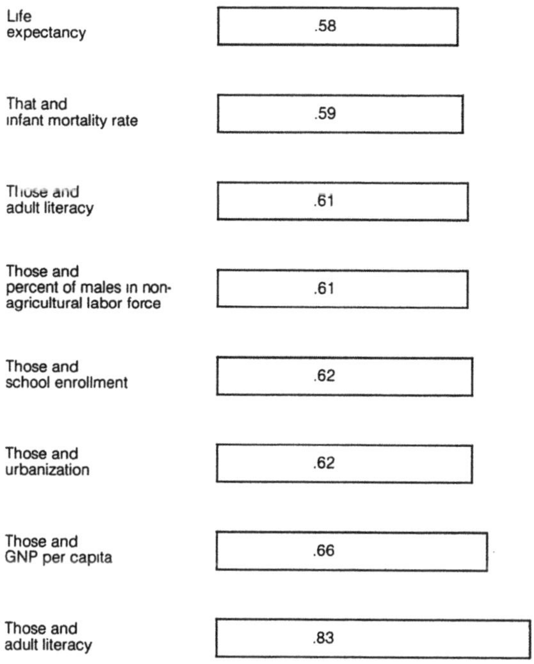

FIGURE 15.2. Multiple correlations (R^2's) of demand (socioeconomic) and supply (program) variables with 1965–75 crude birth rate declines.

able. The R^2 of rank order on socioeconomic variables plus program effort with CBR declines is .82. The Beta coefficient for socioeconomic factors is .23 and for program effort, .75. Each contributes to the overall result, but in different degree; and the relative contributions to the discerned association are consistent throughout.

If we start with the R^2 for the seven socioeconomic variables and CBR decline, in the traditional way, we then add about 25 percent to explained variance when we add program effort (i.e., from .66 to .83). The analysis indicates that both social setting ("modernization") and program effort make a difference and that program effort adds substantially to fertility decline when combined with the social variables.

A replication of the regression analysis of similar character reported in an earlier study,[35] based on the same general concepts but utilizing data for fewer countries (3 social setting indicators and 29 countries in the earlier study, compared with 7 social setting indicators and 89 countries in this study for which data were available on all seven socioeconomic variables) and dealing with a different period (1960–73), provides an interesting comparison:

Variable	Percent of CBR decline associated with variable: Freedman and Berelson	This study
1. Social setting alone	51.3	66.1
2. Program effort alone	60.7	78.5
3. Social setting and program effort	68.1	83.1
4. Net effect of social setting (3–2)	7.4	4.6
5. Net effect of program effort (3–1)	16.8	17.0
6. Joint effect (3 – [5 + 4])	43.9	61.5

Although the values are somewhat higher in the present case, the pattern is on the whole the same: substantial joint effect and similar contributions from the component elements.

Further Modes of Analysis

The above type of correlational analysis, as shown in the literature review, is commonly used. In addition, we utilized other modes of analysis to explore specific aspects of the intricate relationships among demand, supply, and fertility decline.

Path Analysis

This procedure, itself a type of regression analysis, allows us to explore the consequential question: To what extent is program effort itself a function of modernization, of the socioeconomic factors used in the analysis? Program effort is significantly affected by socioeconomic development; the seven demand variables produce a multiple R^2 of .60 with program effort as the dependent variable. Thus, 60 percent of the variance in program effort is "explained" by socioeconomic factors, with 40 percent left to be accounted for by other considerations.

A convenient way of showing the interrelationship among the socioeconomic factors, program effort, and CBR decline is path analysis. In the following model we assume that both social setting and program effort exert a direct impact on fertility decline and that the socioeconomic factors themselves influence program effort.

Path analysis is a statistical model in which "each dependent variable must be regarded explicitly as *completely* determined by some combination of variables in the system. In problems where complete determination by measured variables does not hold, a residual variable uncorrelated with other determining variables must be introduced."[36] A path coefficient is the Beta coefficient in a regression analysis and "gives the expected effect of a change in one standard deviation in the explanatory variable (holding other variables constant); this expected change is expressed in terms of the standard deviation of the predicted variable."[37]

In order to use path analysis we must select a given variable or combine the socioeconomic variables into a single variable—in this case our index of social setting. For convenience we label CBR decline as variable 0, social setting as variable 1, and program effort as variable 2. The correlations and path coefficient values for these variables are:

Variable	Correlation coefficient	Path coefficient
01 Crude birth rate decline and social setting	.67	.23
02 Crude birth rate decline and program effort	.89	.75
21 Program effort and social setting	.58	.58

It should be noted that the R^2 between the socioeconomic variables and CBR decline decreases from .66 to .44 when the seven factors are collapsed into a single variable.[38]

In the graphic presentation of path analysis below, the arrows indicate the assumed direction of effect, with the vertical arrows indicating unexplained or residual effects.

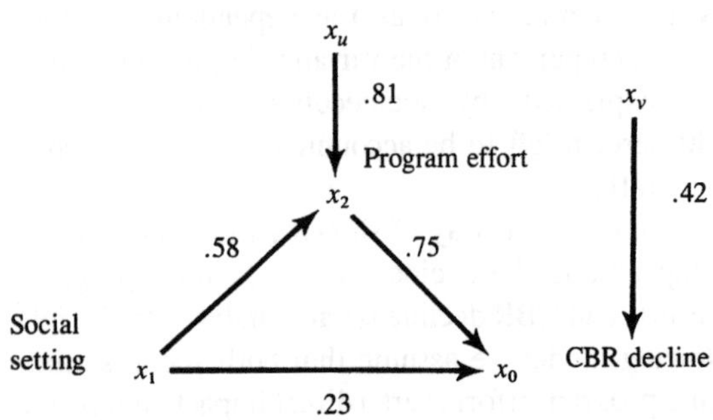

According to this model, program effort has more *direct* effect on CBR decline (.75) than do the socioeconomic variables (.23). But this understates the total effect of the socioeconomic variables inasmuch as they also operate through program effort. Their indirect effect is estimated by multiplying the path value from demand to program effort, expressed as p_{21} (with a value of .58) by p_{02} (with a value of .75), or .44. Thus, the combined direct and indirect effect of the demand variables is .23 + .44, or .67. The diagram shows the direct effect of program effort (.75), but its total effect is given by the correlation coefficient of program effort and CBR decline, .89; thus, the joint and indirect effect of program effort is .14 (.89 − .75). Again, both factors are important, but in this analysis two-thirds of the total effect of social setting is filtered through program effort, and the total effect of program effort is more than that of social setting in a ratio of 89:67, or 4:3.[39] It is worth noting that the path coefficients of unexplained variance are significant, .42 for CBR decline and .81 for program effort. Thus a considerable part of program effort is not associated with socioeconomic status, important though those variables are.

Interaction Effects

To the best of our knowledge, there is no wholly satisfactory way of disentangling the interaction effects of socioeconomic variables and program effort on fertility decline, although we sought to estimate separate effects by using various methods.

Another approach is to estimate the interrelationship between 1960 socioeconomic values and the 1955–65 CBR decline, and to use the Beta coefficients generated by that analysis to predict the effect of 1970 values on the 1965–75 CBR decline. The R^2 between the seven variables, using 1960 values, and the 1955–65 CBR decline is .57, but this association is based on only 38 cases because of lack of data. (We can increase the number of cases by dropping variables with the smallest number of countries with available data, but at the expense of the R^2 value.) Using the Beta values generated with this analysis, and substituting 1970 values, the R^2 between socioeconomic variables and the 1965–75 CBR decline is.53 for the same 38 countries. If the analysis is extended to all countries for which data are available in 1970, the number of cases is increased to 89, and the R^2 decreases to .47. The addition of program effort raises these last two R^2's to .78 in each case. Thus, this approach suggests that socioeconomic variables were somewhat less closely associated with fertility declines before family planning programs were organized than was the case after they were organized. We interpret these findings as another indication of the importance of the interrelationship between program effort and socioeconomic setting.

Change Analysis

On the hypothesis that it is the change in the socioeconomic variables over time that makes for fertility reduction rather than their state at a given time (in our case, the mid-point of the period, circa 1970), we undertook analysis of changes[40] of the following character:

Literacy: percentage increase 1960–70
Education: proportionate increase in the percentage enrolled in primary and secondary schools 1960–70
Life expectancy at birth: percentage increase 1960–70
Infant mortality: percentage decline 1960–70
Nonagricultural labor force: percentage increase for males aged 15–64 1960–70
GNP per capita: annual percentage increase in GNP per capita 1965–70
Urbanization: proportionate increase in percentage of population living in cities of 100,000+ 1960–70

These data are unfortunately not complete. We have data for as few as 57 countries (for the 1960–70 percentage decline in infant mortality) to all 94 countries (for percentage change in life expectancy and males aged 15–64 employed in the nonagricultural labor force). But for only 35 countries are there data for all seven of the variables (see Table 15.5). The multiple correlation for those seven changes with CBR decline is .74, and the R^2 is .55; if program effort is added, the multiple R^2 becomes .84. As is readily noted, the change values alone are slightly smaller than those produced by the initial analyses in which the same factors were measured circa 1970, but of course there is some selectivity in the countries for which values are available for all the factors.

If we use change in six factors (omitting literacy), the number of cases increases from 35 to 46 but with a loss in the association (multiple R^2 of .48); with five factors (also omitting infant mortality), the number of cases is increased to 69, but the multiple R^2 drops to .29; with only three or four change measures, the number of cases can be increased to 85–91, but the multiple R^2's decrease to values of .09–.41, far below the corresponding R^2's for the measures as of 1970.

In general, the countries with better statistical systems and available data tend to be countries that are relatively more advanced than the others in the developing category. (For example, the unweighted average CBR decline for the 35 countries is 16 percent as against about 11 percent for the others.) The two factors with the smallest number of cases are change in infant mortality and change in percentage literate, and both have a moderately high correlation with fertility decline. Overall, this analysis suggests that changes in the social factors have almost as much explanatory power as do the 1970 levels, but lack of data prevents a definitive analysis.

Lag Analysis

It is often put forward that whereas socioeconomic factors are prime determinants of the level of fertility, there is a lag of some years between achievement of a given level of socioeconomic status and the reduction of fertility to a corresponding level. The period of that lag is usually unspecified. For our purposes, we also analyzed the relationship between socioeconomic variables in 1960 and the 1965–75 CBR decline.

The R^2 between the seven socioeconomic variables with 1960 values and 1965–75 CBR decline is .72, slightly higher than with 1970 values (.70 for the same 48 countries, .66 for the 89 countries for which 1970 data are available). Infant mortality rates are less available than the other variables for 1960, and if that variable is dropped from the analysis the number of cases increases to 66, but with a slight decrease in the degree of association with CBR decline, to an R^2 of .69. (The association is trivially increased to .70 by using the logarithm

TABLE 15.5. Program (supply) variable and change in socioeconomic (demand) variables as predictors of crude birth rate declines: 94 developing countries, 1965–75

Item	Multiple regression 1	2	3	4	5	6
Multiple R	.74	.92	.69	.53	.66	.30
Multiple R^2	.55	.84	.48	.29	.44	.09
Socioeconomic (demand) variable	*Beta coefficients*					
Proportion increase in adults literate	.20	.18			.33	
Proportion increase in primary and secondary school enrollment	−.01	−.00	−.03	−.05	.02	.10
Percent change in life expectancy	−.32	−.17	−.44	−.33	−.32	−.28
Percent decline in infant mortality rate	.39	.13	.32			
Increase in percent males aged 15–64 in nonagricultural labor force	−.09	−.11	.02	−.01	−.13	.05
Annual percent increase in GNP per capita, 1965–70	.16	−.09	.16	.30	.23	
Proportion increase in population in cities of 100,000+	.04	.08	.15	.22	.07	
Program (supply) variable		.71				
Number of cases	35	35	46	69	52	86
Degrees of freedom	27	26	39	63	45	82
F-statistics	4.736	17.231	5.884	5.037	5.900	2.783
Significance level: P = <	.05	.01	.05	.05	.05	N.S.

of GNP per capita rather than absolute values, and with no loss in the number of cases.) The comparable figures with 1970 values are .70 and .64, for the same 66 countries and for all countries, respectively. If program effort is added to the six socioeconomic variables (omitting infant mortality), the R^2 with the 1965–75 CBR decline is .87. The comparable R^2 using 1970 data, and restricting the analysis to the same countries for which data were available in 1960, is .86 (and .82 for the 89 countries for which data are available in 1970).

The R^2's obtained using 1960 and 1970 values of socioeconomic factors as dependent variables and CBR declines as the dependent variable are almost identical. Thus, this analysis does not provide a basis for choosing between the two theories or hypotheses (lag as against current development). On empirical grounds we have chosen to use 1970 values inasmuch as data are available for a much larger number of countries than for 1960.

Absolute CBR Decline

Some analysts think that percentage CBR declines are less pertinent to both scientific and policy considerations than absolute declines in CBR; they say, for example, that a 10 percent decline in a CBR of 45—4.5 points—is more pertinent than a 10 percent decline in a CBR of 25—2.5 points. Clearly there is a "floor effect" in that wherever CBRs have declined to a low level, further decline is less likely. At the same time, we know that initial fertility declines may be slower and more difficult to achieve than is the case once fertility has dropped, say, into the mid-30s.

Analyses based on the absolute differences between 1965 and 1975 CBRs show about the same relationships as have been presented for percentage declines in CBRs, but with R^2 values being somewhat lower. For example, using 1960 data, the R^2 with the seven socioeconomic variables and absolute change in the 1965–75 CBR is .64 as compared with .72 for the same countries and time period using the percentage decline for 1965–75. If program effort is added to the former multiple correlation, the R^2 becomes .81 as compared with .86 for the latter, a rather small difference. Comparable figures using 1970 socioeconomic values are .61 for absolute CBR decline and .66 for percentage CBR decline and, with the addition of program effort, are .79 and .83, respectively. Thus, the pattern of relationships is quite similar whether the analysis is based on percentage or on absolute CBR declines from 1965 to 1975. Although the R^2's

TABLE 15.6. Index of correspondence among development indicators

	Index range										
Indicators	0	10	20	30	40	50	60	70	80	90	100
Crude birth rate	48.50	46.75	44.87	44.79	43.67	40.23	35.04	27.25	20.88	17.15	16.50
Infant mortality rate	161.70	148.60	135.67	125.87	106.84	86.32	64.35	45.47	32.48	21.52	13.86
Life expectancy	41.34	44.10	47.05	48.77	52.48	57.79	62.41	66.87	69.44	71.49	72.94
Animal protein consumption per capita per day	9.68	11.27	11.59	12.41	14.04	18.07	24.01	35.98	45.98	53.36	63.16
Percent literate, ages 15+	23.65	32.31	37.07	39.87	47.75	60.07	72.14	85.04	92.76	97.78	101.11
Percent aged 5–19 enrolled in primary and secondary school	23.50	26.80	31.08	35.67	43.76	50.69	56.49	63.27	69.33	75.15	80.68
Percent of dwellings with electricity	23.18	27.43	33.37	37.20	38.24	46.66	58.61	78.25	93.83	98.92	99.78
Newspaper circulation per 1,000 population	4.79	7.35	11.41	17.61	32.41	55.09	83.69	133.10	208.89	290.55	356.82
Telephones per 100,000 population	136.50	205.82	348.34	607.26	1,088.23	2,011.51	3,768.04	6,768.05	12,193.11	22,482.20	41,192,50
Automobiles per 1,000 population	1.88	3.21	4.81	7.05	8.58	13.22	23.07	46.12	92.52	166.79	299.65
Males in agriculture as percent of total male labor force	91.37	81.85	71.04	64.02	57.22	52.16	42.28	29.68	20.96	13.85	8.29
Steel consumption per capita (kg.)	3.68	5.66	8.63	14.85	26.67	43.56	73.67	143.68	275.05	442.57	571.69
Energy consumption per capita (kg.)	37.15	73.22	118.58	201.02	351.72	524.39	871.88	1,600.78	2,837.27	4,389.17	6,608.19
Percent GDP from manufacturing	9.79	10.16	10.46	11.62	14.47	17.92	19.49	22.22	27.18	30.54	33.26
GNP per capita (US $)	72.00	90.29	117.95	163.10	230.46	304.09	464.77	727.58	1,081.07	1,675.49	2,500.47
Crude birth rate	48.50	46.75	44.87	44.79	43.67	40.23	35.04	27.25	20.88	17.15	16.50

Source: United Nations Research Institute for Social Development.

Special thanks are due D. V. McGranahan and his colleagues at the United Nations Research Institute for Social Development for preparing this table.

are lower for the latter as compared with the former, the differences are not large.

Correspondence Analysis

We have been impressed with the work of McGranahan and colleagues at the United Nations Research Institute for Social Development (UNRISD)[41] in generalizing the interrelationship of selected socioeconomic variables in the form of a series of "correspondence points." At our request they developed correspondence points for a variety of available factors, including levels of crude birth rates and infant mortality rates, as shown in Table 15.6.

We appreciate that there is a conceptual problem in using levels of independent variables to explain changes in fertility. But if the model is perfectly general, cross-sectional data for a number of different countries can be viewed as a proxy for a time series for an average country. This correspondence table provides a revealing description of what goes along with what in the process of development, and at what quantitative values, without reference to "cause," only to association. Thus a country with a crude birth rate of 48.5 (first column, Table 15.6) would be expected to have an infant mortality rate of 161.7, a life expectancy of 41.3 years, more than 90 percent of males in the agricultural labor force, GNP per capita of US$72, and so on. With a crude birth rate of 35 (column 7), the infant mortality rate would be expected to have fallen to 64, life expectancy would have risen to 62.4, well below half of employed males would be working in agriculture, and the GNP per capita would be $465. There is, to be sure, considerable variation in the relationship between any two or more variables for a given country, but the UNRISD analyses for 1960 and 1970 provide an interesting, and we think useful, analysis of the relationship among a number of variables—and, in a general sense, is consistent with our results.

Moreover, if the "threshold" range for fertility reduction is defined as between the 50 and 70 correspondence lines, representing CBRs of approximately 40 and 27, then there is considerable agreement between this analysis and that summarized from the literature and supporting text for similar factors:

Variable	From summary	From correspondence analysis (CBRs 40 and 27)
Nonagricultural labor force	50–65 percent	48–70 percent
Life expectancy	65 years	58–67 years
Female literacy	65–75 percent	60–85 percent (adult literacy)
Newspaper circulation	70–100	55–133

There are additional overlaps with single studies, for example, infant mortality of 44–78 in the UN analysis and 45–86 in the UNRISD analysis.

Cross-Tabulational Analysis

Let us now look at the relationship between social setting, program effort, and fertility decline within individual countries, with particular reference to the place of family planning programs in fertility decline relative to the social context within which they operate.

Social Setting and Program Effort

We begin with a cross-tabulation of the demand and supply factors as expressed by the indexes of social setting and of program effort previously described (Table 15.7). Through the number of entries within cells, the tabulation indicates the moderately strong relationship between social setting and program effort, as noted in the correlational analysis. As has been suggested on several occasions,[42] and as we noted in the path analysis above, the social setting as defined has not only a direct effect on fertility reduction in increasing motivation for family limitation but also an indirect effect in facilitating the implementation of family planning programs themselves (through better-trained people, facilitating infrastructures, administrative efficiencies, organizational skills, logistic and evaluational capabilities, etc.).[43]

The salient findings of Table 15.7 are summarized as follows:

1. The relationships of demand and supply to CBR declines are immediately apparent in the marginal figures, with a rather steady progression by demand (social setting) and a sharp break (between

moderate and weak) on the supply side (program effort). By this initial measure, both sets of factors matter. Either index alone differentiates fertility decline on these four-point classifications but program effort does so more than social setting (by a factor of 15 as against 10, in the marginals). There is a strong progression from the upper left cell to the lower right, with about 15–20 times as much fertility decline in the former as in the latter, with other values ranging regularly in between.

2. The single cells at upper left and lower right set the upper and lower limits of fertility reduction for developing countries in this period. The upper limit, by category,[44] is about 30 percent, or 10 points, off the CBR. In this analysis the upper left countries had the dual advantages of fast modernization and strong family planning programs. In sharp contrast, the countries in the lower right cell, with virtually no fertility reduction, had almost no advantages in this respect: little or slow modernization, weak or no family planning efforts.

3. On the whole the intermediate cells reflect the same situation: the layer of countries with a CBR reduction in the 15–30 percent range on average, represented by such countries as Colombia, Chile, Philippines, China, Thailand, Malaysia, and Sri Lanka, is marked by substantial modernization and for the most part moderate family planning programs. And the other cells toward the lower right essentially resemble those in the corner cell: low social setting, weak or no program effort—and, on the whole, small fertility reductions.

4. The only countries with lower middle or low social setting and a fertility reduction above 10 percent, or about 5 points off the CBR, are those with strong or moderate program effort—North Vietnam, India, and Indonesia. Their counterparts, with high or upper middle social setting but with weak or no program effort, had on the average only about one-third as much fertility reduction in this period. This suggests that such countries as Mexico, Venezuela, Brazil, Peru, Zaire, and Ghana could have reduced fertility more sharply with a substantial program effort.

5. The major deviants or "outliers" in this array are three: Iran has "too little" fertility reduction for its location in the tabulation, Turkey and Egypt perhaps "too much." In Iran the actual implementation of the program, as against the policy intent, may be overrated in our index; in Turkey and Egypt the critical factors may be the fast modernization of the former and the unsettled, war-related situation of the latter.

This analysis indicates that the two indexes—social setting and program effort—organize the observed declines quite well.

Qualitative Factors

In addition to the socioeconomic factors we have identified, there are others of a demand character that are often asserted to be associated with fertility behavior, which we briefly note here. They are the ethnic status of a society, island or quasi-island character, and the pace of social change. In order to explore these associations we analyzed the CBR decline in the 94 countries for these factors.

Ethnic Status

Three religious or cultural traditions are associated with higher fertility: Catholic on doctrinal grounds; Muslim through subordination of women in cultural traditions; and black African because of traditional status within the society. Chinese and Chinese-related ethnic groups are associated with lower fertility through pragmatic response to changing conditions.[45]

Island Status

Although often considered as unserious, the notion dies hard that island residence affects fertility[46]—or more precisely, that a community situated and required to live within a restricted space tends to exert a special control over fertility, through the psychology of "being on our own" or "being pushed into the sea" or "having nowhere to go." That response, however, may come not from island residence as such but from the population density associated therewith, for islands are on average relatively densely populated.

Social Change

According to Irene Taeuber, "precipitant social change, disrupted traditions, and cultural shock are more conducive to family restriction than social adjustments that preserve continuities."[47] In the

TABLE 15.7. 1965–75 crude birth rate declines (in percents), by social setting and program effort: 94 developing countries

Social setting	Program effort: Strong (20+) Country	Decline	Moderate (10–19) Country	Decline	Weak (0–9) Country	Decline	None Country	Decline	Total
High	Singapore	40	Cuba	40	Venezuela	11	Korea,		
	Hong Kong	36	Chile	29	Brazil	10	North	5	
	Korea,		Trinidad and		Mexico	9	Kuwait	5	
	South	32	Tobago	29	Paraguay	6	Peru	2	
	Barbados	31	Colombia	25			Lebanon	2	
	Taiwan	30	Panama	22			Jordan	1	
	Mauritius	29					Libya	−1	
	Costa Rica	29							
	Fiji	22							
	Jamaica	21							
	Mean	30	Mean	29	Mean	9	Mean	3	19
	Median	30	Median	29	Median	9.5	Median	2	22
Upper middle	China	24	Malaysia	26	Egypt	17	Mongolia	9	
			Tunisia	24	Turkey	16	Syria	4	
			Thailand	23	Honduras	7	Zambia	−2	
			Dominican		Nicaragua	7	Congo	−2	
			Republic	21	Zaire	6			
			Philippines	19	Algeria	4			
			Sri Lanka	18	Guatemala	4			
			El Salvador	13	Morocco	2			
			Iran	2	Ghana	2			
					Ecuador	0			
					Iraq	0			
	Mean	24	Mean	18	Mean	6	Mean	2	10
	Median	24	Median	20	Median	4	Median	1	7
Lower middle	Vietnam,		India	16	Papua		Angola	4	
	North	23	Indonesia	13	New Guinea	5	Cameroon	3	
					Pakistan	1	Burma	3	
					Bolivia	1	Yemen,		
					Nigeria	1	P.D.R. of	3	
					Kenya	0	Mozambique	2	
					Liberia	0	Khmer/		
					Haiti	0	Kampuchea	2	
					Uganda	−4	Ivory Coast	1	
							Senegal	0	
							Saudi Arabia	0	
							Vietnam,		
							South	0	
							Madagascar	0	
							Lesotho	−4	
	Mean	23	Mean	14	Mean	1	Mean	1	3
	Median	23	Median	14.5	Median	0.5	Median	1.5	1

(*Table 15.7 continued on next page*)

TABLE 15.7. *Continued.*

Social setting	Program effort: Strong (20+) Country	Decline	Moderate (10–19) Country	Decline	Weak (0–9) Country	Decline	None Country	Decline	Total
Low					Tanzania	5	Laos	5	
					Dahomey	3	Central African Republic	5	
					Bangladesh	2	Malawi	5	
					Sudan	0	Bhutan	3	
					Nepal	−1	Ethiopia	2	
					Mali	−1	Guinea	2	
					Afghanistan	−2	Chad	2	
							Togo	2	
							Upper Volta	1	
							Yemen	1	
							Niger	1	
							Burundi	1	
							Sierra Leone	0	
							Mauritania	0	
							Rwanda	0	
							Somalia	0	
					Mean	1	Mean	2	2
					Median	0	Median	1.5	1
Mean		29		21		4		2	9
Median		29		22		2		2	3

absence of objective indicators of the pace of social change, we identified such countries only on the basis of common knowledge—swift modernization (e.g., Singapore, South Korea, Taiwan), rapid increase of per capita income (e.g., Brazil, Mexico, Venezuela, Jamaica), revolutionary political and social change (e.g., China, Cuba), stress of war (e.g., the Vietnams, Egypt).

In these cases, within the four social-setting categories, there is an additional differentiation by these factors (Table 15.8): by ethnic status, in which Muslim and black African average declines are uniformly low, Catholic averages are intermediate, and Chinese and other averages are equivalently high; by island and quasi-island status and by density, (which are closely related) with a clear differentiation except at the bottom of the social scale, so perhaps "the psychology of being crowded in" does break through into conscious control of fertility; and by social change, where a fast pace is associated with fertility decline. Moreover, such influences may be shining through Table 15.7 as well: of the 23 countries in the four upper-left cells, 18 are islands or quasi-islands, 15 experienced fast social change in this decade, and only 1 was Muslim or black African (and it, Iran, was far out of line); of the 43 countries in the lower right cells, 35 were Muslim or black African, only 4 were islands or quasi-islands, and only 4 experienced fast social change.

Duration and Type of Program Effort

Our classification of program effort is meant as an average estimate over the duration of the family planning program, within the indicated period. But given the sharp increase in such policies in recent years, the programs analyzed are of varying durations: some were in operation throughout the decade, some for half the time, some only for a year or two. Let us see how that consideration can be taken into account.

TABLE 15.8. Mean 1965–75 crude birth rate declines (in percents) by ethnic status, island status, density, and pace of social change, by social setting: 94 developing countries

Status	Social setting: High	Upper middle	Lower middle	Low
Ethnic				
African		2 (4)	0 (12)	2 (15)
Muslim	2 (4)	9 (8)	4 (4)	0 (4)
Catholic	16 (9)	10 (7)	1 (2)	
Chinese	29 (5)	21 (4)	8 (3)	5 (1)
Other	29 (6)	18 (1)	8 (3)	1 (2)
Island				
Island	31 (9)	17 (2)	9 (2)	
Quasi-island	23 (5)	13 (6)	8 (3)	
Other	7 (10)	4 (15)	2 (18)	2 (24)
Density				
High	26 (10)	17 (3)	10 (4)	1 (3)
Medium	21 (5)	15 (11)	2 (7)	1 (6)
Low	12 (9)	3 (10)	2 (12)	2 (14)
Pace of social change				
Fast	26 (15)	20 (5)	12 (3)	5 (2)
Not fast	8 (9)	8 (19)	2 (20)	1 (21)

Note: Number of countries is shown in parentheses.

A clear correlation between policy duration and program effort is indicated by the tabulation below, which shows the number of countries in each category of program effort by the year in which their policy was established (38 countries had no family planning policy by 1974).[48] The table suggests that it takes five years or more to develop a moderate or strong effort:

Program effort	Number of countries: 1965 or earlier	1966 -68	1969 -72	1973 -74	Mean number of years since policy established to 1975
Strong	8	3	0	0	11.5
Moderate	4	9	2	0	8.3
Weak	5	8	13	4	5.5
Total	17	20	15	4	

A cross-tabulation of duration of family planning policy and CBR decline confirms that it takes at least five years before a program is effective enough to substantially influence the birth rate, as is demonstrated by the data in Table 15.9.

TABLE 15.9. 1965–75 mean crude birth rate declines and range of declines by year policy was established: 94 developing countries

Year policy established	Country	Mean 1965–75 CBR decline (in percents)	Range of CBR declines (in percents)
1965 or earlier	Hong Kong, Singapore, Taiwan, South Korea, Fiji, China, North Vietnam, Cuba, Tunisia, India, Pakistan/ Bangladesh, Venezuela, Mauritius, Sri Lanka, Turkey, Morocco, Egypt	24.1	1–40
1966–67	Jamaica, Chile, Malaysia, Honduras, Kenya, Nepal, Barbados, Trinidad and Tobago, Colombia, Thailand, Iran, Nicaragua	16.7	−1–31
1968–69	Costa Rica, Panama, Dominican Republic, Ecuador, El Salvador, Guatemala, Indonesia, Ghana, Bolivia, Papua New Guinea	11.1	0–29
1970–71	Philippines, Algeria, South Vietnam, Tanzania, Nigeria, Sudan, Haiti, Afghanistan	3.4	0–19
1972–73	Mexico, Paraguay, Iraq, Zaire, Dahomey/Benin, Liberia, Jordan, Laos, Mali, Uganda, Khmer, P.D.R. of Yemen	2.5	−4–9
1974 or later, or no policy	Remaining 32 countries	1.9	−4–10

Because the dates that policies were established may simply reflect differences in social setting, we cross-tabulated social setting and program duration to show mean percentage of CBR declines (with number of countries shown in parentheses, and data grouped for roughly equivalent numbers by column):

Social setting	Mean 1965–75 CBR decline (in percents) and year program established 1965 or earlier	1966 –68	1969 –72	1973 or later, and no program
High	30 (8)	27 (6)	14 (2)	4 (8)
Upper middle	20 (5)	11 (9)	6 (5)	3 (5)
Lower middle	13 (3)	5 (4)	−1 (3)	1 (13)
Low	2 (1)	−1 (1)	1 (5)	2 (16)

Within our four categories of social setting, the association with policy (program) duration consistently shows through—and again quite strikingly so given the small numbers involved. Not only did countries in the two higher social setting categories adopt such policies (programs) earlier—58 percent by 1968 as against 20 percent for those in two lower social setting categories—but CBR declines are larger with longer program duration, except in countries with low social setting.

Next we examine the relationship between program duration and our measure of program effort, in a tabulation similar to the previous one:

Program effort	Mean 1965–75 CBR decline (in percents) and year program established 1965 or earlier	1966 –68	1969 –72	1973 or later, and no program
Strong	29 (8)	27 (3)		
Moderate	24 (4)	20 (9)	20 (2)	
Weak	10 (5)	3 (8)	1 (13)	6 (4)
None				2 (38)

Here again the findings are striking: duration consistently matters; there are only two strong or moderate programs established as late as 1969 (Philippines and Panama); most weak programs have little impact even with long operation (e.g., Pakistan/Bangladesh, Morocco, Kenya). Indeed, only three weak programs of long duration are in countries with CBR declines of over 10 percent—Egypt, Turkey, and Venezuela.

Family planning programs may be differentiated not only by level of program effort and duration, but by the objectives of the program. By a traditional classification, programs can be grouped into two categories, according to the nature of the population policy they are intended to implement: (1) "official policy to reduce the population growth rate. In addition to supporting family planning to implement this policy, countries in this category also support family planning for reasons of health and as a human right;" and (2) "official support of family planning activities for other than demographic reasons. Countries in this category usually support family planning for reasons of health and as a human right, but any antinatalist effect is a by-product, not an objective."[49] Grouping countries by this classification demonstrates an even sharper correlation with program effort:

Program effort	Number of countries and family planning policy: To reduce population growth rate	For other than demographic reasons	No policy and policy unknown
Strong	9	2	0
Moderate	12	3	0
Weak	10	20	0
None	0	30	38
Total	31	25	38

About two-thirds of the countries with policies to reduce population growth have either strong or moderate programs as against less than one-fifth of those with policies adopted for other than demographic reasons. Demographic motivation for policy appears to make a substantial difference in the degree of implementation of program effort. Here too, the stronger policy position is associated with CBR decline, when social setting is controlled:

Social setting	Mean 1965–75 CBR decline (in percents) and nature of family planning policy: To reduce population growth rate	For other than demographic reasons	No program and unknown
High	28 (11)	21 (7)	3 (6)
Upper middle	15 (14)	4 (6)	2 (4)
Lower middle	7 (4)	4 (8)	2 (11)
Low	1 (2)	1 (4)	2 (17)

Only a high social setting substantially overcomes the weaker policy position; and in the lower right-hand combinations of the tabulation, as demarcated, little CBR decline occurs.

As we have noted, social setting and program effort are themselves correlated: 41 of the 94 countries fall on the diagonal of this classification, and thus provide no independent information on the relative impacts of the two sets of factors. How does the cross-tabulation look without them—that is, when limited to countries differentially located on the demand and supply sides as measured? The mean percentage declines for the countries that remain are:

Social setting	Mean 1965–75 CBR decline (in percents) and program effort: Strong	Moderate	Weak	None	Total
High	X	29	9	3	13
Upper middle	24	X	6	2	6
Lower middle	23	14	X	1	5
Low	–	–	1	X	1
Total	24	25	5	2	

Note that the differential effect of program effort remains—essentially between the upper and lower half—but that the effect of social setting is somewhat attenuated. We have boxed the combinations that yield essentially similar CBR declines; in this complex tabulation of several variables across many developing countries, only three such combinations remain when the diagonal cases are removed—with average CBR declines of about 27, 8 and 2 percent.

In a further compression, which minimizes borderline problems of classification on both sides of the table, we show the same countries (diagonals removed) reduced to a 2 × 2 array:

Social setting	Mean 1965–75 CBR decline (in percents) and program effort: Strong and moderate	Weak and none	Total
High and upper middle	28	5	10
Lower middle and low	17	1	3
Total	22	3	

Here the differential impact is even more striking: a ratio of about 7:1 for program effort as against 3:1 for social setting, or a CBR decline three times as great in low setting/high effort countries as in high setting/low effort countries (17 percent as against 5 percent). In short, with the diagonal countries removed the relationship of program effort to CBR decline by no means disappears: it remains strong, and indeed stronger than social setting.

Summary and Conclusions

Let us start with the briefest distillation of our central findings:

Correlation and Regression Analysis

A series of correlations and multiple regressions were performed using various techniques and different sets of data on social setting, program effort, and fertility decline.

Though done in a variety of analytic ways and with different sets of data, these analyses all reveal a quite consistent overall result: the social setting factors, however measured, correlated around .65 with the 1965–75 CBR decline, and program effort adds another .15–.20, or about 25 percent, to the correlations (somewhat more in those analyses with fewer cases).

Major Analysis

1970 socioeconomic factors, program effort, and 1965–75 CBR declines using:

		R^2
From 1-7 socioeconomic factors		.58–.66
Program effort alone		.78
Socioeconomic factors plus program effort		.83
Net effect of social setting	.05	
Net effect of program effort	.17	
Joint effect	.58	

Summary

Analysis found strong association of CBR decline with socioeconomic factors, with even a few socioeconomic variables indicative of the complex whole. Significant additional association was found with addition of program effort (about 25 percent). Most of the effect was found to be joint, essentially in conformity with earlier study by Freedman and Berelson.

Further Modes of Analysis			
1. Path analysis			
Social setting	.67		A causal model was constructed in which social setting affects fertility decline directly and also through program effort. The indirect effect of social setting was found to be twice as large as its direct effect. The direct effect of program effort is quite large; its indirect effect is modest.
Direct effect	.23		
Joint and indirect effect	.44		
Program effort	.89		
Direct effect	.75		
Joint and indirect effect	.14		
2. Interaction effects			
1960 socioeconomic values and CBR declines, 1955–65 (38 cases)		.57	Analysis assumed relationship between socioeconomic variables and CBR decline is best reflected in Beta coefficients found before family planning programs were significant. Social setting found slightly less important than above; program effort very important.
Using those Beta coefficients:			
1970 socioeconomic values with CBR declines, 1965–75 (38 cases)		.53	
1970 socioeconomic values with CBR declines, 1965–75 (89 cases)		.47	
The last two, plus program effort		.78	
3. Change analysis			
Change in socioeconomic factors, 1960–70 with CBR declines, 1965–75 (35 cases)		.55	Analysis obtained approximately same level of association as using 1970 values, but data availability limits number of cases. Fewer variables permit more cases, but the R^2 values fall.
That plus program effort		.86	
4. Lag analysis			
Socioeconomic factors for 1960 with CBR declines, 1965–75 (48 cases)		.72	Essentially the same correlations were obtained as using 1970 values: for the 48 countries with 1970 data, .70; for the 66 countries adding program effort, .86.
That plus program effort, 1970–72 (66 cases)		.87	
5. Absolute CBR declines, 1965–75			
7 socioeconomic values, 1970 (89 cases)		.61	Results are essentially the same as for percentage decline.
7 socioeconomic values, 1960 (38 cases)		.64	
1970 socioeconomic values plus program effort		.79	

Cross-Tabulational Analysis

Now for the summary of the cross-tabulational analysis of the two indexes for the individual countries:

Social Setting and Program Effort	*Summary*
Differentiation of CBR decline by the two indexes of social setting and program effort in 4 categories each	Both differentiate: social setting by a factor of about 10 in the marginals, program effort by a factor of 15. There was a strong progression from upper left of table (high social setting, strong program effort) to lower right: 15–20 times as much fertility decline was found in the former as in the latter, with other values ranging rather regularly in between. Upper-left and lower-right cells set upper and lower limits of CBR reduction in developing countries for this period: from a high of about 30 percent, or 10–12 points off the CBR, to a low of essentially zero. These are the cells, of course, with the widest disparity in both modernization and program effort (not to mention ethnic differences also involved).
Qualitative factors	With the social setting index controlled, there is a clear relationship between CBR decline and ethnic status of the country (Muslim and African, low; Chinese, high), its island/density status, and its pace of social change.
Supplementary Analyses	
Duration of family planning program	The older the family planning program, the larger the CBR decline: countries with programs in place by 1965 had average declines of 22 percent, those with policies established during 1966–68 average declines of 14 percent, and those with policies established later (or not at all) average declines of 0–2 percent.

(Table continued)

Nature of family planning policy	Countries with policies to reduce population growth rates averaged about 18 percent in CBR decline; those with family planning programs for other than demographic reasons averaged only about 8 percent CBR decline; and those without programs had almost no fertility decline, perhaps 2 percent.
Exploratory data analysis	Using methods developed by Tukey and applied to the cross-tabulation of CBR declines by social setting and program effort, a special analysis by Zenas Sykes found that both factors are important but program effort "explains" much more of the CBR declines than does social setting, by a factor of about 4.

Accounting for the Fertility Decline

Let us try to take the summary one further step, in view of the policy issues and scientific disputes involved. Precisely how much of the observed fertility decline can be allocated to one or another influence—setting or program—cannot now be said with much assurance, given technical limitations in the state of the art and even basic conceptual differences as to how to go about providing an answer. There is a clear and present danger that even the degree of quantitative specifications we estimate below may be misunderstood, may be "taken too seriously," so we wish to preface the presentation with the caution that we are pushing against the limits of analysis—though these orders of magnitude may not be ludicrously removed from the truth, were that capable of being known.

So how account for the 1965–75 CBR decline? We take off from the way demographers decompose the crude birth rate into three components or major intermediate variables in order to account for fertility change up or down: change brought about by the age structure, by marriage patterns (mainly age at marriage), or by marital fertility itself. During the 1965–75 period, changes in age structure tended to increase the CBR somewhat, perhaps as much as 5–10 percent. Changes in age at marriage were quite significant upward, and, if we generalize from the relatively few countries for which we have adequate data (which are small numerically and unrepresentative as well, as in Table 15.3), then rising age at marriage accounted for rather more than one-third of the total decline, say, about 40 percent. Changes in marital fertility themselves accounted for the remainder of the decline, that is, about 70 percent.

How do we account for those shifts in magnitudes? Here again, definitive answers are not forthcoming, but some reasonable approximations can be offered based on our study—to be considered not as certain designations but rather as first orders to be tested and refined again, often in specific countries of some size, as we show below.

Major intermediate variables	Approximate contribution in 1965–75 CBR decline	Comment
Age structure	Slight negative contribution, say—5–10 percent	A single decade is a short time for substantial change in age structure, but because of the high fertility of earlier decades the proportion of married women of reproductive age in the population increased slightly, thus contributing to higher fertility, other things being equal.
Marital patterns	Substantial, say 35–45 percent	
attributable to changes induced by social setting	25 percent	Modernization tends to delay marriage; $R^2 = .62$ with our seven social setting variables.
attributable to legal sanctions and organized pressure (i.e., deliberate program), mainly in China	5–10 percent	Assumes that about one-fourth of China's decline comes from this campaign, with a slight addition from Tunisia on marriage age and perhaps one or two other places.
unattributed causes	5–10 percent	

(*Table continued*)

Marital fertility	Major, say 55–70 percent	
attributable to changes induced by social setting in fertility norms and with fertility control services provided from nonprogram sources	40–45 percent	The direct effect of the basic determinants of traditional demographic analysis, that is, the $R^2 = .66$ of the 55–70 percent.
minus a small effect from lessened lactation as a result of increased modernization	−5 percent	Shorter postpartum lactation has a slight tendency to raise fertility; indeed it appears to be the only important proximate determinant of fertility in addition to those mentioned above.[51]
attributable to organized family planning program effort (contraception, sterilization, abortion)	10–15 percent	Total explained minus that attributed to SES × percent due to change in marital fertility $(.83 - .66) \times (.55 - .70)$.
unattributed	10–15 percent	Unexplained × percent due to change in marital fertility $(1.00 - .83) \times (.55 - .70)$.

By this sort of accounting, then, the "credit" or source of the fertility decline analyzed here would come down to something like this:

Variable	Age structure	Marital patterns	Marital fertility	Total
Social setting		25 percent	40–45 percent − 5 percent lactation = 35–40 percent	60–65 percent
Program effort family planning			10–15 percent + 5 percent spillover = 15–20 percent	15–20 percent
legal sanctions and organized pressure		5–10 percent		5–10 percent
Consequence of earlier demographic trends	−5–10 percent			−5–10 percent
Unknown		5–10 percent	10–15 percent	15–25 percent
Total	−5–10 percent	35–45 percent	60–75 percent	approximately 100 percent

Quickly to repeat, these numbers are by no means precisely nor solidly documented; we have pushed them to their limits, well beyond the scientifically provable, in order to give a general idea of how things stand, given the present state of the art. And this of course refers to the total set of countries; such accounting could be different indeed within individual countries.

Actually, in the way our initial regression analyses were done, the correlation of socioeconomic factors with CBR decline ($R^2 = .66$) was maximized since these factors were considered in that model as prior and given, selected empirically as the most powerful and themselves uninfluenced to any degree by program effort (at least as yet, although such influence is the ultimate objective of program effort). Then the correlation with program effort is residually additional (increasing the R^2 by .17), and it adds far more than any socioeconomic factor beyond the first few in combination. Indeed, the Beta values for program effort are much larger than those for the socioeconomic factors. In other words, its values capture a far higher degree of association with CBR decline than do the socioeconomic factors; this is consistent with the cross-tabulational analysis and, as we shall see, with the predictive potential of the values.

That is what the data show from the standpoint of statistical correlation. Is that "explanation" or, even more, "causation"? This raises muddy and obscure epistemological questions on which qualified men of good will can and do differ in interpretation, and for our part we are almost prepared to leave it at that—except that we are persuaded, to repeat, (1) that the joint effect is more effective than either alone; (2) that program effort makes a substantial difference, not merely a trivial one; (3) that for policy purposes, given the wide disparity in developmental and family planning funding, great precision is not required for economic judgments as to policy; and (4) that from the scientific standpoint, it is in any case not attainable at this time. Further to the questions of precision and causation, deponent sayeth not.

A General Summary for the Policymaker

Finally, if we were asked to summarize the whole exercise for the informed policymaker, rather than the scientist, what would we say? Recognizing that to be a most legitimate responsibility (yet claiming all the caveats we can and referring doubts and criticisms to the academic haven of "need for further research"), our reply would go something like this:

- To begin with, there are of course all sorts of problems with data of this kind. Data on fertility and fertility change are far from adequate, but for some countries the data are quite good and where data are really bad they show no change in fertility anyway. No doubt different analysts would come up with a slightly different set of numbers, but it now seems clear that there have been significant fertility declines—some quite spectacular—in a sizable number of developing countries. The socioeconomic and demographic data are not as complete as we would like, and there are always questions of how accurate they are. We consider that large differences are correctly (if not always precisely) reflected in the data and that small differences don't matter much anyway. Our measure of program effort, centered on a given period in time, is essentially based on the subjective judgments of knowledgeable people, but judgments made on 15 different aspects of the program, some of them objective measures. Again, we are confident that those programs getting high scores are better programs, as these things go, and those getting low scores are less good. In the empirical event, a dichotomy of program effort captures the major discrimination, and program duration does reasonably well by itself.
- We studied 94 developing countries, containing 2.8 billion people or 98 percent of the population of all developing countries. We concentrated on the period 1965–75, during which there was substantial fertility decline in Asia (about 17 percent), quite a bit in the Americas (about 12 percent); but almost none in black Africa (though Tunisia, Egypt, and Mauritius did have significant declines on that continent). The large countries, those with populations of 35 million or more, showed greater declines than did smaller countries —13–16 percent as compared with 6–7 percent. China affects that average, to be sure, and we may well be underestimating China's decline (we use a CBR of 26 for 1975), but the conclusion remains essentially the same if China is left out of the analysis. Even so, several large countries have had hardly any change and still have high fertility—Bangladesh, Pakistan, Nigeria—and the changes in Mexico and Brazil are quite recent and still rather small.
- We looked at the data in a variety of ways: simple cross-tabulations of program effort and an index of socioeconomic variables; simple correlations between the variables; multiple regression analyses using both 1970 values of socioeconomic variables and, for the alternative lag theory, the 1960 values; change in the socioeconomic variables over time; a special form of regression analysis called path analysis in which program effort is considered to be partly a function of socioeconomic level; and a relatively new type of analysis called exploratory data analysis.
- From such data and analyses, we found that the level of "modernization" as reflected in our seven socioeconomic factors has a substantial relationship to fertility decline: the better-off countries, particularly those near the top, do better than the less well-off. That was to be expected in sociodemographic theory. But we also find, as a less-expectable finding, that on balance family planning programs have a significant, independent effect over and above the effect of socioeconomic factors. Some of the analyses show program effort to be more important than socioeconomic factors, but even the path analysis, which assumes program effort to be a function of the socioeconomic variables, shows that a good program effort adds substantially to the amount of fertility decline accounted for. Weak programs might as well not exist, so far as fertility reduction is concerned.
- Moreover, the longer a family planning program has existed, the greater its effect (although

there are several weak programs that have existed for many years). In addition, countries that have adopted population policies with demographic goals in order to reduce fertility or rates of natural increase have had much more fertility decline than countries with family planning programs adopted only for health or humanitarian reasons or with none at all.

• The key finding probably is that the two—social setting and program effort—go together most effectively. The joint analysis appears to "explain" or predict about 83 percent of the total variance in fertility decline. Countries that rank well on socioeconomic variables *and also* make substantial program effort have on average much more fertility decline than do countries that have one *or* the other, and far more than those with neither. The policy implications are that, if a country wants to reduce its fertility, it should seek a high degree of modernization (which of course all do, and find costly and difficult) and it should adopt a substantial family planning program; for countries at or near the bottom of the socioeconomic scale, however, the results would probably be slight and the administrative implementation very difficult. In such settings it requires a special kind of determination—as found in India, Indonesia, and China in the early to mid-1970s—to implement a strong program effort in a deprived setting. In short, without wishing to be misunderstood, one could conclude that the Bucharest judgment that family planning effort is of little consequence is itself of little consequence.

Some Final Observations

Assuming for the moment that the data are reasonably valid, what is to be made of all our findings as a prediction or "explanation" of the observed fertility declines?

There are still some conceptual issues in assessing determination of fertility trends that remain muddy. If development increases motivation for fertility control, which is then satisfied by a family planning program in the absence of other sources, how is the credit for the subsequent decline to be allocated? What if under the same social conditions the same decline of fertility would appear in the absence of program effort, but only N years later? What if development establishes a general infrastructural capability that then is utilized to launch a strong program effort, which in turn has a demonstrable effect? Questions of this kind are largely bypassed in the current state of the art.

Given the received wisdom, is our result believable—that program effort has a substantial effect on CBR decline? What are the possible explanations for this result? We can identify five, which need not be mutually exclusive but may be supplementary on such a complex matter:

1. There is the technical dismissal—that the finding is based on faulty data, faulty mode(s) of analysis, and/or faulty classifications. That is of course possible, though we have taken what pains we could on all these counts. If this is the fact, however, it would presumably apply equally to formally similar studies in the scientific literature, as cited above—from which the traditional wisdom has itself emerged.

2. It might be that fertility was already declining in countries undertaking family planning programs and that such programs served merely an expediting or facilitating role, not an initiating one. In the absence of program effort, by this argument, equivalent declines would have occurred, but perhaps in a somewhat longer period of time. Unfortunately, social science does not know how to test for the what-would-have-happened-if condition—and not just in this field—but programs, if economic of resources as weighed against alternatives, can be considered effective even if relegated to a facilitating role. And given the power of demographic momentum, expediting a slower rate of growth is itself a valuable product.

3. If it is development or modernization or some traditional component(s) thereof that lead to (account for, determine, cause) fertility decline, such development also generates not only the establishment of family planning policy but the actual implementation of the program; this is the indirect or infrastructural argument. In this view, the programs arise only in order to satisfy the motivation that development itself creates. Here again there is the question of the quantitative allocation of "credit," in magnitude and time (which we have tried to measure, as reported above). If program effort is simply "another" discriminating factor within social setting, then its additional effect as compared to further socioeconomic factors needs

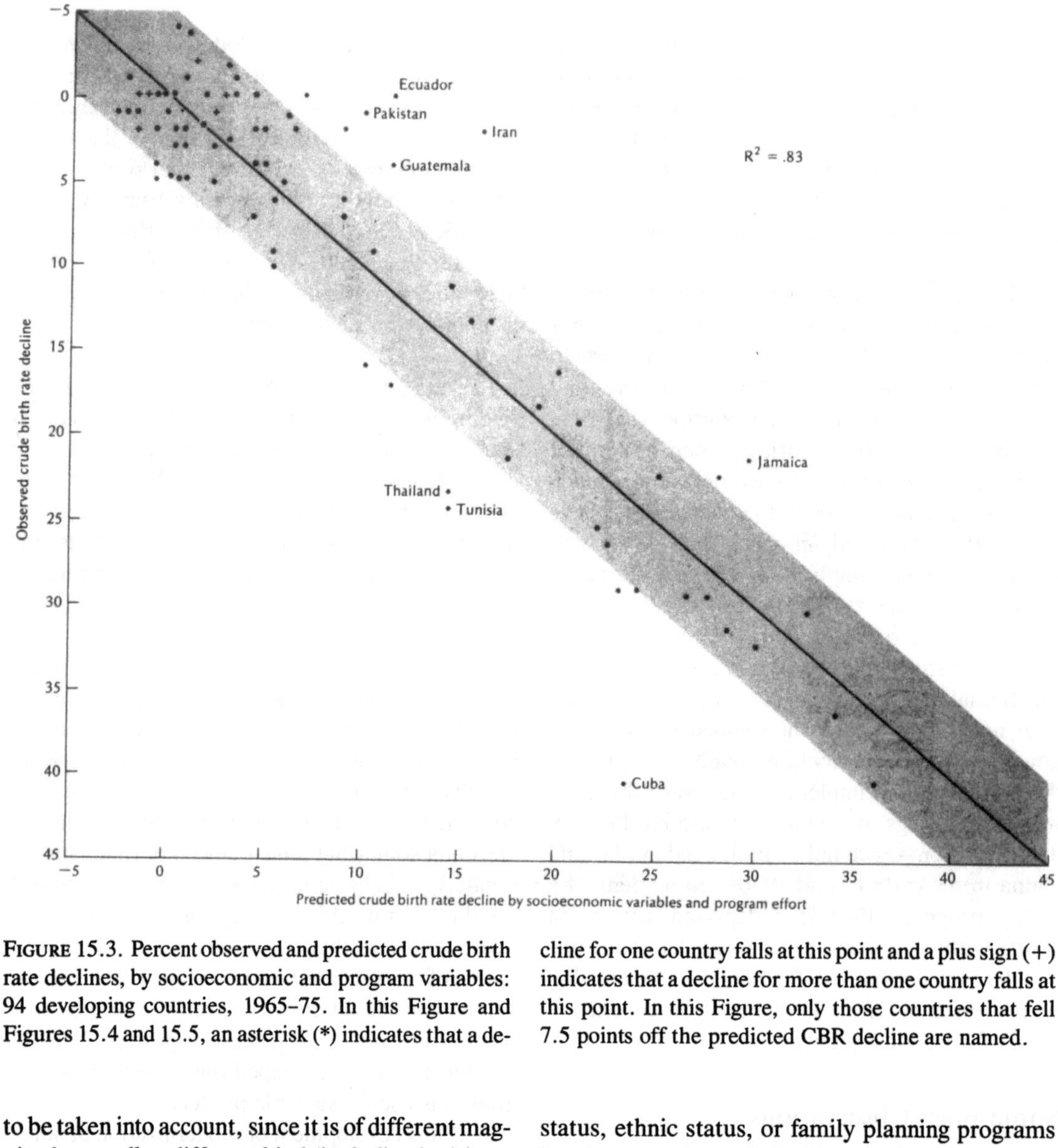

FIGURE 15.3. Percent observed and predicted crude birth rate declines, by socioeconomic and program variables: 94 developing countries, 1965–75. In this Figure and Figures 15.4 and 15.5, an asterisk (*) indicates that a decline for one country falls at this point and a plus sign (+) indicates that a decline for more than one country falls at this point. In this Figure, only those countries that fell 7.5 points off the predicted CBR decline are named.

to be taken into account, since it is of different magnitude as well as different kind (including legitimation and spillover). Moreover, the cases off the diagonal – for example, India and Indonesia in one direction and Mexico and Brazil in the other – need to be explained in this line of argument.

4. Perhaps the determinants of fertility decline, as individually independent, identifiable, and discrete factors, whether of the demand or the supply type, need to give way as concept to the "holistic process" of societal transformation – in which fertility change goes along with all the other changes in a mutually interdependent manner. In this conception,[52] fertility change is not "caused" by education, urbanization, lowered mortality, women's status, ethnic status, or family planning programs but is part of a whole historical movement in which, as someone has said, everything goes over the dam together. This point of view does some violence to the common-sense view, and still one scientific view, that such changes are somehow individually accountable, and in any case does not make obsolete either the question that some factors are more closely associated with fertility change than others, within the "holistic process," or the policy issues of efficient intervention.

5. Perhaps the finding is correct, and program effort does make a substantial difference to fertility decline over the period of a decade, along with social setting.[53]

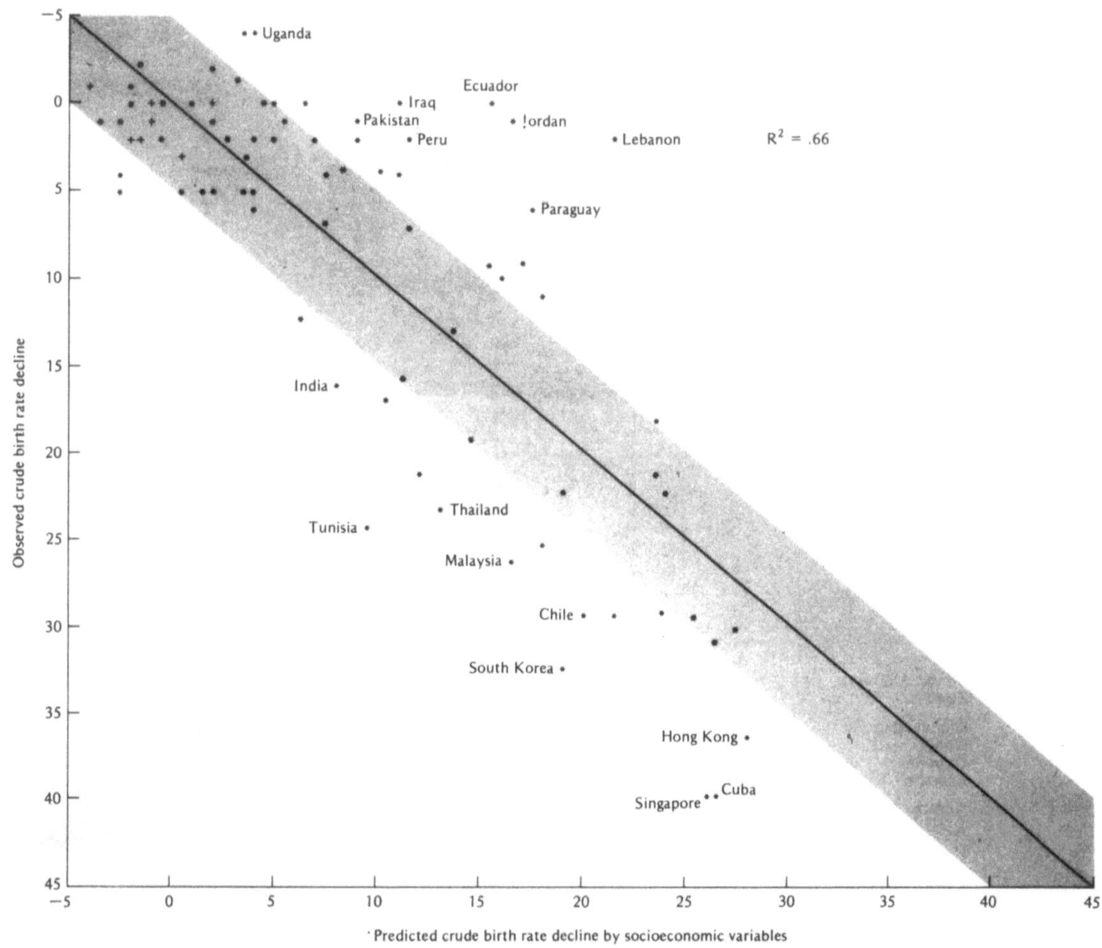

FIGURE 15.4. Percent observed and predicted crude birth rate declines, by socioeconomic variables: 94 developing countries, 1965–75.

We conclude by noting the predictive potential of our analysis—on the ground that prediction has something to do with explanation. The seven socioeconomic factors and program effort together yield a predicted CBR decline quite close to the observed decline (see Figure 15.3), with an R^2 of .83. Outside the shaded area (which includes all cases plus or minus 5 percentage points from perfect correlation) fall only 17 countries, and 9 of them are marginal (i.e., within 6 points of perfect correlation). By this overall measure, the major deviants are Cuba (16 points off), Iran (14), Ecuador and Tunisia (11), Pakistan and Jamaica (9), and Thailand (8). Moreover, as expected from both our correlational and cross-tabulational analyses, this combination does substantially better in predicting CBR decline than either the socioeconomic factors or program effort alone, with the latter being more predictive than the former (Figures 15.4 and 15.5). As is indicated in the table, twice as many countries fall outside the band when only socioeconomic variables are used as compared with the prediction based on the combination, and half again as many as with program effort alone.

It remains for us to emphasize that throughout this paper we have been concerned with the *effectiveness* of influences upon fertility decline, not with the *efficiency* of policy interventions, defined as effectiveness per dollar of investment. From the policy point of view, it is typically efficiency that is at issue since resources are inevitably limited. In this connection a rational approach to policy would

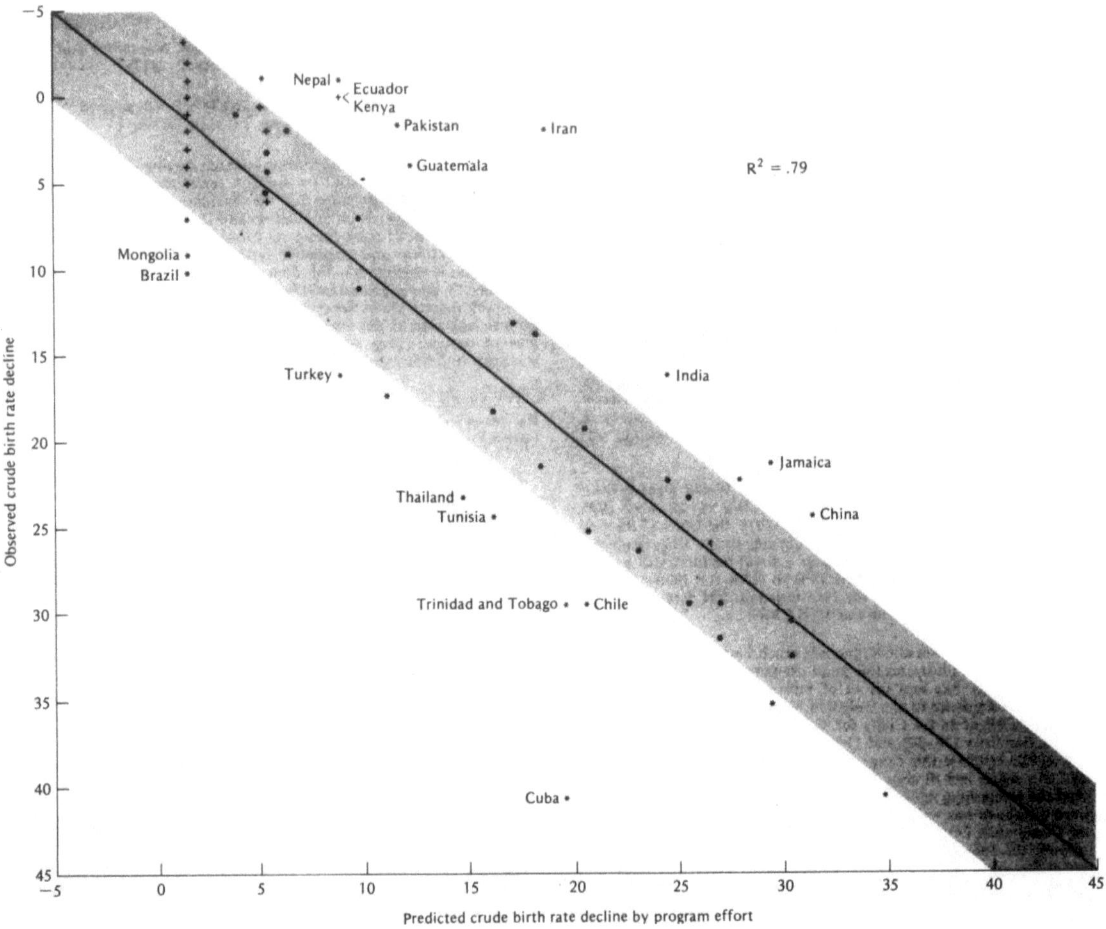

FIGURE 15.5. Percent observed and predicted crude birth rate declines, by program variables: 94 developing countries, 1965–75.

be to ask, for example, how much it would cost to achieve a change in the socioeconomic factors that would result in a fertility decline of x amount as against a change in program effort that would also result in a fertility decline of x amount (assuming that fertility decline is a proximate objective of policy). From this standpoint, a given policy may be most efficient even though not most effective.[54] In the real world, of course, the socioeconomic factors are far more expensive and difficult of realization than is program effort. Policy rests on realizable interventions, not on theoretical explanations.

In any case, the record for the period 1965–75 shows that large CBR declines in developing countries were strongly associated with substantial program effort and high social setting was associated with only modest CBR declines, unless linked with significant family planning effort. Countries with both significant program effort and high social setting had an average CBR decline of about 30 percent; those with only significant program effort, a decline of about 20 percent; those with high social setting alone, a drop of 5 percent; and those with neither, a zero change.

If the past record can be extrapolated to the future, a country that wished to reduce its CBR substantially would be well advised to institute a family planning program of at least moderate strength. Given the existence of a moderate program effort, improving social setting takes precedence; but relying only on enhanced social setting would appear to result in a slower decrease in CBR than could be achieved with explicit attention to the intermediate or instrumental variable of fertility control services, as a supplementing and expediting policy measure.

As always in such analyses, one would like to have more complete, more timely, more appropriate, more valid data—not to mention more incisive methods of analysis. But at least we trust that this analysis suggests how the question of international and cross-cultural determinants of fertility decline can be approached at the macro level. To revert to our title, we hope that we have thus illuminated the conditions of fertility decline in developing countries, 1965–75.

Notes

[1]For example, in France the birth rate began to decline before the end of the 18th century, and in the United States by the beginning of the 19th century. Ansley J. Coale, "The history of the human population," *Scientific American* 231, no. 3 (September 1974):48. A similar decline was noted in Austria-Hungary in the 19th century; see Paul Demeny, "Early fertility decline in Austria-Hungary: A lesson in demographic transition," *Daedalus* (Spring 1968):502–522.

[2]See, for example: Ronald Freedman and Bernard Berelson, "The record of family planning programs," *Studies in Family Planning* 7, no. 1 (January 1976); Ronald Freedman and John Y. Takeshita, *Family Planning in Taiwan* (Princeton University Press, 1969) chapter 13; Tieng Pardthaisong, *The Recent Fertility Decline in the Chiang Mai Area of Thailand*, Papers of the East West Population Institute, no. 47, (Honolulu, 1978); W. Brass, "Impact of the family planning programme on fertility in Mauritius," *IPPF Medical Bulletin* 10, no. 4 (August 1976): 1–2; Terence H. Hull, Valerie J. Hull, and Masri Singarimbun, "Indonesia's family planning story: Success and challenge," *Population Bulletin* 32, no. 6:1–52.

[3]John Bongaarts, "A framework for analyzing the proximate determinants of fertility," *Working Papers* (New York: Center for Policy Studies, The Population Council, January 1978) p. 1.

[4]World Bank, *Population Policies and Economic Development*, a World Bank Staff Report, coordinating author, Timothy King, Appendix B, "The relationship between program inputs, socioeconomic levels, and family planning performance: A regression analysis" (Baltimore: Johns Hopkins University Press, 1974) pp. 149–163; Bernard Berelson, "An evaluation of the effects of population control programmes," in H. B. Parry, ed., *Population and Its Problems: A Plain Man's Guide* (Oxford: Clarendon Press, 1974) pp. 133–168; K. S. Srikantan, *The Family Planning Program in the Socioeconomic Context,* (New York: The Population Council, 1977); Ronald Freedman and Bernard Berelson, 1976, pp. 1–40.

[5]Kingsley Davis, "Population analysis and social behavior," paper presented at the Conference on Research in Human Relations (New York: The Rockefeller Foundation, [early 1950s]) pp. 3–4.

[6]A. J. Coale, "The demographic transition reconsidered," *International Conference, Liege, 1973* (Liege: IUSSP, 1973) vol. 1, p. 65.

[7]For a recent review see Nancy Birdsall, "Analytical approaches to the relationships of population growth and development," *Population and Development Review* 3, nos. 1–2 (March-June 1977):63–102, especially "Macro-determinants research," pp. 79–82.

[8]From another kind of literature, note this observation from *The Forsyte Saga* (from chapter I of *In Chancery*):

> Thus, of the ten old Forsytes twenty-one young Forsytes had been born; but of the twenty-one young Forsytes there were as yet only seventeen descendants; and it already seemed unlikely that there would be more than a further unconsidered trifle or so. A student of statistics must have noticed that the birth rate had varied in accordance with the rate of interest for your money. Grandfather 'superior Dosset' Forsyte in the early nineteenth century had been getting ten per cent for his, hence ten children. Those ten, leaving out the four who had not married, and Juley, whose husband Septimus Small had, of course, died almost at once, had averaged from four to five per cent for theirs, and produced accordingly. The twenty-one whom they produced were now getting barely three per cent in the Consols to which their father had mostly tied the Settlements they made to avoid death duties, and the six of them who had been reproduced had seventeen children, or just the proper two and five-sixths per stem.
>
> There were other reasons, too, for this mild reproduction. A distrust of their earning powers, natural where a sufficiency is guaranteed, together with the knowledge that their fathers did not die, kept them cautious. If one had children and not much income, the standard of taste and comfort must of necessity go down; what was enough for two was not enough for four, and so on—it would be better to wait and see what Father did. Besides, it was nice to be able to take holidays unhampered. Sooner in fact than own children, they preferred to concentrate on the ownership of themselves, conforming to the growing tendency—*fin de siècle,* as it was called. In this way, little risk was run, and one would be able to have a motor car. . . . In the meantime, no more children!

Thus did Galsworthy anticipate Becker and Easterlin!

[9]United Nations, Department of Economics and Social Affairs, *Population Bulletin,* no. 7–1963, "With special reference to conditions and trends of fertility in the world" (United Nations, 1965); Dudley Kirk, "A new demographic transition?" in *Rapid Population Growth; Consequences and Policy Implications* (published for the National Academy of Science by the Johns Hopkins University Press, 1971) pp. 138–145; K. S. Srikantan, 1977.

[10]Kirk, 1971, pp. 145–146.

[11]United Nations, 1965, p. 150.

[12]Paul Gregory, John Campbell, and Benjamin Cheng, "Differences in fertility determinants: Developed and developing countries," *Journal of Development Studies* 9 (1972):233–241; Steven E. Beaver, *Demographic Transition Theory Reinterpreted: An Application to Recent Natality Trends in Latin America* (Lexington, 1975); World Bank, 1974.

[13]The primary sources are the various yearbooks of the UN system, including the *Demographic Yearbook*, the *Statistical Yearbook*, UNESCO's *Statistical Yearbook*, FAO's *Production Yearbook*, and *World Tables* by the World Bank.

[14]Data contained in United Nations' *Selected World Demographic Indicators by Countries, 1950–2000*, ESA/P/WP.55, 28 May 1975, were used to estimate total fertility rates. For 1975, the UN's TFRs were adjusted by the ratio of our 1975 CBR estimates to the UN's projected CBRs. For 1965, the United Nations gave general fertility rates but not TFRs. We assumed that the ratio of TFR to GFR for 1970–1975 was a constant, then estimated TFRs for 1965 based on UN data, and finally adjusted them to correspond with our 1965 CBRs.

[15]To repeat the caution above, there is much uncertainty about some of the figures. China illustrates this point dramatically, since the Chinese have released only bits and pieces of information—and, of course, it contributes substantially to the weighted figures in view of its size. We have used a CBR of 26 for China for 1975, which is consistent with the figures of Bannister (26–30) and Orleans (27), and is somewhat below Aird's middle estimate (his range being 21–34, with the medium value of 28). Our figure is well above the dramatic figure of Brown (CBR of 19) and the astonishing figure of Ravenholt (CBR of 14).

Since the above was written, the Chairman of the Central Committee of the Communist Party in China, Hua Kuo-feng, stated that their goal is to lower the annual rate of population growth to less than 1 percent within three years. That statement was made in March 1978. Assume their goal is an increase of 1 percent in 1981 and that the crude death rate will be 7–8 per 1,000: This would imply a goal of a crude birth rate of 17–18 in 1981. Assume further that their ambitious plans are to at least equal declines experienced in some developing countries of 1–1.5 points per year: This would suggest a crude birth rate of 24–27 for 1975, and 22–24 for 1977. If mortality is falling rapidly, the estimated crude birth rate for 1975 and 1977 would be slightly higher than the figures just quoted.

Similarly, for Brazil we have chosen to base our estimate for 1965 on Carvalho rather than on Merrick or Berquo although a strong case can be made for using either of the latter figures. Similarly, most observers agree that fertility is declining in India, though there is less consensus on the level of fertility; the Indonesian figures are less firm but there is substantial evidence that fertility has begun to decline; and some students of demographic trends in Pakistan argue that fertility has declined in that country but we have yet to see the evidence. For sources, see: Judith Bannister, "Implementing fertility and mortality decline in the People's Republic of China—Recent official data," in *The Current Vital Rates and Population Size of the People's Republic of China and Its Provinces*, Ph.D. dissertation, Food Research Institute, Stanford University, 1977, paper presented at the Annual Meeting of the Population Association of America, St. Louis, April 1977; Leo A. Orleans, "China's birth rate, death rate, and population growth: Another perspective," in Report Prepared for the Committee on International Relations, US House of Representatives, by the Congressional Research Service, Library of Congress, September 1977; John Aird, Letter to *People* 4, no. 2 (1977):49–51; Lester R. Brown, "World population trends: Signs of hope, signs of stress," *World Watch Paper* 8 (October 1976); R. T. Ravenholt, Letter to *People* 3, no. 4 (1976):51; J. A. M. Carvalho, "Regional trends in fertility and mortality in Brazil, *Population Studies* 28, no. 3 (August 1974); Thomas W. Merrick, "Interregional difference in fertility in Brazil, 1950–1970," *Demography* 11, no. 3 (August 1974); Elsa S. Berquo, "Fecondite," in *La Population du Bresil*, CICRED Series, 1974.

[16]M. Badrud Duza and C. Stephen Baldwin, *Nuptiality and Population Policy* (New York: The Population Council, 1977).

[17]J. C. Caldwell, "Fertility decline and female chances of marriage in Malaya," *Population Studies* 17, no. 1 (1963):20–32.

[18]Gavin W. Jones, "Social science research on population and development in East and South-East Asia: A review and search for directions," Draft report prepared for the International Review Group of Social Science Research on Population and Development (Mexico City, January 1978) p. 21, and James A. Palmore and Ariffin bin Marzuki, "Marriage patterns and cumulative fertility in West Malaysia," *Demography* 6, no. 4 (1969):383–401. Jones points out that marriage patterns also vary by ethnic groups in Indonesia and Thailand. Moreover, there are many reports about the emphasis the mainland Chinese have placed on late marriage; if this strong campaign has had even a moderate degree of success, rising age at marriage probably has contributed substantially to fertility decline in China.

[19]John Knodel, *Fertility and Family Planning in Thailand: Results of the Second Round of a National Survey*, Paper no. 19 (Bangkok: Institute of Population Studies, Chulalongkorn University, 1977).

[20]Ansley J. Coale, "The demographic transition," *The Population Debate: Dimensions and Perspectives* (United Nations, 1975) p. 353.

[21]Paul Demeny, 1968, p. 510.

[22]N. B. Ryder, "Fertility" in Philip M. Hauser and Otis Dudley Duncan, eds., *The Study of Population* (University of Chicago Press, 1959) p. 410.

[23]Economic Commission for Europe, "Recent demographic trends in Europe and the outlook until the year 2000," in *The Population Debate: Dimensions and Perspectives,* (United Nations, 1975) p. 277.

[24]For a sample of recent reviews on the matter, see Bernard Berelson, "Social science research on population: A review," *Population and Development Review* 2, no. 2 (June 1976):219–266; Bernard Berelson, "Social science research for population policy," paper prepared for The International Review Group of Social Science Research on Population and Development, June 1977; Nancy Birdsall, "Analytical approaches to the relationship of population growth and development," *Population and Development Review* 3, nos. 1–2 (March-June 1977); John C. Caldwell, "Toward a restatement of demographic transition theory," *Population and Development Review* 2, nos. 3–4 (September-December 1976):321–366; Robert H. Cassen, "Population and development: A survey," *World Development* 4, nos. 10–11 (1976):785–830; Coale, 1973, pp. 53–72; Susan H. Cochrane, "Education and fertility: What do we really know?", Population and Human Resources Division, World Bank, March 1977; Interdisciplinary Communications Program, *The Policy Relevance of Recent Social Research on Fertility,* an ICP Staff Report (Washington, D.C.: Smithsonian Institution, September 1974); Research Triangle Institute, *Social and Economic Correlates of Family Fertility: A Survey of the Evidence,* prepared by Karen Oppenheim Mason and Abraham S. David, project leaders, September 1971; Nwanganga Shields, "Female labor force participation and fertility: Review of empirical evidence from L.D.C.," Population and Human Resources Division, World Bank, February 1977; Michael Teitelbaum, "Relevance of demographic transition theory for developing countries," *Science* 188 (2 May 1975):420–425.

[25]Infant mortality rates are not available for many of the developing countries and, where not available, are inferred from model life tables. This procedure leads to a high correlation between the two measures, but we have retained both inasmuch as separate data are available for a number of countries.

[26]For further discussion along this line, see Ronald Ridker, ed., *Population and Development: The Search for Selective Interventions* (Baltimore: Johns Hopkins University Press, 1976).

[27]A recent publication of the World Fertility Survey, for example, found that the average "time of travel to perceived nearest outlet" for methods of fertility regulation was as follows (in minutes):

Area	India	Panama	Turkey
Medians			
Urban	15	15	10
Rural	30	30	30
Means			
Urban	26	19	13
Rural	51	31	57

Source: German Rodriguez, "Assessing the availability of fertility regulation methods: Report on a methodological study," *World Fertility Survey, Scientific Report no. 1,* February 1977, Table 3.9.1, p. 52. The data are taken from in-depth pilot studies designed to determine the feasibility of obtaining information on household and community availability of fertility control methods. Accordingly, the data should be considered as illustrative.

[28]As initially presented in Robert J. Lapham and W. Parker Mauldin, "National family planning programs: Review and evaluation," *Studies in Family Planning* 3, no. 3 (March 1972):31–34 and Table 2.B. The same index was used in Bernard Berelson, 1974, pp. 133–168; and in Freedman and Berelson, 1976.

[29]Twenty countries were included in the original Lapham-Mauldin list; another 23 were added in the Freedman-Berelson extension; and a final 11 were added for this paper: China, North Vietnam, Cuba, Panama, Brazil, Iraq, Nicaragua, Bolivia, Papua New Guinea, Uganda, and Mali. Since the original classification was done around 1970–71, the ratings of a few countries were revised in the light of later developments—Pakistan/Bangladesh downward in view of the suspension of program activities associated with the 1970–71 civil war and its aftermath; the Philippines and Indonesia upward in view of their intensified efforts as of about 1970–72. In general, as will be seen later, this classification correlates strongly with both duration of program effort and demographic commitment in policy (as against health or human rights). Furthermore, 17 of the 26 strong and moderate programs had numerical demographic targets around 1969–70 as against only 3 out of 29 weak programs (counting Pakistan/Bangladesh as one).

[30]For further detail on several countries, see Freedman and Berelson, 1976, pp. 20–29.

[31]We have benefited in this analysis from the consultation and advice of Professor Leo Goodman of the University of Chicago, to whom we express our gratitude.

As a technical reminder, we briefly describe the measures utilized in this section.

Coefficient of Correlation. Where the relationship between two variables is found or assumed to be a straight line, the value of $\sigma'/\sigma y$ is termed the coefficient of correlation. The symbol R is used to represent it. When values of *Y* are estimates from values of *X* according to a straight-line equation, then the proportion of the variation in *Y* which is so accounted for is indicated by the notation R_{yx}' which is read "the coefficient of correlation between *y* and *x*." The coefficient of correlation may therefore be defined:

$$R_{yx} = \frac{\sigma y'}{\sigma y}$$

Coefficient of Determination. Where both *X* and *Y* are assumed to be built up of simple elements of equal variability all of which are present in *Y* but some of which are lacking in *X,* it can be proved mathematically that R^2

measures that proportion of all the elements in *Y* which are also present in *X*. For that reason, in cases where the dependent variable is known to be causally related to the independent variable, R^2 may be called the coefficient of determination. It may be said to measure the percentage to which the variance in *Y* is determined by *X* since it measures the proportion of all the elements of variance in *Y* which are also present in *X*. Since the coefficient of determination is the most direct and unequivocal way of stating the proportion of the variance in the dependent factor which is associated with the independent factor, it should be used in preference to the correlation coefficient.

Partial Correlation. Coefficients of partial correlation measure the correlation between the dependent factor and each of the independent factors, while eliminating any (linear) tendency of the remaining independent factors to obscure the relation. The other factors are "held constant," that is, are assumed to have the same values. The partial correlation coefficient $R_{12.3}'$ or $p_{12.3}$ is the correlation between variables 1 and 2 in a cross section of individuals *all having the same values of variable 3.* "Partial correlation does not involve the notion of independent and dependent variables; it is a measure of interdependence. On the other hand, the *multiple correlation coefficient* applies to the situation in which one variable, say *Y*, has been singled out to examine its joint relation with the other variables. In the population, the multiple correlation coefficient between *Y* and X_1, X_2 $\ldots X_k$ is defined as the simple correlation coefficient between *Y* and its linear regression $B_1X_1 + B_2X_2 \ldots + B_kX_k$ on $X_1 \ldots X_k$. Since it is hard to attach a useful meaning to the sign of this correlation, most applications deal with its square." George W. Snedecor and William G. Cochran, *Statistical Methods* (Ames: The Iowa State University Press, 1967), p. 402.

The Beta Coefficient. The coefficient of regression measures the slope of the regression line; that is, it shows the average number of units of increase or decrease in the dependent variable that occur with each increase of a specified unit in the independent variable. When each value of a variable is expressed in deviation from the standard deviation of that variable, the Beta coefficient shows the average number of units of increase or decrease. Partial correlations measure how much a given variable reduces the variation in the dependent variable after all the other variables except it are taken into account. Partial correlations and Beta coefficients are two different measures of the relative importance of different factors. Their exact values differ but usually the rank and relative size of the two measures are similar.

[32]Substituting percentage urban for percentage of population living in cities of 100,000+ does not affect the R^2 value with this set of socioeconomic variables.

[33]In such correlations, the results depend upon where one starts. For example, the correlation between program effort and CBR decline (R^2) is .74 (thus more predictive than the 7 socioeconomic factors taken together), and as from one to all seven of those factors are added, the R^2 increases to between .82 and .83.

[34]Here again, another multiple R^2 plateau asserts itself: when program effort is combined with from one to six of the demand variables, the R^2's all fall within the range .821 to .828. Only when the "intensifier" variable of newspaper circulation is added does it increase, and then to only .843 for the entire array.

[35]Freedman and Berelson, 1976, Table 10 and the tabulation on p. 19. The replicated method is reported on p. 40 of that publication.

[36]Otis Dudley Duncan, "Path analysis: Sociological examples," *American Journal of Sociology* 72, no. 1 (July 1966):3.

[37]M. G. Kendall and C. A. O'Muircheártaigh, *Path Analysis and Model Building*, No. 2/Tech 414, World Fertility Survey, Technical Bulletins, March 1977.

[38]The path coefficients for each of the seven socioeconomic variables and CBR declines range from .08 to .30 (GNP per capita and life expectancy), and the corresponding path coefficient between program effort and CBR decline range from .88 to .69. The indirect effects of the socioeconomic variables through program effort range from .05 to .46.

[39]For a similar analysis of direct and indirect effects, see Srikantan, 1977.

[40]There are several different measures of change that can be used, and we have used three. First, the difference in percentages in 1960 and 1970: for example, for school enrollment we subtracted the percentage enrolled in 1960 from the percentage enrolled in 1970. Second, the percentage change in the variable between the two dates: for example, life expectancy at birth in 1960 was subtracted from life expectancy at birth in 1970, and that figure multiplied by 100 was divided by life expectancy at birth in 1960. Third, in the case of literacy, the difference in percentage literate 1960 to 1970 as a ratio of the proportion illiterate at the earlier date and multiplied by 100; we label this as proportionate increase 1960–70. More generally, we sought the measure of change that was most closely associated with CBR decline, and for each variable used the measure that could explain the largest amount of variance in the CBR decline.

[41]D. V. McGranahan, C. Richard-Proust, N. V. Sovani, and M. Subramanian, *Contents and Measurement of Socioeconomic Development*, (New York: Praeger Publishers, 1972), and *Research Data Bank of Development Indicators* prepared by the Statistical Unit of the Institute, United Nations Research Institute for Social Development, Report No. 76.3, Geneva, 1976.

[42]Srikantan has analyzed fertility decline as a function of family planning programs and socioeconomic factors for 20 program countries and for 10 countries in East and Southeast Asia (with an overlap of 8 countries in the two groups). He employed a variety of statistical tech-

niques, including correlations, partial and multiple correlations, path analysis, and principal component analysis. He identifies five types of effects, namely, direct socioeconomic effects, direct program effects, infrastructural effects on program inputs of socioeconomic factors, spillover of program inputs to the nonprogram sector, and substitution of program services for nonprogram birth control. He summarizes his major findings as follows:

> Analysis of 20 program countries drawn from different cultural regions indicates that the direct effects of the socioeconomic indicators and the program outputs were substantial and about equal. The infrastructural effect was about one-half as large, and the spillover effect about one-fourth as large. An analysis of a more homogeneous group of ten countries in East and Southeast Asia in greater depth showed that the direct effect of the socioeconomic indicators is about as large as the program spillover effect, while the indirect effect of the socioeconomic indicators was three-fourths as large and the program output effect one-half as large (pp. 232–233).

[43]Under some conditions, as our colleague Anrudh Jain reminds us, "improvements in social setting may also increase the birth rate especially if there are changes in breastfeeding, abstinence, occupational related separation, and mortality. Thus the total and relative contributions of demand and supply factors may be underestimated in this analysis" (personal communication, 1978).

[44]As against individual country, where the range is from 40 percent decrease (Singapore and Cuba) to 4 percent increase (Lesotho and Uganda).

[45]For example, see Dudley Kirk, "Factors affecting Moslem natality," in Bernard Berelson et al. (eds.), *Family Planning and Population Programs* (The University of Chicago Press, 1966), pp. 561–579; and Irene B. Taeuber, "Policies, programs, and the decline of birth rates: China and the Chinese populations of East Asia," in Minoru Muramatsu and Paul A. Harper (eds.), *Population Dynamics* (Baltimore: Johns Hopkins Press, 1965), pp. 99–104. Note also that ethnic differences—linguistic and cultural—are closely associated with fertility rates in developed countries as well, e.g., in Belgium (R. Lesthaeghe and E. Van de Walle, "Economic factors and fertility decline in France and Belgium," in Ansley J. Coale (ed.), *Economic Factors in Population Growth,* (New York: Macmillan, 1976); or in Spain (Ansley J. Coale, "The demographic transition reconsidered"); or other countries (Bernard Berelson, "Ethnicity and fertility: What and so what," Working Paper, Center for Policy Studies, Population Council, 1978).

[46]For example, see *People* 4, no. 2 (1977) on "Aspects of islands." And this notion may apply not only to islands in the literal sense; reports from China remark the same effect from restrictions on outmigration from villages.

[47]Taeuber, 1965, p. 100. Note that this measure of "precipitant social change" differs from the more gradual changes in exclusively socioeconomic factors reviewed in the correlational material. When the latter are classified into a 4-part index, it does not differentiate well among CBR declines—not nearly so well as the social-setting index.

[48]The dating and duration of programs is taken from Walter B. Watson (ed.), *Family Planning in the Developing World: A Review of Programs*, A Population Council Factbook, (New York: Population Council, 1977), footnote to Table 1, p. 2; and from Dorothy Nortman, assisted by Ellen Hofstatter, "Population and Family Planning Programs: A Factbook," *Reports on Population/Family Planning,* no. 2, eighth ed. (October 1976): Table 6.

[49]Nortman and Hofstatter, 1977, p. 21.

[50]Because these methods may be unfamiliar to many readers, we have included brief explanations of them as they arise in the analysis. For a complete description, see John W. Tukey, *Exploratory Data Analysis* (Reading, Mass.: Addison-Wesley, 1977). For an introductory summary, see Donald R. McNeil, *Interactive Data Analysis* (New York: Wiley, 1975).

[51]Bongaarts, 1978.

[52]This is the case in the following conclusions by Frank Wm. Oechsli and Dudley Kirk, "Modernization and the demographic transition in Latin America and the Caribbean," *Economic Development and Cultural Change* 23, no. 3 (April 1975):391–419. These conclusions do, however, put aside the questions of "causation":

> In fact, we cannot easily distinguish between cause and effect in the complex of changes we label 'modernization.' We can say that modernization, at some level, is associated with a given mortality level, and we can say that the birth rate tends to stay high until some critical level of development is reached and then tends to decline as development proceeds, but we cannot say that development 'causes' declining birth and death rates; rather, certain patterns of change in these vital rates are parts of the process of development.
>
> Similarly, we might argue that one or the other of the variables is the key element in causing, say, birth-rate declines, but such an argument, at present levels of understanding, often seems to be more an exercise in developing intuitively pleasing and plausible explanations than a serious research aim.
>
> Thus, the theoretical basis for the present study avoids attempts to outline specific causal chains and, instead, proceeding from the postulate that development is an orderly holistic process with some empirically determinable consistencies, attempts to fit changes in birth and death rates into the process (pp. 403–404).

[53]Our colleague Geoffrey McNicoll made the following comment on an earlier version. We include it with his permission and our thanks in view of its intrinsic value:

> I take it as tautology that (marital) fertility declines when there is an appropriate shift in the micro-level calculus encompassing perceived benefits and costs of having children or endeavoring not to have them. Effective antinatalist-policy measures must impinge on this micro-setting. At the national level, policies tend to be either focused directly on fertility (propaganda about

family size, subsidizing contraceptives, etc.) or focused indirectly (i.e., have other primary goals, such as educating women, but incidentally change the micro-setting of fertility decision making). Looked at from this level, then, it is hardly surprising at least in the early stages of transition to find a measure of "program effort" (directly addressing fertility) more closely tied to a fertility change than is a broad-based measure of development.

But there is another dimension involved in addition to 'breadth' of policy content: this is closeness to the individual decision making setting. Pulling a lever at the national level—say, pouring money into a family planning program or into an educational system—may have virtually any outcome depending on the internal workings of that program or system. What matters is how things change at the bottom. Your index of program effort spans both national and local levels (e.g., customs regulations on the one hand, home visits on the other)—with more emphasis on the latter than is the case with your components of development (although certainly this is a matter of judgment). In a sense, then, there is more scope for slips twixt cup and lip on the development side than on the program effort side. (Personal communication.)

[54]For an exploration along this line, see Robert Haveman and Bernard Berelson, "Intervention strategy and resource allocation for fertility reduction." Chapter 6 and see Bibliography entry on p. 264 in this volume.

Appendix: Status of Women

There is some agreement that the position of women in society is significantly related to the level of fertility, though there is substantial difference about specifics. For example the World Population Plan of Action states that one important way to moderate fertility is through "the full integration of women into the development process, particularly by means of their greater participation in educational, social, economic and political opportunities, and especially by means of the removal of obstacles to their employment in the nonagricultural sector wherever possible" (para. 32).

We searched for but did not find an accepted index of women's status in developing countries. There are many possible indexes of women's position within a country[1] and some useful analyses of appropriate indicators,[2] but data are rarely available in a reliable form or quantity.

In view of its special interest in connection with fertility decline, we include here a more detailed consideration of the status of women—which might have been included as another socioeconomic variable had sufficient data of a suitable measure been available. Female enrollment in school and female employment in nonagricultural occupations correlate highly with male enrollment and employment, and thus reflect educational and industrial status rather than female status. As noted, we looked for but did not find a valid index of female status in developing countries with reasonably available data.

The one indicator of female status we found to be distinctive was the percentage of young women never married, particularly for the 20–24 age group. The zero order correlation of this variable with the 1965–75 CBR decline for the 56 countries for which data are currently available is .56, higher than the corresponding correlations of percent of population living in cities of 100,000 or more (.45) or GNP per capita (.11) with CBR decline. Similarly, in a multiple regression analysis in which the percentage of women aged 20–24 never married is added to the seven socioeconomic variables we used earlier, the Beta coefficient for CBR decline is larger than that for school enrollment and is equal to literacy. Thus, female status would have been included if more data had been available and if the same relationship were to hold for a larger number of countries. However, we apparently "recapture," in the magnitude of the R^2, what is lost by omission of female status by adding other variables.

The list of variables for which a moderate amount of data are available includes:

percentage of women aged 15–19 never married
percentage of women aged 20–24 never married
percentage of adult women who are literate
percentage of women of relevant ages who are enrolled in primary and secondary school
life expectancy at birth for females
percentage of women aged 15–64 employed in the nonagricultural labor force

In addition, we examined the changes of these variables over time, in this case changes from 1960 to 1970. And finally, we constructed indexes of male/female differences for these variables, except for age at marriage. We shall examine the relationship of these variables to fertility decline,

[1] Elise Boulding et al., *Handbook of International Data on Women,* (Sage Publications, New York: John Wiley and Sons, 1976).

[2] Constantina Safilios-Rothschild, "A cross-cultural examination of women's marital, educational and occupational options," *Acta Sociologica* 14, no. 1-2 (1971), and "Methodological problems involved in the cross-cultural examination of indicators related to the status of women," manuscript, 1972.

TABLE 15.A1. Status of women variables as predictors of crude birth rate declines: 94 developing countries, 1965–75

	Beta coefficients												
	Percent females never married												
Regression number	Aged 15–19	Aged 20–24	Adults literate	Primary and secondary school enrollment	Life expectancy	Percent aged 15–64 in nonagricultural labor force	Program effort	R	R^2	N[a]	Degrees of freedom	F-statistics	Significance level
	Using 1970 female values												
1	.24	−.05	.03	−.06	.34	.28		.70	.50	40	33	5.44	<.05
2		.11	−.01	.06	.37	.25		.70	.49	40	34	6.49	<.05
3		−.06		.12	.53	.23		.75	.56	56	51	16.44	<.01
4				.01	.70	.14		.78	.61	91	87	46.21	<.01
	1970 female level		Substituting 1970 male values										
5	.19	.14	.24	−.02	.11	.14		.72	.51	39	32	5.63	<.05
6		.25	.25	.03	.16	.11		.71	.51	39	33	6.79	<.05
7		.19		.02	.54	.04		.73	.54	52	47	13.56	<.01
8				.02	.73	.07		.77	.59	85	81	39.26	<.01
	Using 1960–70 change in female levels												
9	−.05	.06	.20	−.18	−.02	.40		.53	.28	24	17	1.11	NS
10	−.01	.25		−.08	.16	.47		.58	.34	33	27	2.77	NS
11				−.16	.10	.36		.39	.15	75	71	4.14	<.01
	1970 female level		Male minus female 1970 levels										
12	.29	.37	.14	−.00	.13	−.02		.70	.48	38	31	4.87	<.05
13		.43		−.14	.17	.16		.66	.43	52	47	9.01	<.01
14		.46			.17	.18		.61	.37	56	52	10.36	<.01
15		.46			.21			.59	.34	56	53	13.94	<.01
	1960–70 change in female level		Male minus female 1970 levels										
16	−.02	.56	.37	−.33	.20	−.09		.81	.65	25	18	5.64	<.05
17	.25	.23		−.75	.02	−.07		.79	.62	39	33	10.87	<.01
18		.55	.36	−.34	.21	−.10		.81	.65	25	19	7.14	<.05
19		.35		−.30	.36	.03		.74	.55	37	32	9.66	<.01
20			.06	−.13	.41	.19		.55	.30	39	34	3.64	NS
21				−.20	.40	.29		.60	.35	76	72	13.13	<.01
22	.08	−.08		−.02	.29	.11	.81	.93	.87	37	30	33.80	<.01
23				.02	.18	.10	.82	.93	.86	76	71	107.62	<.01

[a]Number of countries.
NS = Not significant at .05 level.

first looking at the levels of the female indicators, then at their change over time, and finally at male/female differentials (Table 15.A1).

The R^2 between the level of the above variables around 1970 and fertility decline is .50, which indicates an appreciable relationship but less than some of the sets of variables considered earlier. Moreover, if one substitutes male indicators for literacy, school enrollment, life expectancy at birth, and labor force participation in nonagriculture, the result is about the same (.51), and similarly for various combinations—all of which suggests to us, as noted, that female and male indicators for these variables are a reflection of the degree of development in these respects rather than a singular indication of female or male status.

Data on changes in the above variables are available for relatively few countries (24–33) and produce R^2's that are quite low (.28–.34). Male minus female indicators for literacy, secondary school enrollment, life expectancy at birth, participation in the nonagricultural labor force, and change in percentage of young women never married (15–24) gives a relatively high R^2 of .65, but we have data for only 25 countries for this set of variables. Finally, the ratio of female to male values on the different socioeconomic variables seems a promising approach but is flawed because constant differences at different levels (e.g., 80/95 versus 30/15) give quite different values and often are unrelated to level of development generally, as well as to changes in CBR.

In conclusion, female and male measures on the typical socioeconomic variables appear to reflect level of development rather than sex status as such; the most distinctive measure we could find for a reasonable number of countries did not add to the overall correlation of CBR decline with "modernization"; it still may be that, as differences between men and women narrow with regard to literacy, primary plus secondary school enrollment, life expectancy (with female life expectancy surpassing that of males), and participation in the nonagricultural labor force and as the proportion of women marrying at early age decreases, fertility declines.

Bibliography

We have attempted to trace all of Berelson's published writings on population. The following bibliography arranges items in reverse chronologic order under each topic. Reprinted or closely similar items are given together. A number of items were issued also in The Population Council's Working Paper Series; these are designated by "PCWP." Items included as chapters in this volume are preceded by an asterisk.

Contraceptive Technology

Demographic Requirements of Fertility Control Technology: 15 Propositions. Seattle, Washington: *PIACT Papers*, 20 p; 1978.

*The impact of new technology. *Proceedings of the Royal Society of London*; 1976 December 10; B 195(1118):25–35.

With Campbell AA. Contraceptive specifications: report on a workshop. *Studies in Family Planning*; 1971 January; 2(1):14–19.

Application of intra-uterine contraception in family planning programs. In: *Proceedings of the Second International Conference on Intra-Uterine Contraception*; 1964 October; New York: 9–13. Excerpta Medica International Congress Series No. 86.

Ethics

*With Lieberson J. Government efforts to influence fertility: the ethical issues. *Population and Development Review*; 1979 December; 5(4): 581–613. Also *PCWP.*

Ethnicity

Ethnicity and fertility: what and so what. In: Himmelfarb M, and Baras V, eds., *Zero Population Growth: For Whom? Differential Fertility and Minority Group Survival*. Westwood, Connecticut: Greenwood Press; 1978:74–118. Also *PCWP.*

Field Strategies for Family Planning Programs

With Taylor HC Jr. Comprehensive family planning based on maternal/child health services: a feasibility study for a world program. *Studies in Family Planning*; 1971 February; 2(2):22–54.

With Taylor HC Jr, Helbig DW, and Chen K. Requirements for the extension of maternity care and family planning through countries of the developing world. *International Journal of Gynaecology and Obstetrics*; 1970 September; 8(5) (Pt. 2):718–723.

Preface. In: Zatuchni GI, ed., *Post-partum Family Planning: A Report on the International Program*. New York: McGraw-Hill; 1969:v-viii.

National population programs and the medical community. *Journal of Medical Education*; 1968 September; 43(9):953–960.

*With Taylor HC Jr. Maternity care and family planning as a world program. *American Journal of Obstetrics and Gynecology*; 1968 April 1;100(7):885–893. Also published in Zatuchni GI, ed., *Post-partum Family Planning: A Report on the International Program*. New York: McGraw-Hill; 1969:385–399.

The Population Council communication suitcase. In: Bogue DJ, ed., *Mass Communication and Motivation for Birth Control.* Chicago: Community and Family Study Center, University of Chicago; 1967:168–170.

Family planning programs: the place for research. *International Understanding*; 1967 Spring; 4.

*National family planning programs: a guide. *Studies in Family Planning*; 1964 December; 5(Suppl): 1–12.

*With Freedman R. A study in fertility control. *Scientific American*; 1964 May; 210(5):3–11.

On family planning communication. *Demography*; 1964;1(1):94–105. Also published in Bogue DJ, ed., *Mass Communication and Motivation for Birth Control*. Chicago: Community and Family Study Center, University of Chicago; 1967:42–57.

Communication, communication research, and family planning. In: *Emerging Techniques in Population Research, Proceedings of a Round Table at the Thirty-Ninth Annual Conference of the Milbank Memorial Fund, September 18–19, 1962*. New York: Milbank Memorial Fund; 1963:159–171.

National Family Planning Program Assessments

Where are we going? An outline. In: *Bellagio IV Population Conference, June 7–9, 1977*. New York: Rockefeller Foundation; 1977:98–113. Also *PCWP.*

*With Freedman R. The record of family planning programs. *Studies in Family Planning*; 1976; 7(1):1–40.

An evaluation of the effects of population control programs. *Studies in Family Planning*; 1974 January; 5(1):2–12. Also published in Parry HB, ed., *Population and Its Problems: A Plain Man's Guide.* Oxford: Clarendon Press; 1974:133–168.

The present state of family planning programs. *Studies in Family Planning*; 1970 September; 57:1–11. Also published in Singer SF, ed., *Is There an Optimum Level of Population? Appendix D,* New York: McGraw-Hill; 1971:336–363.

National family planning programs: where we stand. Behrman SJ, Corsa L Jr, and Freedman R, eds., *Fertility and Family Planning: A World Review.* Ann Arbor: University of Michigan Press; 1969:341–387. Also published in *Studies in Family Planning*; 1969 March; 39(suppl.): 341–387. See also Editorial in *Science*, 1970 Sept. 4;169(3949):931.

World-wide trends in family planning programmes. In: Sadik N, Anderson JK, Siddiqi KA, Ahmad B, Butt MN, Samad S, and Sharih K, eds., *Population Control Implications, Trends and Prospects: Proceedings of the Pakistan International Family Planning Conference, Dacca, January 28-February 4, 1969*. Lahore, West Pakistan: Sweden Pakistan Family Welfare Project, Communication Media Section; 1969:40–44.

Family planning programs and population control. In: Berelson B, ed., *Family Planning Programs: An International Survey.* New York: Basic Books; 1969:291– 303.

Ed., *Family Planning Programs: An International Survey.* New York: Basic Books; 310 p; 1969.

A review of major governmental programmes. In: United Nations Dept. of Economic and Social Affairs. *Proceedings of the World Population Conference, Belgrade, 30 August-10 September 1965. Vol.* 2. Selected papers and summaries: fertility, family planning, mortality, (E/CONF. 41/3); New York: UN; 1967:253–256.

Family planning programs in Taiwan. In: Muramatsu M and Harper PA, eds., *Population Dynamics: International Action and Training Programs.* Baltimore, Maryland: The Johns Hopkins Press; 1965:87–97.

Family planning programs throughout the world: a geographic and strategic survey. *The New England Assembly on the Population Dilemma;* 1964. Also published in Moran WE Jr, ed., *Population Growth—Threat to Peace?*, and excerpted in *Development Digest.*

Population Overviews

With Mauldin WP and Segal SJ. Population: current status and policy options. *Social Science and Medicine. Medical Economics*; June 1980;14C(2):71–97. Also *PCWP.*

1966–1977: a look at the record. *Family Planning Perspectives;* 1978 January/February; 10(1):20–22.

With Freedman R. The human population. *Scientific American*; 1974 September; 231(3):31–39.

World population: status report 1974. A guide for the concerned citizen. *Reports on Population/Family Planning*; 47 p; 1974 January: No. 15.

Status report on population developments. In: *Rockefeller Foundation. Working Papers: Third Bellagio Conference on Population, May 10–12, 1973.* New York; 1974 June: 1–12.

With others, eds., *Family Planning and Population Programs: A Review of World Developments.* Chicago: The University of Chicago Press; 848 p; 1966.

Population Policy: Developed Nations

Foreword. In: Friedlander D and Goldscheider C. *The Population of Israel.* New York: Columbia University Press; 1979: xiii–xix.

*Romania's 1966 anti-abortion decree: the demographic experience of the first decade. *Population Studies*; 1979;33(2):209–222. Also *PCWP.*

Introduction, and Summary. In: Berelson B, ed., *Population Policy in Developed Countries.* New York: McGraw-Hill; 1974:1–7 and 771–789.

Ed., *Population Policy in Developed Countries.* New York: McGraw-Hill; 793 p; 1974.

Toward a policy for an optimum population. In: Singer SF, ed., *Is There an Optimum Level of Population?* New York: McGraw-Hill; 1971: 302–306.

American attitudes on population policy. *Studies in Family Planning*; 1966 January; 1(9):5–8.

Population Policy: Developing Nations

*Paths to fertility reduction: the "policy cube." *Family Planning Perspectives*; 1977 September-October; 9(5):214–219.

The world population plan of action: where now? *Population and Development Review*; 1975 September; 1(1):115–146.

**The Great Debate on Population Policy: An Instructive Entertainment.* New York: The Population Council; 32 p; 1975.

Bucharest, the Council, and the fourth world. *The Population Council Annual Report 1974.* New York: The Population Council; 1974:19–24.

The difficulty of being earnest. In: *Readings on Population Information and Education.* Background papers for a Ford Foundation Meeting on Population, Elsinore, Denmark, June 1972. New York: Ford Foundation; 1973 June:23–25. Also in *The Population Council Annual Report 1970.* New York: The Population Council; 1970:15–20.

Formulation of population policy. *Perspectives in Biology and Medicine*; 1973 Spring; 16(3): 446–456.

Positions on population growth. *The Population Council Annual Report 1973.* New York: The Population Council; 1973:19–27.

Population policies: conceptions and misconceptions. In: Lewit S, ed., *Advances in Planned Parenthood. Proceedings of the Tenth Annual Meeting of the American Association of Planned*

Parenthood Physicians, Detroit, MI, 1972 April 6–7; Amsterdam: Excerpta Medica Foundation; 1973:3–8.

The population problem: conceptions and misconceptions. *Anesthesia and Analgesia*; 1971 July-August; 50(4):481–489.

Population policy: personal notes. *Population Studies*; 1971 July; 25(2):173–182.

*18–35 in place of 15–45? *The Population Council Annual Report 1971*. New York: The Population Council; 1971:19–27.

With Wood FC, Mastroianni L, Guttmacher AF, and Viel B. Population avalanche. *Transactions and Studies of The College of Physicians of Philadelphia*; 1969 July; 37(1):1–28.

*Beyond family planning. *Science*; 1969 February 7;163(3867):533–543. Also published in *Studies in Family Planning*; 1969 February; 38:1–16, and in Chaplin D, ed., *Population Policies and Growth in Latin America*. Lexington, Massachusetts: D.C. Heath; 1971:71–108.

With McElroy WD, Coale A, Duffy B Jr, Folkers K, Freedman R, Kety S, Markert CL, Snyder J, and Taylor HC. Family planning and other population controls. (Letter). *Science*; 1968 February 23;159(3817): 827.

Resource Allocation

With Haveman RH. On allocating resources for fertility reduction in developing countries. *Population Studies*; 1980 July; 34(2):227–237.

*With Haveman RH. On the efficient allocation of resources for fertility reduction. *International Family Planning Perspectives*; 1979 December; 5(4):133–142. Also published as Toward efficient allocation of fertility reduction expenditures. *Evaluation Review*; 1981 April; 5(2):147–167, and as Intervention strategy and resource allocation for fertility reduction in developing countries. *Working Paper Series*. Center for Demography and Ecology, Madison, Wisconsin: University of Wisconsin; (78–29); 88 p; 1978. Also *PCWP.*

Social Science Research

Social Science Research for Population Policy. Appendix 1 of the Final Report. International Review Group of Social Science Research on Population and Development. Mexico City: El Colegio de Mexico; 47 p.; December 1978.

Social science research on population: a review. *Population and Development Review*; 1976 June; 2(2):219–266.

The social science of population. In: *Organisation for Economic Cooperation and Development (OECD). Development Center. Population: International Assistance and Research. Proceedings of the First Population Conference of the Development Center, Paris, December 3–5, 1968.* Paris: OECD; 1969:153–156.

Sociology in action: in population and in general. In: Shostak AB, ed., *Sociology in Action*. Homewood, Illinois: Dorsey Press; 1966.

Special Studies

*Prospects and programs for fertility reduction: what? where? *Population and Development Review*; 1978 December; 4(4):579–616. Also *PCWP.*

With Mauldin WP. Reply [to Ruth Dixon's "On drawing policy conclusions from multiple regressions. . ."]. *Studies in Family Planning*; 1978;9(10–11):288.

*With Mauldin WP and Sykes Z. Conditions of fertility decline in developing countries 1965–75. *Studies in Family Planning*; 1978 May; 9(5):89–147. Preliminary version published as: Cross-cultural review of the effectiveness of family planning programs. *National Population Conference/Congress International de la Population (IUSSP), Mexico*: 1977; 3:163–185.

The value of children: a taxonomical essay. In: Talbot NB, ed., *Raising Children in Modern America: Problems and Prospective Solutions.* Boston: Little, Brown and Co.; 1976:11–24. Also in *The Population Council Annual Report*

1972. New York: The Population Council; 1972: 19–27.

KAP studies on fertility. In: Berelson B, et al. eds., *Family Planning and Population Programs: A Review of World Developments*. Chicago: The University of Chicago Press; 1966:655–668.

Turkey: national survey on population. *Studies in Family Planning*; 1964 December; 5:1–5.

Work of The Population Council

Report of the President. A day in the life. *The Population Council Annual Report 1969*. New York: The Population Council; 1969:13–23.

The Work of The Population Council. In: Organisation for Economic Cooperation and Development (OECD). Population: International Assistance and Research. *Proceedings of the First Population Conference of the Development Centre, Paris, December 3–5, 1968*. Paris: OECD; 1969:141–150.

Report of the president. Where we are, where we are going. *The Population Council Annual Report, 1968*. New York: The Population Council; 1968:13–19.

Miscellaneous

With Sekhar AC, Freedman R, Ohlin G, and Sai FT. *Final Report of the External Advisory Panel on Population*. Washington, D.C.: The World Bank; 70 p.; 1976 August.

John D. Rockefeller 3rd, 1906–1978: In Memoriam. *Studies in Family Planning*; 1978 July; 9(7):178–179.

Paul Preston Hartman, 1911–1968. [Obituary]. *Studies in Family Planning*; 1968; 35:12.

Index

Abortion, induced, 20–21, 34, 45, 47, 95, 111, 116, 117, 133, 134, 135, 147, 160, 209
  delegalization of, 6, 21, 59–69, 160, 162, 163
  ethics and access to, 160
  free, 51
  legalization of, 21, 67
  resources allocation to programs including, 83, 84
  see also Spontaneous abortion
Academic critic, *see* AcCrit position in population debate
Acceptability of paths to fertility reduction, 37, 38, 39
Acceptance of family planning
  contraceptive technology, and fertility reduction, 118–20, 135, 136, 138
  performance of programs, 127–28
    strength of program, social setting, and, 138–42
  populations with highest, 87
  by postpartum women, 102–3
  Taichung experiment results, 184–89
    cost per acceptance, 189
Acceptors, characteristics of, 128–34
  in Taichung experiment, 187–89
Access to means of fertility control, 33, 34, 39
  government manipulation of, ethics of, 158, 163
  in national family planning program, 86
Accessibility of postpartum population, 102
AcCrit position in population policy debate, 12–28
  basic beliefs of, 12
  on merit of family planning programs, 18–21
  on population in context of development, 13–18
  on strategies of intervention, 23–27
  summary, 27
Administration and organization of national family planning program, 90
Administrative feasibility of proposals beyond family planning, 47–48, 52
Afghanistan, prospects and programs for fertility reduction in, 191, 193, 197, 198, 199–202, 203, 206, 211
Africa, 25, 131, 217
  see also individual countries
Age at marriage, *see* Marriage, age at
Age of acceptors, 128–30, 180, 188
Age of mother, limiting to 18 to 35-year-olds, 109–14
Age structure, 224, 246
Agriculture
  nonagricultural labor force, 220, 221
  productivity of, 16
Algeria, prospects and programs for fertility reduction in, 191, 193, 197, 198, 199–202, 203, 206, 211
Allocation of resources, *see* Resource allocation for fertility reduction
Asia, 217
  see also individual countries
Attitudes toward family planning, 85–6
  desired family size, *see* Desired family size
  Taichung survey, 180–82
  women wanting no more children but not using contraception, 131–33
Australia, 65
Austria-Hungary, 15
Autonomy, *see* Freedom, concepts of

"Baby boom," 65, 66, 67, 68
Bali, 131, 134, 161
Bangladesh, 24, 37, 119, 135
  prospects and programs for fertility reduction in, 191, 193, 197, 198, 199–202, 203, 206, 211
Birth control, *see individual methods of birth control*
Birth intervals, 112
  see also Spacing of births
Birth payments, 160
Birth quotas, 161
Birth rates, 22, 115
  crude, *see* Crude birth rate
  in developed countries, 25, 115
  goals for, in developing countries, 42–43
  record of family planning programs in affecting, 142–46
  Romanian delegalization of abortion and, 6, 59–69
  see also individual countries

Bongaarts, John, 205
Brazil, prospects and programs for fertility reduction in, 191, 192, 196, 198, 202–4, 211
Breastfeeding, 102
Bucharest World Population Conference of 1984, 12, 13, 14, 18, 20, 25, 36, 67, 69, 123, 209, 218
Budgets
for maternal health care/family planning services, 107–108
for national family planning programs, 96
see also Resources allocation for fertility reduction, efficient
Bulgaria, 126, 160
Burma, 127, 191

Canada, 65
Ceylon, *see* Sri Lanka
Change analysis, 235, 245
Child assistance subsidies, 158, 160
Childbearing years, limiting, to ages 18 to 35, 4, 109–14
Children, 22
health care for, *see* Maternal and child health (MCH) programs, family planning attached to
labor by, 16, 51
mortality of, 103, 147, 158
reduction of, to reduce birth rates, 34, 44
rights of, 16
Chile, prospects and programs for fertility reduction in, 191, 192, 194–96, 198, 202, 203, 211
China, 24, 130
abortion in, 134, 135
access to fertility control methods in, 34
community pressure to limit family size in, 35, 37
disincentives used in, 161
incentives used in, 35, 158
legal age of marriage in, 161
propaganda used in, 35, 160
prospects and programs for fertility reduction in, 191, 192, 196, 198, 202–4, 211
sanctions used in, 36, 37, 151, 158, 161
"Circulation effect," *see* Diffusion principle
Coale, Ansley, 126
Coercive measures, *see* Sanctions (coercion) and pressures
Colombia, 119
prospects and programs for fertility reduction in, 191, 192, 196, 198, 202–4, 211
Community
development program, access to fertility control methods in, 34, 147
incentives and disincentives to influence fertility behavior, 35, 37, 39, 84, 116, 158
small-family norms, creating, 35, 37, 39, 84, 116, 166
Taichung experiment's involvement in, 183
see also Sanctions (coercion) and pressures
Complications of pregnancy, age of mother and, 110
Condom, 94, 95, 116, 134, 135, 160
distribution of, 95–6
in Taichung experiment, 184, 187
Congenital abnormalities, age of mother and, 111
Content and design of national family planning programs, 88–90
Continuation of contraceptive use
contraceptive technology improvements and, 117–20, 135, 138
in Taichung experiment, 187
Contraception, 47
access to, *see* Access to means of fertility control
advances in, *see* Technological advances in contraception
distribution methods, 95–6
methods for national planning programs, 92–4, 134
motivation and contraceptive technology, 93–4
women wanting no more children but not using, 131–33
see also individual methods of contraception
Coombs Number Scale, 137
Coombs preference scale, 132, 133
Correlation analyses of demand and supply variables linked with fertility decline, 230–33, 244–45, 247
Correspondence analysis, 238
Cross-tabulation analysis of factors related to fertility decline, 238–44, 245–46
Crude birth rate, 20, 115, 208, 222
absolute declines in, 236–38
CBR 20 by year 200 for developing countries, prospects and programs for reaching, 190–212
in developed countries, 114
in Eastern Europe, 61–64
in Japan, 67
as measure of fertility change in study of developing countries, 222–53 *passim*
program strength, and social setting, 142–46
in Romania, 59–60, 61–64
"30/30 rule," 145–46, 151
Cultural milieu and fertility behavior, 159, 165
Czechoslovakia, 160

Death rate, 179
Debate on population policy, 5–6, 11–29
introduction, 12–13
merit of family planning programs, 18–22
population in context of development, 13–18
strategies of intervention, 22–7
summaries of positions, 27–9
Demographic gap, 157
Design and content of national family planning programs, 88–90
Desired family size, 17, 21, 86, 131, 149
changes in, and acceptance of contraception, 133–34
community small-family norms, 35, 37, 39, 84, 116, 166
first-preference statements, 137
incentives and, 23–4
see also Incentives to affect population policy

information programs reinforcing, 89
in Taichung, 180, 181
women wanting no more children but not using contraception, 131–33
see also Unwanted births
DevDev position in population policy debate, 12–28 *passim*
basic beliefs of, 12
on merit of family planning programs, 18–22
on population in context of development, 13–18
on strategies of intervention, 23–27
summary, 27
Developed countries, 25, 115, 116, 125, 129, 134
see also individual countries
Developing countries
conditions of fertility decline in, 1965–75, 9, 217–53
with family planning programs, 126–27
prospects and programs for fertility reduction in, 191–217
see also individual countries
Development, 71, 116, 121, 125, 133, 147, 151, 160–61
advocates of, as answer to population problem, *see* DevDev position in population policy debate
fertility decline in developing countries, 1965–75 and level of, 9, 217–53
population programs as component of, 14
prospects and programs for fertility reduction in developing countries and, 208–209
threshold factors and, *see* Threshold factors in fertility reduction
Diaphragm, 94, 95, 184
Diffusion principle, 89
Taichung experiment and, 179, 183, 186–87
Directors of national family planning programs, 90
Disincentives to affect population policy, 158
ethics of, 160–61, 164
as path to fertility reduction, 35, 39
see also Incentives to affect population policy
Distribution of contraceptives, 95–6
Divorce, 23, 60

East Germany, 160
East Java, 131, 161
Eastern Europe
crude birth rates in, 61–64
incentives in, 160
sterilization in, 60
see also individual countries; Europe
Economic capability of proposals beyond family planning, 48–49, 52
Economic development, *see* Development
Economic status, variables leading to fertility decline, 226–29
Economic Survey of Europe, 61
Ecuador, 115
Education, 15, 18, 26, 147, 149, 150, 158
acceptors and level of, 130–31, 187, 188, 189
compulsory, 51
as path to fertility reduction, 35, 36, 39, 220
population, in school curricula, 35, 36, 43, 48, 54, 92–3, 147
of postpartum women, 102
by satellite television, 43, 48, 54
in Taichung
acceptors and, 187, 188, 189
contraceptive use and, 182
family size and, 182
variables leading to fertility decline, 226, 227–29
Effectiveness
of contraceptives, 117, 118, 119, 135, 138
of paths to fertility reduction, 37–8, 39
presumed, of proposals beyond family planning, 50–2
Egypt, 105, 119, 134
prospects and programs for fertility reduction in, 191, 193, 196–98, 203, 204–5, 206, 211
Emigration, 33, 42, 157
see also Migration
Employment, opportunities for, 16, 18
for women, 16, 26, 147
Energy consumption per capita, 221
England, 126
Ethics of measures to influence fertility, 8–9, 24–25, 49–50, 52, 86, 157–73
conclusion, 172–73
ethical framework used to assess policies, 166–72
decision not system, 166–67
ethical consistencies, 171–72
procedural and substantive criteria, 167–69
settlement through informed judgment, 169–71
incentives, 163–65
introduction, 157–59
limitations on access to methods of fertility control, 163
Ethics of measures to influence fertility
the policy situation, 159–62
official promotion of propaganda, 160–61
pressures and sanctions, 161–62
politically organized peer pressure, 165–66
Ethiopia, 127, 191
Europe, 145
family allowance programs in, 51
fertility decline in, 15, 125–26
see also individual countries; Eastern Europe; Western Europe
European Fertility Study, 125–26

Family allowances, 160
Family planning programs, 116, 121
attached to maternal and child health (MCH) programs, 34, 47, 48, 51, 54, 88–89, 101–8
advantages of, 101–3

Family planning programs (*cont.*)
attached to maternal and child health (MCH) programs (*cont.*)
present distribution of institutionalized maternity care, 103, 104–5
project requirements for, 105–8
a guide to national, 85–100
budget and costs, 96
contraceptive methods, 93–5
design and content, 88–90
field workers, 90–2
medical community, 93
organization and administration, 90
records, 96–9
special publics, 92–3
strategy, 85–8
summary, 99–100
time-table, 99
merit of, 18–22, 42, 52–3, 150–51
criticisms of, 124–25, 150
proposals beyond, 42–55
conclusion, 52–5
the proposals, 43–5, 146–47
review of the issues, 45–52
prospects and, for fertility reduction in the developing world, 10, 190–212
the certain, 191, 192, 194–96, 198, 202, 203, 208–12
the possible, 191, 193, 196–98, 203, 204–5, 206, 208–12
the probable, 191, 192, 196, 198, 202–4, 208–12
the programs, 202–5
the prospects, 191–202
proximate determinants, 205–7
summary and conclusion, 207–10
targets for, 190–91
the unlikely, 191, 193, 197, 198, 199–202, 206, 208–12
record of, 5, 123–52
by acceptors, 128–34
alternative means of fertility intervention, 146–47
conclusion and commentary, 148–52
by effect on birth rates, 142–46
introduction, 123–26
by methods, 134–38
need for fuller knowledge of, 152
preface, 123
program and performance, 126–46
by setting and effort, 138–42
strength of, and social setting
acceptance and, 138–42
crude birth rates and, 142–46
fertility decline in developing countries, 1965–75, 9, 217–53
Family size, 179
community small-family norms, 35, 37, 39, 84, 116, 166
desired, *see* Desired family size
limitations placed on, 36, 37, 161
see also Parity
Family structure, direct manipulation of, 26, 44, 53
FamPlan position in population policy debate, 12–28 *passim*
basic beliefs of, 12
on merit of family planning programs, 18–22
on population in context of development, 13–18
on strategies of intervention, 22–7
summary, 27–8
Farmers' associations, family planning as part of health program of, 93
Feasibility of paths to fertility reduction, 37, 38, 39
administrative, 47–8
Fertility decline, 17–18
conditions of, in developing countries, 1965–75, 9, 217–52
correlation and regression analyses, 230–38, 244–45, 247
cross-tabulational analyses, 238–44, 245–46
introduction, 217–19
the literature on, 219–21
the measures and the data, 221–30
summary and conclusions, 244–53
development and, 14–15, 16, 17, 20
differences for developing countries from Western experience, 149
family planning programs and, 18–22
historically, 14, 15, 20, 125–26, 148, 149
strategies to hasten, debate on, 22–7
coercion, 24
incentives, 23–4
manipulation of family's role, 26
motives of, 25
research, 23
social revolution, 25–6
workable vs. acceptable, 23
threshold factors, *see* Threshold factors in fertility reduction
Fertility rate in Taiwan, 179–80, 181
Taichung results, 184
Fertility reduction
ethics of measures to bring about, *see* Ethics of measures to influence fertility
limiting childbearing years to 18 to 35 and, 113
by methods beyond family planning, 42–55
new technology and, *see* Technological advances in contraception
paths to, *see* Paths to fertility reduction
prospects and programs for, in the developing world, 10, 190–202
the certain, 191, 192, 194–96, 198, 202, 203, 218–12
the possible, 191, 193, 196–98, 203, 204–5, 206, 208–12
the probable, 191, 192, 196, 198, 202–4, 208–12
the programs, 191–202
the prospects, 191–202
proximate determinants, 205–7
summary and conclusion, 207–10

targets for, 190–91
the unlikely, 191, 193, 197, 198, 199–202, 203, 206, 208–12
record of family planning programs, *see* Family planning programs, record of
resource allocation for, 8, 71–84
Taichung experiment, 2–3, 179–89
Fertility transition, 115, 125, 126, 128, 149–50, 226
Field workers
background of, 91, 92
incentives for, 92
for national family planning programs, 90–2
number of, 92
supervisors of, 92
in Taichung experiment, 183, 184
training of, 91–2
Fiji, 138–39, 146, 225
Foam tablet, contraceptive, 94, 184, 187
France, 15, 126, 160
Freedman, Ronald, 2, 5, 123–52, 179–89
Freedom, concepts of, 168–69, 170

Geneva Conference of 1965, 123
Germany, 126
Ghana, 105, 115
Government policies, *see specific policies and countries*
Group meetings, 88
Guatemala, 145
Guide to national family planning programs, *see* Family planning programs, a guide to national

Haveman, Robert H., 71–84
Health services, 16, 18, 19, 226, 227
access to fertility control methods through, 34
variables leading to fertility decline, 226, 227–29
Health variables leading to fertility decline, 226, 227–29
History of fertility decline, 14, 15, 20, 125–26, 148, 149
Home delivery
with qualified and/or supervised personnel, 103, 104–105
without qualified supervision, 104
Home visits, 88
in Taichung experiment, 183, 184, 186
Hong Kong, 135, 225
Hospital deliveries, 103, 104, 105
Hospital services, 220, 221
Housing, 16, 158
incentives related to, 160, 161
Hungary, 126, 132, 160
Husbands
family planning program efforts aimed at, 88
Taichung experiment and
effort directed at, 183, 186, 187
survey data, 180
Hutterites, 15

Illegitimate children, 111
Incentives to affect population policy, 23–4, 158
economic cost of, 49
ethics of, 160–61, 163–65
for fertility increases, 60, 160
for fertility reduction, 35, 36–7, 39, 43, 44, 48, 49, 52, 116, 128–29, 147, 160–61
prospects and programs for fertility reduction in developing countries and, 208–9
resources allocation to, 83
see also Disincentives to affect population policy
Income equalization, 16, 17, 18, 35, 147, 158
Income per capita, 221, 222
India, 14, 26, 46, 53, 134, 135
compulsory sterilization proposal, 45
incentives used in, 35, 36, 46, 158, 160, 161, 164
propaganda in, 160
prospects and programs for fertility reduction in, 191, 193, 196–98, 203, 204–5, 206, 211
sanctions used in, 36, 37, 158, 162
Indonesia, 149, 158
propaganda in, 160
prospects and programs for fertility reduction in, 191, 193, 196–98, 203, 204–5, 206, 211
sanctions and pressures in, 161–62
Induced abortion, *see* Abortion, induced
Industrialization, 16, 35, 158
Industry, family planning as part of health programs of, 93
Infant mortality, 16, 182
reduction of, 147, 158, 220, 222
age of mother and, 110, 111
to reduce birth rates, 34, 36, 44
in Taichung, 182
Information programs
in national family planning programs, 86, 88, 89
as path to fertility reduction, 35, 36, 39, 147
resources allocation to, 84
in Taichung experiment, 183, 184
see also Education
Inheritance law reform, 16
Interaction effects of socio-economic variables and program effort, 234–35, 245
International Conference of Family Planning Programs of 1965, 123
International Institute for the Study of Human Reproduction, 108
International Postpartum Program, 51
Intrauterine device, *see* IUD
Involuntary fertility control, 43, 52
see also Sanctions (coercion) and pressures
Iran, 160
prospects and programs for fertility reduction in, 191, 193, 197, 198, 199–202, 203, 206, 211
Iraq, 191
Israel, 61, 160

IUD, 45, 60, 95, 116, 134, 135, 160
distribution of, 95
insertion, 93
Taichung experiment and, 184, 187

Japan
abortion in, 21, 51, 67, 160
crude birth rate in, 67
the pill in, 160
Jelly, contraceptive, 184

Kenya, 119, 134
prospects and programs for fertility reduction in, 191, 193, 197, 198, 199–202, 203, 206, 211
Kerala, 149
Korea, North, 191
Korea, South, 35, 119, 120, 132, 134, 135, 136, 146, 225
acceptors in, 131
continuity of contraceptive use in, 135
propaganda in, 160
prospects and programs for fertility reduction in, 191, 192, 194–96, 202, 203, 211

Labor unions, family planning as part of health program of, 93
Lag analysis, 235–36, 245
Land reform, 16
Latin America, 105, 217
see also individual countries
Legal s.•nctions, *see* Sanctions
Lieberson, Jonathan, 8–9, 157–73
Life expectancy, 158, 179, 220, 221, 222
Literacy, 220, 221, 222
see also Education
Living standards, *see* Standard of living
Low birth-weight infants, age of mother and, 111

Mailings, 88
in Taichung experiment, 183, 186
Malaysia, 132, 137, 224, 225
prospects and programs for fertility reduction in, 191, 193, 196, 198, 202–4, 211
Marriage
age at, 221, 246
fertility decline and, 224–26
higher, 51, 53, 149, 224
incentives for higher, 23, 44, 48, 161
legal, 23, 36, 37, 44, 116, 147, 161
fertility in, 226, 247
promotion of "childless," 44
Marriage licenses, conditions attached to granting, 161
Married women of reproductive age (MWRA), acceptors as percentage of, 127–28
in Taichung, 184–86, 188
Maternal and child health (MCH) programs, family planning attached to, 3, 34, 47, 48, 51, 53, 54, 88–9, 101–8
advantages of, 101–3
present distribution of institutionalized maternity care, 103, 104–5
projected requirements for, 105–8
Maternal mortality, 109–10
Maternity leave, 60, 158, 160, 161
Maternity payments, 160
Mauldin, W. Parker, 9, 217–53
Mauritius, 105, 225
Media, mass, 88
satellite television, 43, 48, 54
see also Information programs
Medical community's role in national family planning programs, 93
Mexico, 119
prospects and programs for fertility reduction in, 191, 192, 196, 198, 202–4, 211
Midwives, 89, 92
see also Nurse-midwives
Migration, limitations on, 36, 37
see also Emigration
Military, information program for, 92
Ministry of Health, 93
Mobile informational teams, 89
Mobile maternal health and family planning services, 106
Modernization, *see* Development
Morality, *see* Ethics
Morocco, 115, 145
prospects and programs for fertility reduction in, 191, 193, 197, 198, 199–202, 203, 206, 211
Mortality decline, 19, 133, 149, 150, 179
Mortality rate, 130, 131
fetal, 110
infant-child, 34, 36, 44, 103, 110, 111, 147, 158, 182, 220, 222
maternal, 109–10
perinatal, 111
raising the, 33, 42, 157
Motivation, 116, 120, 218
contraceptive technology and, 93–4, 120, 136–38
of postpartum women, 102
Taichung experiment's findings on, 179

National Academy of Sciences, 19
National family planning programs, *see* Family planning programs
Nepal, 105, 145
prospects and programs for fertility reduction in, 191, 193, 197, 198, 199–202, 203, 206, 211
New Zealand, 65
Newspaper circulation, 220, 221
Nigeria, 119
prospects and programs for fertility reduction in, 191, 193, 197, 198, 199–202, 206, 211
Nurse-midwives, 91
see also Midwives
Nursing, 102

Old-age benefits, 16, 23, 35, 37, 47
Oral pill, *see* Pill, birth control

Organization and administration of national family planning programs, 90

Pakistan, 119
prospects and programs for fertility reduction in, 191, 193, 197, 198, 199-202, 203, 206, 211
Parity, 226
high, population with
acceptors among, 128–29, 134, 187–89
family planning programs aimed at, 87
sterilization and, 95
low
acceptors among, 129–30, 188
reaching postpartum women of, 102
see also Family size
Path analysis, 223–24, 245
Paths to fertility reduction, 33–41
criteria for choices, 37–8
on demand side, 36–7
evaluated against criteria, 38–41
Policy Cube, 6, 40–1
on supply side, 33–6
Peer pressure, *see* Sanctions (coercion) and pressures
Peru, prospects and programs for fertility reduction in, 191, 193, 196–98, 203, 204–5, 206, 211
Philippines, 119, 131, 132, 161
population education in, 36
prospects and programs for fertility reduction in, 191, 192, 196, 198, 202–4, 211
Pill, birth control, 45, 60, 94–5, 116, 134, 135, 160
in Taichung experiment, 184, 187
Policy Cube, 6, 40–1
Political channels and organization used to reduce fertility, 44, 52
Political viability of proposals beyond family planning, 46–7, 52
Politics, international, 25
Polygamy, 16
Population Council, 104, 108, 179
Population Council Fact Book, 211
Population distribution, allocation of resources by, 80–2, 84
see also Rural areas; Urban areas
Population growth, 20, 22, 71, 149, 157
academic critic's views on, 13–14, 15, 17
development's and family planning's roles in curbing, 13–18
zero, 18, 42, 44, 46, 130
see also Fertility decline
Population Policies and Economic Development (World Bank Staff Report), 140
Population policy debate, *see* Debate on population policy
Postpartum programs, *see* Maternal and child health (MCH) programs, family planning attached to
Poverty, development's role in alleviating, 13, 16, 17, 27
Premature births, age of mother and, 111
Pressure, *see* Sanctions (coercion) and pressures
Program implementation strength, efficient allocation of resources for fertility reduction and, 72, 73–84
Propaganda, 35, 116, 158
ethics of government promotion of, 160
Proximate determinants, prospects and programs for fertility reduction in developing countries and, 205–7, 210–11

Racism, 25
Radio receivers per 1,000 population, 221
Recordkeeping
for national family planning programs, 96–9
of pregnancies and births, 106
Regression analysis, 140, 141, 142–45, 150, 230–33, 244–45, 247
absolute CBR decline, 236–38
change analysis, 235, 245
correspondence analysis, 237
interaction effects, 234–35, 245
lag analysis, 235–36, 245
path analysis, 233–34
Replacement fertility, 130, 134
see also Zero population growth
Reproduction period, confining, to 18 to 35-year-olds, 4, 109–14
Research on population policy, 23, 27, 44-5, 51, 52, 53
specificity of proposals for, 53–4
Resources allocation for fertility reduction, efficient, 8, 71–84, 86, 121
basis of the study, 71–3
effectiveness ratings, 72–3
matrix of cells, 72
the participants, 73
program implementation strength, 72
social setting, 72
strategies for fertility reduction, 72
by clusters of respondents, 79–80
diffusion principle, 89–90
effectiveness ratings, 72–6
profile of, 76
implications of responses for, 76–9
in the past, 76
by population distributions, 80–2, 87
summary, 82–4
urgency of need and, 81, 82
see also Budgets
Rhythm method, 94, 116, 184
Road improvements, 16
Romania, delegalization of abortion in, 6, 21, 59–69, 160, 162, 163
conclusion, 68-69
Rural areas
acceptors from, 131, 188
family planning programs in, 87
combined with maternal care, 106–8
Rural modernization, 16, 36

Sanctions (coercion) and pressures, 24, 27
as path to fertility reduction, 36, 37, 39, 84, 116, 147, 151

Sanctions (coercion) and pressures (*cont.*)
as path to fertility reduction (*cont.*)
ethics of, 161–62, 165–66, 168, 169, 170–71
politically organized peer pressure, 165–66
prospects and programs for fertility reduction in developing countries and, 208–9
Schools, *see* Education
Select Committee on Population of U.S. House of Representatives, Report of, 158–59
Semantics of family planning, 87–88
Singapore, 162, 225
incentives used in, 35, 36, 161
propaganda used in, 35
Social mobility, 16
Social revolution, 25–6
see also Development
Social security benefits, 16, 35, 37, 47, 48, 116, 147
Social setting
efficient allocation of resources for fertility reduction and, 72, 73–84
program strength and
crude birth rates and, 142–46
fertility decline in developing countries, 1965–75, 9, 217–53
record of family planning programs by, 138–42
Socioeconomic conditions, changes in, *see* Development; *specific changes, e.g.* Education; Women, equality for
Sons, number of, acceptors and, in Taichung experiment, 187, 188
Soviet Union, 15, 126
Spacing of births, 102
family planning programs aimed at, 87
see also Birth intervals
Spontaneous abortion, 110
Sri Lanka, 19, 119, 134, 149, 224, 225
prospects and programs for fertility reduction in, 191, 192, 196, 198, 202–4, 211
Standard of living, 16, 18, 36, 149, 220
in Taiwan, 179, 189
Sterility, 22
Sterilization, 34, 45, 60, 87, 95, 116, 134, 135, 147, 209
ethics and access to, 160
incentives for, 23, 36, 161
resources allocation for programs including, 83, 84
see also Vasectomy
Strategy of national family planning program, 85–8
Substitution of contraceptive methods, 118, 135
Sudan, prospects and programs for fertility reduction in, 191, 193, 197, 198, 199–202, 203, 206, 211
Supplies for national family planning programs, 95–6, 133
Sweden, 160
Switching contraceptive methods, 118, 135

Taichung experiment, 2–3, 179–89
baseline survey, 180–82
effectiveness of, 184–86
the experiment, 183–84
findings of, 184–89
objective of, 183
setting for, 179–80
Taiwan, 2–3, 14, 119, 120, 134, 135, 136, 137, 146, 179–89, 225
acceptors in, 131, 133–34
birth rate in, 179, 180, 181
contraceptive use and attitudes prior to Taichung experiment, 180–82
continuity of contraceptive use in, 135
death rate in, 179, 180
fertility rates in, 179–80, 181
incentives used in, 35, 36, 161
population studies center, 180
prospects and programs for fertility reduction in, 191, 192, 194–96, 198, 202, 203, 211
supervised home delivery in, 105
Taichung experiment, 2–3, 179–89
women wanting no more children but not using contraception in, 132–33
Tanzania, prospects and programs for fertility reduction in, 191, 192, 197, 198, 199–202, 203, 206, 211
Target populations
for maternal health care/family planning programs, 101–102
for national family planning programs, 86–7
Tax benefits and penalties, 158
for fertility increases, 60
for fertility reduction, 43, 46, 47, 52, 53, 161
Taylor, Dr. Howard C., Jr., 101–8
Technological advances in contraception, 6–7, 21, 22, 115–21
as path to fertility reduction, 33, 34, 36, 39, 51, 115–21, 134–38
proposals beyond family planning and, 45–6, 51, 52
resources and time factors, 121
trade-offs in, 118–21
ways to improve technology, 117–18
see also Acceptance of family planning; Continuation of contraceptive use; Effectiveness, of contraceptives
Teenage pregnancies, 4, 109–14
Television satellite, education programs on, 43, 48, 54
Thailand, 119, 131, 134, 135, 225
acceptors in, and desired family size, 134
prospects and programs for fertility reduction in, 191, 192, 196, 198, 202–4, 211
Threshold factors in fertility reduction, 15–16, 19, 34–5, 36, 145, 149–50, 220–21, 222
prospects and programs for fertility reduction and, 191, 194, 202–5, 206, 210

Time factor
contraceptive technology and, 121
short- and long-term views of family planning programs, 152
Time-table for national family planning program, 99
Total fertility rate, 222–23
Tunisia, 36, 224
Turkey, 225
prospects and programs for fertility reduction in, 191, 192, 196, 198, 202–4, 211

Uganda, 191
UNICEF, 47
United Arab Republic, *see* Egypt
United Nations, 157
Bucharest conference, *see* Bucharest World Population Conference of 1974
United Nations Development Programme, 14
United Nations Fund for Population Activities, 14, 157
United States, 132, 133
abortions in, 111, 133, 160
age of women giving birth in, 112
"baby boom" in, 65, 66, 67, 68
crude birth rate in, 115, 145
hospital deliveries in, 105
University of Michigan, 180
Unwanted births, 21
in Taichung, 182
Unwanted pregnancy, 111
Urban areas
acceptors from, 188
contraceptive use in, 182
family planning programs in, 104, 105
hospital deliveries in, 104, 105
Urbanization, 16, 35, 158, 220, 222
variables leading to fertility decline, 227–29
U.S.S.R., *see* Soviet Union

Vasectomy, 36, 45, 94, 95
compulsory, 45
incentives for, 49, 160
see also Sterilization
Venezuela, prospects and programs for fertility reduction in, 191, 193, 196, 198, 202–4, 211
Vietnam, 191
Voluntary fertility control, 43, 50–1, 52

Welfare, concepts of, 169
Welfare benefits and penalties for fertility reduction, 43–4, 52
West Malaysia, 134
Western Europe
crude birth rate in, 115
fertility decline in, 15, 125–26, 128
see also individual countries; Europe
Withdrawal, 94, 116, 184
Women
confining reproduction to 18 to 35-year-olds, 4, 109–15
employment opportunities for, 16, 26, 147
equality for, 15, 35, 147, 158
family planning as liberating factor for, 22, 25, 26
in labor force, 51, 220, 222
required participation, 44, 46–7
literacy of, 220, 221
postpartum, *see* Maternal and child health (MCH) programs, family planning attached to
variables for status of, and fertility decline, 227–29, 258–60
Women's organizations, involvement of family planning programs of, 93
Word-of-mouth, *see* Diffusion principle
World Bank Staff Reports, 140
World Health Organization, 47
World Population Conference in Bucharest, *see* Bucharest World Population Conference of 1974

"Youth corps," 35, 44, 48, 147

Zaire, prospects and programs for fertility reduction in, 191, 193, 197, 199–202, 203, 206, 211
Zatuchni, Dr. Gerald, 101
Zero population growth, 19, 42, 44, 46, 130

MIX
Papier aus verantwortungsvollen Quellen
Paper from responsible sources
FSC® C105338

If you have any concerns about our products,
you can contact us on
ProductSafety@springernature.com

In case Publisher is established outside the EU,
the EU authorized representative is:
Springer Nature Customer Service Center GmbH
Europaplatz 3, 69115 Heidelberg, Germany

Printed by Libri Plureos GmbH
in Hamburg, Germany